"Facing unprecedented chal[illegible]care leaders need practical and insightful guidanc[illegible]is book delivers a vital and timely intervention, weaving together systems thinking, psychological insights, and real-world examples to illuminate the multifaceted nature of contemporary leadership. A must-read for navigating the complexities of today's organisational environment. Congratulations to the contributors for this excellent work—it will be a very helpful source for teachers, students, practitioners, and leaders now and into the future. This book delivers a vital and timely intervention, weaving together systems thinking, psychological insights, and real-world examples to illuminate the multifaceted nature of contemporary leadership."

Professor John Connolly, *Vice Dean and Professor of Public Policy, Glasgow School for Business & Society, Glasgow Caledonian University*

"Dr Amra Rao has assembled an excellent group of scholars who have explored a number of complex issues of leadership and organisational dynamics of relevance to psychologists. You learn a great deal from this book, and I thoroughly recommend it. It brings a much-needed lens to leadership, bridging theory and practice in ways that are both insightful and applicable. A valuable resource for those navigating leadership in complex systems.

Professor Mark Stein, *Emeritus Professor of Leadership and Management, University of Leicester*

"Amra Rao's book *Rethinking Leadership for Clinical, Counselling and Health Psychologists* is an outstanding and much needed resource. It highlights such issues like leading clinical change, the political skills needed in everyday leadership, the importance and role of business skills in strengthening psychological leadership, wellbeing as leadership, and many more skills to be an effective leader in the fields of applied psychological practice. The contributors to this volume are first rate, and the contributions are innovative. A must buy for psychologists working across a range of contexts. An outstanding and much-needed resource highlighting skills to be an effective leader in the fields of applied psychological practice. A must buy for psychologists working across a range of contexts."

Professor Sir Cary Cooper, *CBE, 50th Anniversary Professor of Organizational Psychology & Health, Alliance Manchester Business School, University of Manchester*

"We need to bring a more psychological approach to leadership in a complex, uncertain, and rapidly evolving world. *Rethinking Leadership for Clinical, Counselling and Health Psychologists* shows us how. It provides a distinctive and timely addition to the leadership literature, bringing together psychological insights into a comprehensive volume to guide how we understand and practise leadership, whatever our role."

Dr Adrian Whittington, *National Clinical Lead for Psychological Professions, NHS England*

"This book, *Rethinking Leadership for Clinical, Counselling and Health Psychologists*, offers a multi-dimensional approach drawing on a wealth of material from different schools of thought to capture the complexity and nuance of modern organisational life and how leadership can be thought about and practised within it. Rather than offering easy or quick-fix answers, this book takes seriously the tensions, costs, and risks inherent in the leadership task, but persistently engages with thinking that re-orients leadership towards relationship, inclusion, care, and flexibility.

With case studies throughout, focusing on the realities of leadership in the current NHS, there are contemporary accounts of leaders and what they have done in the situations they faced, including situations of relational conflict and rupture, managing organisational change, facing ethical dilemmas and moral distress, and using political and business perspectives to navigate difficulties. Whatever your own history in both leadership and psychology you will find a perspective and insight that will resonate with you.

A critical, essential text that draws together diverse, rich contributions into a proposal for generative leadership—this book offers both companionship and hope to those seeking leadership roles and those working to co-enact leadership with integrity and equity for the good of the health systems in which they seek to make a difference. There is a space here for creative thinking, and an invitation to all readers to make sense of complex systems and at the same time consider what is essentially psychological in leadership, as well as to find their own place and use within the leadership domain."

Dr Robyn Vesey, *Consultant Clinical Psychologist, Programme Director of the Henley Advanced Personal Leadership Programme*

"As a Health Psychologist, I welcome this book on leadership in practice, which includes insights from a broad, diverse range of experts working in applied practice. It opens up questions around context and systems, what impactful practice looks like, and the role of self and identity in leadership. It covers a range of topics of fundamental importance, including understanding what leadership is, how leaders can foster change and collaboration, navigating complex organisational change whilst fostering resilience, addressing identity and power dynamics, and leadership in an era of uncertainty, and is enhanced by case studies of practice. This book is particularly to be lauded for including a section on cultivating an organisational culture that prioritises wellbeing and describing wellbeing as essential. I would recommend the book as required reading for practitioner psychologists across the career span, whether they work in the NHS or private firms, as a guide for what they have to offer to leadership and how they can maximise their leadership skills."

Dr Emily Arden-Close, *Professor of Health Psychology, Principal Academic in Psychology, Department of Psychology, Bournemouth University*

"If you are a psychologist who has a leadership position (or are considering going down this road) this book will make you rethink how you view leadership. The different authors take us on a journey of exploration across the many areas that psychologists must navigate in the ever-changing landscape of leadership. Across the chapters they invite us to consider the impact of context, complexity, and human connection on how we lead. The book draws together key evidence and experience to provide a valuable guide to being a psychology leader in these fast-changing times, where leaders must be dynamic, adaptive, and socially responsible. A thoughtful and insightful read."

Dr Heather Buchanan, *Associate Professor in Health Psychology, Faculty of Medicine & Health Sciences, University of Nottingham*

Rethinking Leadership for Clinical, Counselling and Health Psychologists

This pioneering book offers a bold, psychologically informed take on leadership for today's complex and evolving systems. Written for clinical, counselling, and health psychologists, it challenges traditional models and reframes leadership as a dynamic, adaptive, and systems-aware practice.

With a distinctive triadic lens—looking within, between, and across systems—it integrates psychological theory, organisational insight, and systems thinking to explore how identity, emotion, power, and context shape leadership and followership in real-world environments. It offers practical tools to navigate relational challenges, manage work pressures, foster psychological safety, and lead with purpose through conflict, change, and uncertainty.

Grounded in lived experience and learning-in-action, this book shows how leadership is co-created through reflective and reflexive practice, inclusive collaboration, and ethical influence. It argues that sustainable, transformational change requires strategic focus, courageous engagement with power dynamics, and support for leadership at all levels.

Essential reading not only for psychologists, managers, and aspiring leaders but for anyone interested in creating healthier, more equitable workplaces and leading with courage, compassion, and systemic insight.

Dr Amra Saleem Rao is Consultant Clinical Psychologist, Organisational and Leadership Development Consultant, and Director of Psychological Horizons: a London-based psychological therapies and organisational consultancy. With more than 30 years of experience across UK healthcare and other sectors, and international contexts, she brings a distinctive integration of psychological depth, systemic awareness, and lived leadership to inspire change in people and organisations.

BPS Professional Practice and Development Series

British Psychological Society

In partnership with the British Psychological Society (BPS), Routledge is pleased to present *BPS Professional Practice and Development*, a series of inspiring books designed to support continuing professional development. Offering accessible, evidence-based guides to deepen understanding, develop expertise and improve techniques and strategies, books in this series address key topics and challenges faced by psychologists in their research and practice, and include case studies and real-life examples in relevant contexts.

Each book strikes a careful balance between research and practical strategies, as well as resources for implementation and opportunities for reflection. Covering a broad range of subject areas for practitioners in a range of roles, titles may also be accompanied by digital resources to support professionals in employing new strategies and practices in their work.

Reimagining Race in Psychology
Challenging Narratives and Widening Perspectives in Training and Practice
Edited by Yetunde Ade-Serrano and Ohemaa Nkansa-Dwamena

Rethinking Leadership for Clinical, Counselling and Health Psychologists
Managing Complexity and Change for Thriving Workplaces
Edited by Dr Amra Saleem Rao

For more information about this series, please visit: BPS Professional Practice and Development Series - Book SeriesRoutledge & CRC Press

Rethinking Leadership for Clinical, Counselling and Health Psychologists

Managing Complexity and Change for Thriving Workplaces

EDITED BY DR AMRA SALEEM RAO

Routledge
Taylor & Francis Group
LONDON AND NEW YORK

Designed cover image: Getty Images

First published 2026
by Routledge
4 Park Square, Milton Park, Abingdon, Oxon OX14 4RN

and by Routledge
605 Third Avenue, New York, NY 10158

Routledge is an imprint of the Taylor & Francis Group, an informa business

British Library Cataloguing-in-Publication Data
A catalogue record for this book is available from the British Library

ISBN: 9781032794976 (hbk)
ISBN: 9781032794952 (pbk)
ISBN: 9781003492399 (ebk)

DOI: 10.4324/9781003492399

Typeset in Dante and Avenir
by Deanta Global Publishing Services, Chennai, India

Access the Support Material: www.routledge.com/9781032794976

Dedication and Acknowledgement

To my father—a prolific writer, profound thinker, and steadfast thought leader, whose curiosity, courage, and conviction continue to inspire new ways of seeing, leading, and being.

With deepest gratitude to my husband—whose unwavering support and steady presence have nurtured the ground from which new ideas take root and grow.

And to my mentors, colleagues, and those I've worked alongside—
Thank you for the shared ideas, questions, and challenges that have shaped my thinking and strengthened my resolve to reimagine leadership in today's complex world. Together, you have shown me the power of growth through ongoing learning and lived experience.

Contents

Foreword

The purpose of leadership is to bring people together to work on a shared endeavour. We live in divided and atomised times where people need to be connected beyond the echo chambers of like-thinking and like-feeling others. This makes the task of bringing people together to achieve collective purposes more challenging, not helped by the scepticism and suspicion of leaders, resulting in plummeting levels of trust caused by their perceived failure to respond adequately to the various financial, health and environmental challenges of our times. This collection of chapters by experts on the topic of leadership, and in particular its psychological foundations, is therefore timely. It also provides a comprehensive overview of current thinking and approaches to leadership in the psychology profession. Amra Rao is chair of the BPS Leadership and Management Faculty, whose purpose is to champion, support and develop psychologists and psychological leadership. As such, she is well placed to bring together the impressive contributors to this book.

Those currently in leadership roles in psychology grew up in a different era and need to reflect on and adapt their style of leadership to the current context with changed attitudes to power and authority. Leadership is a practice which can only be learned on the job, learning by doing. Whilst much written and many theories generated every year, none will be exactly right for you in your context; that book hasn't been written, and if it is to be written, you will need to write it yourself! In other words, every leader has to develop their own model of leadership, albeit drawing on the ideas and experiences of others. Leaders have to own and inhabit the role if they are to be convincing. Furthermore, what may seem like good leadership to some will be seen as bad by others. The idea that good leadership must result in ethically good outcomes is a common confusion in the field. Ethically poor leadership can lead to good outcomes – victory in war, profit in commerce. Ethically good leadership may simply lead to contented followers, but not necessarily to effective outcomes.

Academic research on leadership can be enlightening, but despite claims to the contrary by the psychometrics industry and the multitude of providers of leadership training, there are few sound generalisations that can be made. Definitions of leadership abound, and perhaps the only certainty is that leadership entails inspiring others to go in a certain direction, generating the energy to do so, and helping the organisation adapt to its environment. Leadership is best viewed not as a characteristic of an individual but as an emergent property of the interaction between an individual, a group and its environment. Several of the chapters in the book expand on this view of leadership as an emergent practice in relation to a complex, fast-changing environment. In conditions of radical uncertainty, the assumption that it is possible to predict the future, analyse the risks and therefore determine one's responses based on what has been done in the past is mistaken. To be effective, leaders have to learn to tolerate states of uncertainty long enough for novel solutions to emerge.

Leadership exists not in an individual person, but in their relationships with others. Like beauty, leadership exists in the eye of the beholder. Disconcertingly, you are not who you think you are, but who they think you are. Organisational culture and environmental context eat leadership development programmes for breakfast. So it is fitting that the first section of this book addresses understanding leadership in context. Other sections cover topics such as the political skills of leadership, the nature of strategic leadership, navigating change, fostering workplace well-being, as well as race, culture, and identity.

The reader will find in this book a multiplicity of perspectives on important leadership topics and the psychology profession, which, whilst not promising all the answers, will certainly stimulate your thinking. Whilst the book is targeted at psychologist leaders, its insights will also resonate with other professionals interested in psychologically informed leadership.

Jon Stokes, Associate Scholar, Said Business School, University of Oxford. Director, Stokes & Jolly Limited. www.stokesjolly.com

About the Editor

Dr Amra Saleem Rao is Consultant Clinical Psychologist, Organisational and Leadership Development Consultant, and Director of Psychological Horizons: a London-based Psychological Therapies & Organisational Consultancy. With Extensive experience spanning more than 30 years across the NHS and international contexts, she brings a distinctive integration of psychological depth, organisational insight, and lived leadership to her work.

She currently chairs both the *British Psychological Society's Division of Clinical Psychology Faculties Network* and the *DCP Leadership & Management Faculty*. She has led the *National Psychological Professions Wellbeing Programme* and the *Developing Leaders* initiative, shaping inclusive, reflective, and purposeful leadership across complex systems.

Dr Rao brings extensive lived experience of leadership in healthcare and beyond. Decades of mentoring, coaching, and consulting—including healthcare, finance, law, politics, and management—have deepened her understanding of the emotional demands, paradoxes, and systemic forces that shape leadership. She is committed to advancing equity and engaging with dynamics of difference, not as a policy fix, but as a deeply human, relational, and developmental imperative.

She has honorary academic roles and consults at Group Relations conferences in the UK and internationally. She is an experienced supervisors clinical supervisor and has led the adaptation of Dynamic Interpersonal Therapy (DIT) pilot for complex presentations.

Dr Rao has published widely across clinical, personal, and organisational domains—including on leadership, workforce, wellbeing, organisational change, and the challenges of cross-cultural leadership. She is co-editor of *Mentoring in Health, Social Care and Beyond* (2024). She advocates for leadership that is relationally attuned, psychologically informed, socially conscious, sustainable, and collectively courageous—capable of responding to human complexity while staying alert to the political, economic, and global forces shaping our shared future.

Contributors

Dr Sarina Afzali Shamsabad completed her doctoral training at Royal Holloway University and went on to study Clinical Neuropsychology at the University of Bristol. She is particularly interested in widening access to neuropsychological testing for individuals from diverse backgrounds and keen to develop culturally appropriate assessments. With ten years of experience working in the NHS, she currently works in a dementia and cognitive impairment service in West London and proactively seeks to reduce barriers in accessing services for minoritised communities and enhancing the level of support offered to carers. She is passionate about increasing the presence of under-represented groups within the clinical psychology profession and has been involved in multiple widening access and mentoring schemes over the years. She is committed to equity in healthcare and continues to advocate for inclusive and accessible services for all.

Professor Aimée Aubeeluck is Chartered Psychologist (British Psychological Society) and Registered Practitioner Health Psychologist (HCPC). She holds a BA (Hons) in Psychology, an MSc in Health Psychology, a PGDip in Higher Education, and a PGCert in Leadership and Management. She is also Principal Fellow of Advance HE, reflecting her sustained commitment to academic leadership and student experience. Professor Aubeeluck was awarded a PhD in Health Psychology in 2005 for her research on the impact of spousal caregiving in Huntington's disease. Her scholarly and research activity continues to evolve, with a focus on student-centred education, the psychological experiences of learners (including impostor phenomenon), and health psychology research spanning chronic illness, quality of life, psychometrics, and behaviour change. She is passionate about the transformational nature and culture of good leadership and committed to generating new evidence through research activity to improve population health and wellbeing.

Clare Baguley was Programme Manager for the Psychological Professions Network in the North West between 2013 and 2022. She trained as Cognitive Behaviour Therapist at the Oxford Centre for Cognitive Therapy in 1998, having previously worked as a community psychiatric nurse in Tameside, Greater Manchester. In 2004, she joined the University of Manchester and led the post-graduate education programme for Psychological Wellbeing Practitioners under the Department of Health's Improving Access to Psychological Therapies (IAPT) programme, which latterly developed to incorporate pathways in dementia care and psycho-social interventions for psychosis. Subsequently, Clare Baguley became the IAPT North West Education Programme Lead with responsibility for managing and developing the interface between universities in the NW region of England and their clinical practice partners. She has contributed regionally, nationally, and internationally to publications, training, and conferences on primary care mental health with a particular interest in the use of psychological approaches in physical health care settings.

Dr Charlotte Baribeau is a trainee clinical psychologist in her final year at Royal Holloway, University of London. She has eight years of experience working in NHS mental health services across a range of settings, including staff wellbeing, children and young people's mental health, neurodevelopment, psychosis rehabilitation inpatient, and clinical health psychology. Charlotte completed a service-related research project on the application of the Power Threat Meaning Framework within a specialist women's health psychology service. Her doctoral thesis explores experiences of couples-based motivational interviewing for heavy alcohol use for people living with HIV. Charlotte is committed to supporting the NHS workforce and reducing inequalities experienced by staff and patients through a compassionate leadership approach.

Gita Bhutani trained and worked as a clinical psychologist in Glasgow and subsequently in North West England. From 2006 to 2023, Gita Bhutani was the director for Psychological Professions at Lancashire & South Cumbria NHS Trust, with professional responsibility for psychological professions staff across the lifespan and a range of settings. Alongside this role within the Trust, Gita Bhutani implemented a supervision system for all staff, developed the staff wellbeing portfolio, and during Covid, set up the county-wide staff wellbeing service/resilience hub. Gita Bhutani is a founding member and co-chair of the Psychological Professions Network (PPN), which started in the North West in 2013. From 2018 to 2023, she undertook a range of projects and roles with Health Education England, including National Psychological Professions Development Lead. She is Honorary Research Fellow at the University of Manchester. Gita Bhutani has contributed to and chaired committees for the National Institute of Health & Care Excellence (NICE), including Quality Standards, and as a member of the Guideline Development Group for the PTSD Guidelines update. She has been a member of a number of the British Psychological Society's Division of Clinical Psychology Faculties and Groups over the past 25 years.

Dr Rachel Bradley is a consultant clinical psychologist with over 20 years' experience of working clinically with children, young people, and families, primarily in CAMHS (Child and Adolescent Mental Health Services) and in therapeutic services for children in care or adopted. She has worked in clinical leadership roles in a variety of settings for many years and enjoys the challenges of developing services, improving team cultures, and leading on organisation-wide projects. Dr Bradley has also been Workforce Lead for Psychological Professionals at an ICS (Integrated Care System) level, bringing together consideration of workforce issues and system-wide developments in relation to clinical services. Alongside her NHS roles, she chairs the British Psychological Society's Faculty for Children, Young People and their Families within the Division of Clinical Psychology.

Yoyo King-Yin Chan is a trainee counselling psychologist at The University of Manchester. She has worked as a registered social worker in Hong Kong with clinical experiences in cancer care, working with patients, caregivers, and families, particularly with individuals from marginalised populations. Her experience in the UK involved working with cancer patients and families, individuals affected by ME/CFS, and university students. Yoyo's research interests lie in the field of social justice, racial equality, and anti-oppressive practice, with the aim of examining the training gaps and curriculum development to improve anti-oppressive practices in counselling psychology.

Dr Arshia Choudhury is a clinical psychologist and lecturer. She completed her Doctoral Training in Clinical Psychology from Royal Holloway in 2024. Arshia has over 4 years of experience working in NHS and non-NHS services across a range of settings, including children and young people's mental health, rare dementia, primary care talking therapies, and a research and innovation consultancy. She has also lectured on developmental psychology and research modules for over 2 years. Arshia's doctoral thesis focused on developing a cognitive-behavioural model of women's experiences of coercive control. She currently works in a neurodevelopmental team within a Central London CAMHS service.

Jeremy C. Clarke CBE is Psychoanalytic Psychotherapist registered with the British Psychoanalytic Council and British Association for Counselling and Psychotherapy, and an Accredited Supervisor in Dynamic Interpersonal Therapy with Anna Freud Centre. He is Clinical Director at Albany Trust and Chair of the Association for Psychoanalytic Psychotherapy in the Public Sector. Formerly, he was a National Adviser to the IAPT programme, an expert member on the NICE

Depression guideline for adults, 2009 and 2022, and helped design and evaluate Greater Manchester's Working Well programme. Jeremy C. Clarke co-led the Staff Wellbeing project with Dr. Amra Rao. He was awarded the title CBE in 2012 for his contribution to mental health.

Dr Esther Cohen-Tovée is a consultant clinical psychologist and a director of AHPs and Psychological Services at Cumbria, Northumberland Tyne & Wear NHS FT, with over 35 years of NHS service. She has worked in a series of leadership and management roles since 1996. Dr Cohen-Tovée has served as a trustee of the British Psychological Society (2019–2022) and as a chair of the BPS Division of Clinical Psychology (2016–17; 2019–21). She was the chair of the DCP Leadership & Management Faculty from 2014 to 2016. Dr Cohen-Tovée was a co-founder and a co-chair of the BPS & Royal College of Psychiatrists' Accreditation Programme for Psychological Therapies Services (2014–2023). She was the BPS representative on the Five-Year Forward View for Mental Health & NHS Long Term Plan Independent Oversight & Advisory Group (2016–2021). Dr Cohen-Tovée's clinical field is in adult mental health, with a special interest in Eating Disorders. She has provided training in this field nationally and internationally.

Dr Rajinder Dhanjal works as Principal Clinical Psychologist in Leeds and York Partnership Foundation Trust. With over 20 years of experience, she has a particular interest in Cognitive Analytical Therapy (CAT), complex trauma, community psychology, race, and equity. Alongside this, she is interested in research and development in psychotherapy and mental health.

Amy C. Edmondson is the Novartis Professor of Leadership and Management at Harvard Business School, renowned for her research over the last 20 years on psychological safety and teaming. Her award-winning work has appeared in *The New York Times*, *The Wall Street Journal*, the *Financial Times*, *Psychology Today*, *Fast Company*, *Harvard Business Review*, and more. Named by Thinkers 50 in 2021 as the #1 Management Thinker in the world, Amy's TED Talk "How to Turn a Group of Strangers into a Team" has been viewed over three million times. She is the author of *The Fearless Organisation*, *Teaming*, and most recently, *Right Kind of Wrong: The Science of Failing Well.*

Dr Rosie Gilderthorp is a clinical psychologist, coach, and military spouse. Since founding Know Your Mind Consulting and Psychology Business School, she has moved house four times, solo-parented three neurodivergent children, and somehow survived on coffee while juggling two businesses and completing an MBA from Warwick Business School. With 16 years of experience in the NHS, HM Prison Service, and private practice, Dr Gilderthorp is passionate about helping parents thrive through adversity. Her research interest is in Hyperemesis Gravidarum and transforming women's health through innovation. She provides practical, free support for parents through her *Know Your Mind* newsletter on Substack and the Pregnant and Sick podcast. When she's not seeing clients, teaching, coaching other therapists, recording The Business of Psychology podcast, or running in the rain, she's in her garden office in Tunbridge Wells—often interrupted by her two oversized cats.

Dr Lorraine Gordon has worked in the UK National Health Service for over 25 years. She is a consultant counselling psychologist and head of psychology and psychotherapy for a South London borough's adult mental health service. Dr Lorraine is a member of the UK Association of Black Psychologists and the Black, African, and Asian Therapist Network. She is a British Association of Behavioural and Cognitive Psychotherapy accredited cognitive behavioural therapist and an advanced accredited schema therapist, supervisor, and trainer. She completed a course in Black Psychology and African Centred Therapy. She was also awarded an MA in Business and Management with distinction. Lorraine teaches post-graduate students on topics such as antiracism. Dr Lorraine was the staff senior lead for the Patient and Carer Race Equality Framework (PCREF) in a South London borough, and for a few years, was Psychology and Psychotherapy PCREF lead for the mental health Trust where she is based.

Dr Maryam Haghiran is a clinical psychologist and advocate for racial equity in mental health care. She completed her Doctoral Training in Clinical Psychology at Royal Holloway in 2025 and is dedicated to improving access to care and enhancing the quality of services for marginalised communities. With over a decade of experience across NHS and non-NHS settings—including adult forensic services, child and adolescent mental health services, primary care talking therapies, and specialist trauma services—she is passionate about driving meaningful change. Her doctoral research focused on the effects of racial trauma in forensic settings and how social and ethnic identity can be better embedded in care. She currently works in a leading role within a Community Mental Health Team in North East London, where she continues to push for more inclusive and effective mental health support.

Joanne Hemmingfield is CEO and Founder of Hemmingfield Consultancy. An expert in Coproduction, she advises on how to hear from the widest community in shaping mental health services. She is interested in how people who use services can influence board-level decision-making, including governance and strategic development. With lived experience of using services, she has served on senior committees within the British Psychological Society, including the Executive Committee and the Leadership and Management Faculty of the Division of Clinical Psychology. Joanne is currently Coproduction Consultant working on a strategy to improve care in an NHS Trust and a Trustee at C3 Hope. Ambitious, with a can-do attitude, Joanne believes that despite the many obstacles, there is hope for us to provide better care for those with mental distress. A thought-leader in this area, she consults with organisations to build confidence and develop their approach to Coproduction.

Dr Kerry Hinsby is Lead Consultant Clinical and Forensic Psychologist. She has over 25 years of experience working across a range of forensic settings. During this time, she became interested in the impact of trauma both within the lives of the service users and within the staff working in the area. Having qualified as a coach, she moved fulltime into staff wellbeing roles. She is now Clinical Lead at the West Yorkshire Staff Mental Health and Wellbeing Hub. The duality of her background has allowed her to build services that are genuinely trauma-informed and responsive to both the needs of the service user and the staff. Dr Hinsby has published articles and spoken widely on these topics. She is currently leading the project focused on building a trauma-informed Critical Incident Staff Support Pathway (CrISSP) across the West Yorkshire Integrated Care System.

Professor Jan Hughes is the joint director of the clinical psychology training programme at the University of Leeds. She was Joint Chair of the Group of Trainers in Clinical Psychology and continues to have a national role in the DCP Workforce and Training Sub Committee. Her clinical interest in the last few years has been around staff support in the NHS.

Dr Elizabeth Jenkinson Associate Professor in Health Psychology, UWE, Bristol & National Training Director in Health Psychology for Workforce Redesign, NHS England Workforce Training and Education. Dr Jenkinson is an experienced registered practitioner health psychologist (HCPC), chartered psychologist (BPS) and senior academic (SFHEA), skilled in clinical applications of health psychology, research, teaching, supervision and practice. Liz currently leads research, teaching and knowledge exchange at UWE, Bristol as an Associate Professor, and leads innovation in Health Psychology at NHS England as the National Training Director for Health Psychology in Workforce Redesign.

Liz Kell is a qualified psychological wellbeing practitioner, initially training as a primary care graduate mental health worker in 2004. Liz Kell has worked in primary mental health services and NHS Talking Therapies (previously IAPT) services as a PWP, supervisor, and PWP lead, including developing and launching a new Standalone PWP IAPT service as Clinical Service Manager within a Public Health Management Team, before moving to the University of Central Lancashire as course leader for the PWP training (2016–2023) and Principal Lecturer leading the Psychological Therapies portfolio. She is Associate Professor,

Co-Director of the Low Intensity CBT Portfolio within Cedar at the University of Exeter. Throughout her career, Liz Kell has been involved in multiple regional and national networks supporting PWPs and other new roles within the psychological professions. Liz Kell has actively campaigned for and supported the recent practitioner registration developments. She is the co-chair of the BPS PWP Training Committee, the previous chair of the BABCP Low Intensity Special Interest Group, where she remains as an active committee member and a member of the BPS Wider Psychological Workforce Advisory Group. Liz Kell represents Wellbeing Practitioners on the BABCP Practitioner Accreditation and Registration Committee and is chair of their Wellbeing Practitioner sub-committee. Liz Kell has been part of the Psychological Professions Network in the Northwest since its launch in 2013, initially representing the PWP workforce, chairing the first PWP community of practice, and the senior PWP network. She supported the development of Senior PWP networks in the North East and Yorkshire and co-delivered PWP North Conferences. She has been co-chair of the PPN North West since October 2021.

Dr Saim Kirhan completed his Clinical Psychology training at Royal Holloway, University of London, in 2024. He was actively involved in the Widening Access Committee and Diversity Working Group, addressing racial, ethnic, and cultural disparities for trainee psychologists. His doctoral thesis explored trauma-informed care among male adults with histories of offending and substance use, examining the role of racial identity in therapeutic relationships and care quality. Committed to human rights and social justice, Saim aims to reduce racial disparities for NHS staff and patients. He currently works at a Major Trauma Centre in East London and offers teaching on racial trauma and racial identity development to NHS staff in London.

Kalpita Kunde is Consultant Clinical Psychologist with over 25 years of experience working in the Health Care sector in England, specialising in complex trauma, suicide and prevention, long-term mental health conditions, and wellbeing. Although Kalpita is a strong proponent of evidence-based talking treatments, she is also a keen aerial yoga enthusiast and a ceramicist, and finds that there are many other modalities that can help with recovery from trauma. Kalpita is currently the UK Chair for the Division of Clinical Psychology with the British Psychological Society and is employed by Cumbria Northumberland and Tyne and Wear NHS Trust. Kalpita is passionate about influencing leaders using a relational trauma-informed approach in order to create psychologically safe working cultures and systems for the workforce. Kalpita strongly believes in embedding the values and lessons learned from hardships and lived experiences.

Professor Gary Latchford is the joint director of the clinical psychology training programme at the University of Leeds. He was also Joint Chair of the Group of Trainers in Clinical Psychology and continues to have a national role in the DCP Workforce and Training Sub Committee. His clinical work has been in clinical health psychology, and for many years, he combined a role at the University with being head of Adult Medical Psychology at Leeds Teaching Hospitals.

Professor Tony Lavender is trained in Clinical Psychology at the Institute of Psychiatry and holds a doctorate from Kings College London. He has played a leading role in workforce development nationally with the Department of Health, British Psychological Society, and NHS Digital. He has published extensively on services and therapies for people with psychosis and personality disorder, anorexia, workforce planning, and the history of clinical psychology. He held roles as Dean of a large Faculty and Pro-Vice Chancellor at Canterbury Christ Church University. He directed the Clinical Psychology Programme (Salomons) for 21 years. He retired in December 2016 but continues to maintain an active involvement in research, mentoring, organisational consultancy, and workforce planning. Professor Lavender chairs the BPS's Practice Board and is a member of the Division of Clinical Psychology (DCP) Executive, chairing the DCP Workforce and Training Group. He is on the NHSE/I/HEE National Psychological Professions Workforce Advisory Group.

Dr. David Lawlor is a social scientist and a professional partner at the Tavistock Institute of Human Relations, specialising in organisational consultancy, research, and training. He co-directs the professional development programme *Organisational Consultancy: Working with the Dynamics*, which focuses on applying systems psychodynamic theory to organisational contexts. In his consultancy work, he assists organisations in navigating the technical and emotional challenges of implementing change through reflective practices and systemic interventions. He is the co-author, alongside Dr. Mannie Sher, of a trilogy on systems psychodynamics: *An Introduction to Systems Psychodynamics*; *Systems Psychodynamics: Innovative Approaches to Change* and *Whole Systems & Complexity*, and *Systems Psychodynamics: Theorist and Practitioner Voices from the Field*.These works synthesise decades of Tavistock Institute practice, offering insights into the unconscious dynamics that influence organisational life. Dr. Lawlor's contributions have significantly advanced the understanding of how unconscious processes impact organisational behaviour, making him a leading figure in the field of systems psychodynamics.

Jennifer Lees-Marshment is Professor of Political Marketing and Management at the University of Dundee. She is a research-led but practice-oriented cross-disciplinary academic focused on researching political marketing, political management, and political leadership. She has interviewed over 350 political practitioners, including government ministers and staffers/advisors to Prime Ministers and Presidents, and is author/editor of 19 books. Her most recent edited works are *Political Management in Practice* (2024) and *Political Marketing and Management in the 2020 New Zealand Election* (2021), and her own research *The Human Resource Management of Political Staffers: Insights from Prime Ministers' Advisers and Reformers* (2024), *From Landslide to Mudslide: The Strategic Marketing Mistakes of the 2020–2023 New Zealand Labour Government* (2024) and *Political Management: The Dance of Government and Politics* (2020).

Dr Olga Luzón is Chartered Clinical Psychologist and Senior Lecturer at Royal Holloway, University of London, leading the Academic aspect of the Doctorate in Clinical Psychology course. She holds a Doctorate in Clinical Psychology, a Postgraduate Diploma in CBT, and a Postgraduate Certificate in Academic Practice. She is Associate Fellow of the BPS, Fellow of the Higher Education Academy, and is part of various BPS committees and Faculties. With over 20 years of clinical experience, Olga has worked as a clinical psychologist, supervisor, and trainer across various NHS services. Her research focuses on domestic abuse and its impact on victims and children, and she has supervised over 30 doctoral theses on a range of topics. She is dedicated to promoting diversity and inclusion in higher education and clinical practice, actively contributing to initiatives that foster equity and access. Passionate about shaping the future of the profession, Olga is committed to mentoring and empowering the next generation of clinical psychologists to meet emerging societal challenges with compassion, courage, and innovation.

Ian MacRae is an award-winning author, work psychologist, and director of High Potential Psychology, which focuses on psychological research and developing workplace psychometric assessments that have been completed over one million times since its founding in 2014. He holds a BA in Psychology from the University of British Columbia and an MSc in Research Methods in Psychology from University College London. His expertise covers personality, leadership potential, workplace performance, digital communication, and the psychological effects of emerging digital technologies. He developed the High Potential Trait Inventory (HPTI), and his books include *High Potential: How to Spot, Manage and Develop Talented People at Work*; *Motivation and Performance*; and *Dark Social: Understanding the Darker Side of Work, Personality and Social Media*, which offer research-led, practical frameworks relevant to leadership selection, development, and performance management. He serves on the British Psychological Society's Research Board and the Division of Occupational Psychology committee.

Professor (Emeritus) Reg Morris, BA, PhD, DipPsych, C.Psychol., is a distinguished clinical psychologist and academic with over four decades of experience in clinical practice, training, and research. After completing his PhD in Psychology in 1977, he held several senior academic leadership roles, including Director of the Bristol Clinical Psychology Training Programme (2001–2008), Director of the South Wales Programme (2008–2020), and Clinical Director in Plymouth (2020–2023). Since 1996, Professor Morris has worked extensively in NHS stroke services and with third sector organisations such as The Stroke Association and Bristol after Stroke. His work has focused on face-to-face clinical care, staff training, service development, peer support, and psychological assessment. His primary research interests lie in stroke rehabilitation, with additional contributions in forensic and occupational psychology. He has authored or co-authored numerous peer-reviewed articles and key texts, including *Psychological Management of Stroke* (2012), *Rebuilding Your Life after Stroke* (2017), and *Living Your Life with Cancer through ACT* (2021). A founding member of the OPSYRIS network, Professor Morris has held leadership roles within the British Psychological Society, including co-chairing the Group of Trainers in Clinical Psychology and serving on both the DCP Workforce and Training Subcommittee and the DCP Staff Well-Being Subcommittee.

Stephen Murgatroyd teaches anticipatory studies for leadership in graduate programs at the University of Alberta and Athabasca University. A former Dean of the Faculty of Business at Athabasca and CEO of a large UK-based strategic human resource consultancy, Stephen has worked extensively on change and transformation initiatives for 40 of the Fortune 500 companies, as well as a range of health systems, education systems, and non-profit networks. He is a psychologist and author of over 50 books and 200 papers, book chapters, and articles. He has pioneered approaches to mentoring, coaching, and peer support for leaders facing challenges and change.

Dr Adrian Neal is Consultant Clinical Psychologist with additional Organisational Psychology training and has been Head of Employee Wellbeing at Aneurin Bevan University Health Board since 2014. He has previously held leadership roles within the British Psychological Society's Division of Clinical Psychology, Applied Psychologists in Health Special Advisory Group (Wales), and has worked in both the public and private sectors. Dr Adrian Neal has contributed to NICE Guidelines for Employee Wellbeing, has published and researched widely in the area, and holds a number of honorary academic roles. Dr Neal's primary interests are the psychosocial factors that underpin and shape organisational wellbeing (e.g., leadership, team dynamics, and relational approaches). He firmly believes that 'prevention is better than cure' and that the more we can understand and proactively manage the psychosocial work of our organisations, the more we can improve wellbeing, performance, the experience of our employees, and ultimately the quality of the services we offer.

Dr Charlotte O'Brien, CPsychol, DCounsPsych, AFBPsS, HCPC Reg., is the programme director and lecturer in Counselling Psychology at the University of Manchester and is an associate fellow of the British Psychological Society. Charlotte also works as an HCPC registered Counselling Psychologist in the NHS and in private practice, where she specialises in working with adults who have experienced complex trauma. Charlotte's research interests include working creatively, therapeutically, and in a culturally informed way with vulnerable individuals and groups such as refugees, asylum seekers, and veterans. Charlotte's research focuses on taking a non-pathologising approach to the concept of 'Embodied Trauma', which applies a bio-psycho-social-sexual-spiritual-existential or 'holistic' lens to the conceptualisation of mental health and distress. Charlotte is passionate about anti-oppressive and socially just approaches to therapeutic practice and leadership in psychology and has written a number of academic publications in this field.

Dr Anton Obholzer is a distinguished psychiatrist, psychoanalyst, and organisational consultant known for his pioneering work on the emotional dynamics of leadership and systems. He served as Chief Executive of the Tavistock & Portman NHS Trust in London for over a decade. A Fellow of the Royal College of Psychiatrists, he has brought psychologically informed leadership practices to health, public, and business sectors. Internationally respected as a teacher and consultant, he has worked with senior leaders across government, business, and academia, and is a staff member at INSEAD. He also serves as a Visiting Professor in Vienna and Graz. His co-edited book, *The Unconscious at Work*, is a seminal contribution to systems psychodynamics. Dr. Obholzer continues to influence leaders by integrating emotional intelligence, ethical awareness, and systemic insight in navigating authority, role, and organisational complexity.

Dr Andrew Roberts is Consultant Clinical Psychologist with over 25 years of experience across a wide range of mental health and neurological services, working with both working-age adults and older adults. His interest in leadership developed through participation in a range of leadership programmes and through leading multiple projects and service developments within NHS Trusts. In recent years, Dr Roberts's focus has turned to system leadership—exploring how to influence complex, interdependent systems to deliver improved outcomes and experiences for those who use NHS services. Dr Andrew has been Workforce Lead for Psychological Professionals within an Integrated Care System, and currently works as Lead for Older People's Mental Health Community Services in an NHS Trust.

Dr Hannah Shaw is a clinical psychologist with over eight years of experience in the mental health field, having worked across both NHS and non-NHS settings. Her experience spans a range of services, including eating disorders, sexual health, specialist and forensic inpatient, prisons, youth offending, homelessness, paediatrics, and talking therapies. Hannah completed her doctoral training at Royal Holloway University of London in 2023 and was the first clinical psychology trainee to undertake a leadership placement in the UK Parliament. Her research is centred on the challenges faced by disadvantaged groups in accessing mental health services. Guided by a critical human-rights-based approach, Hannah is committed to challenging discrimination, reducing inequalities, and fostering socially inclusive practices.

Dr Lynne Taylor graduated from the University of Aberdeen with First Class Honours in Psychology and obtained a clinical doctorate in Psychology from the University of Glasgow in 2000. Dr Lynne has held several senior leadership roles, including working as Clinical Director for CAMHS and as Director of Psychology for all cross-system psychological services in a Scottish Health Board. Trained in senior systems leadership, Dr Taylor has led various organisational redesigns. Since February 2021, she has worked full-time within the Scottish Government—first as Principal Psychology Advisor, and now as Principal Psychology Officer. She provides highly specialist psychological advice to Civil Servants, Directors, and Ministers, executive operational leads, and stakeholders by offering expert psychological perspectives on policy and a wide range of issues (e.g., waiting times, veterans, staff wellbeing, refugees, civil contingencies planning, mental health, and complex care). Dr Taylor is deeply committed to delivering high-quality services and positively influencing whole-system strategic change informed by the voices and expertise of those with lived experience. Her key skills span strategic change, leadership, planning, policy, and implementation.

Dr Kathryn Walters is Consultant Clinical Psychologist who jointly leads a service of 300 psychological professionals working across the lifespan in both physical and mental health settings in the NHS in Wales. She began the long training process in 1989 in Oxford and finished it in Guildford in 1996. After qualifying, she worked in central London for 5 years in an adult CMHT before moving to Wales in 2001. Dr Walters has held a senior psychology leadership role for 20 years, and in 2022 was an interim Divisional Director, with responsibility for 1800 staff and a budget of £110 million. She is an advocate for compassionate leadership and believes in the importance of relationships in shaping the experience and meaning of work.

Dr Ashley Weinberg is a chartered occupational psychologist and a senior lecturer in Psychology based at the University of Salford since 2000. He specialises in organisational, job-related, and individual factors contributing to employee well-being. As inaugural Chair of the BPS Political Psychology Section and editor of books with Cambridge University Press titled *The Psychology of Politicians* and *Psychology of Democracy: Of the People, by the People, for the People*, he is keen to promote understanding of the political features of all our working lives with a view to enhancing psychological health. In 2020, Dr. Weinberg was awarded the Occupational Psychology Policy Impact Award, and in 2023, he became a Fellow of the BPS.

Dr Lawrence Welch trained as a psychotherapist at Warwick University, where he also qualified as a Cognitive Analytic Therapist (CAT). He played a key role in developing CAT training and contributed to establishing courses for the Association for Cognitive Analytic Therapy (ACAT). Dr Welch worked in the NHS in Leeds from 1996, later becoming a Consultant Psychotherapist in the NHS in Wallsend, Newcastle—a post he held until his redundancy in 2014. Now retired, he continues to practise privately on a small scale. He has authored several published articles on CAT, supervision, reciprocal roles, organisational dynamics, and the influence of politics and power on dialogue within healthcare settings.

Michael West CBE is Senior Visiting Fellow at The King's Fund, London, and Professor of Organisational Psychology at Lancaster University. He also serves as Visiting Professor at University College Dublin and is Emeritus Professor at Aston University. He has written, edited, or co-edited 21 books and published over 200 articles on teamwork, innovation, leadership, and organisational culture, with a focus on healthcare. Michael West is Fellow of the British Psychological Society, the American Psychological Association, and the Academy of Social Sciences, and an Honorary Fellow of several medical colleges. He co-chaired the UK General Medical Council's inquiry *Caring for Doctors, Caring for Patients* (2019), and led the King's Fund's *The Courage of Compassion* (2020) review. His latest book, *Compassionate Leadership* (2021), explores sustaining humanity in health and social care. He advises health organisations internationally and was appointed CBE in 2020 for services to compassion and innovation in healthcare.

Dr Simon Western is a leading expert in leadership and organisational culture. With a background as a general and psychiatric nurse, clinical manager, and family therapist, Dr Western brings an embodied understanding of leadership in healthcare. He holds a PhD in Leadership and has authored several influential books, including *Leadership: A Critical Text.* He is CEO of the Eco-Leadership Institute, which runs a Diploma in Systems and Depth Coaching for leaders and hosts the popular podcast Edgy Ideas, which explores how to live a good life and create a good society through a psychosocial lens.

Dr Laura Anne Winter is a reader in Education and Counselling Psychology and Director for Equality, Diversity and Inclusion in the School of Environment, Education and Development. She is an HCPC-registered Counselling Psychologist, a BPS Chartered Psychologist, Fellow of the Higher Education Academy, and deputy-chair of the BPS Training Committee in Counselling Psychology. Her research interests centre on social justice, inequality, and politics, and how these are understood by psychologists, as well as how they influence their work as practitioners. Her recent publications include *The SAGE Handbook of Counselling and Psychotherapy* (5th edition with Professor Terry Hanley, 2023) and the *Handbook of Social Justice in the Psychological Therapies* (with Professor Divine Charura, 2023). She is a white, cis woman, and she has three young children.

Introduction

Leadership today is a dynamic and contextually bound process, continually shaped—and often stretched—by the turbulence of our times. From global instability and socio-political polarisation to ecological threats, economic uncertainty, rising work pressures, and shifting workforce expectations, leaders operate within relentless complexity and change. In such precarious conditions, effective leadership requires the ability to make difficult decisions amid ambiguity and volatility, navigating competing stakeholder interests and visible and hidden power structures, while ensuring ethical and equitable outcomes (Snowden & Boone, 2007; Obholzer & Roberts, 1994).

Contemporary leadership demands emotional resilience, adaptability, and the ability to foster psychological safety, environments where individuals feel empowered to speak up, take risks, and innovate without fear (Heifetz, Grashow & Linsky, 2009; Edmondson, 2018). Leaders are called to build cultures of trust, where trust is not merely aspirational but foundational, enabling organisations to navigate uncertainty with shared commitment and purpose.

Leadership transcends individual roles; it is a collective enterprise that inspires and cultivates leadership potential across the entire organisation. Everyone holds the potential to guide, influence, and make valuable contributions (Raelin, 2011; Uhl-Bien, 2006). However, those in formal leadership positions carry the added responsibility of fostering and enabling leadership at all levels. This collaborative and distributed approach is essential for navigating the complexity and uncertainty of today's organisational landscape.

DOI: 10.4324/9781003492399-1

At the same time, leadership cannot be disentangled from issues of identity, power, and privilege. As organisations confront systemic inequities, it becomes essential to understand how race, gender, class, and other intersecting identities shape both access to leadership roles and perceptions of authority (Eagly & Carli, 2007; Bourke & Dillon, 2018). Leadership today must be understood through an intersectional lens, one that recognises how diverse identities impact career trajectories and workplace experience within complex organisational systems. This entails the deliberate unearthing of implicit bias and the intentional design of inclusive systems that elevate and respond to diverse voices and perspectives.

To engage meaningfully with leadership in today's complex and evolving environments, it is essential to reflect on the interplay between three interconnected concepts: leadership (the domain), leading (the process), and leaders (the role) (Samma, 2025). Each offers a distinct lens for understanding how leadership is enacted within organisational life. This interaction is not merely theoretical; it is a lived reality, where every decision reverberates through the organisation and beyond, impacting both individuals and systems. Insights from multiple disciplines affirm that these elements do not operate in isolation; their interaction is dynamic, fluid, and contextually shaped. Making sense of this complexity calls for an integrative perspective, grounded in systems thinking and informed by critical approaches that illuminate the multiple dimensions and tensions influencing leadership practice.

This book invites readers to rethink leadership in all its complexity, examining how systems shape leadership practice, what effective leadership truly requires, and how a reflective stance can foster inclusive, impactful, and thriving workplaces. Through the diverse contributions of its authors, this volume opens up several essential questions:

- Context and Systems: *How do broader systems and organisational dynamics influence leadership roles, behaviours, and decisions?*
- The Leadership Task: *What constitutes leadership, and what does impactful practice look like? How can models and frameworks support leaders in addressing real-world challenges?*
- Self and Identity: *How do identity, authority, and privilege underpin leadership practice, and what risks arise if these forces remain unacknowledged?*

Exploring these domains offers a foundation for understanding contemporary leadership practice—an inquiry that unfolds and deepens throughout the chapters of this book.

Navigating Precarious Times—Context Is Key: Leadership never occurs in isolation. It is embedded within complex systems and organisational environments that shape boundaries, roles, authority, and tasks (Green & Molenkamp, 2005). These systems are influenced not only by internal structures such as culture, hierarchy, and group dynamics but also by external forces, including societal and political instability, economic shifts, and technological disruption (Senge, 2006; Stacey, 2012). Together, these dynamics present both constraints and opportunities, requiring leaders to adopt a systems-informed mindset.

For example, psychologists working in healthcare must understand not only the structure of the health system and current policy drivers but also regulatory expectations, stakeholder dynamics, and the evolving complexities of healthcare delivery. These broader contextual factors shape leadership decisions and demand a nuanced understanding of the operating environment. Without such awareness, leadership risks becoming reactive, disconnected, or misaligned with systemic realities.

Context is not merely background—it is the ground on which leadership stands. Effective leadership involves navigating shifting contexts such as stakeholder demands, regulatory pressures, and societal expectations. Doing so requires political acumen, negotiation skills, and relational intelligence to reconcile competing interests while maintaining legitimacy and trust.

At the heart of organisational life, group dynamics and relational processes silently shape how authority is taken up, resisted, or projected (Obholzer & Roberts, 1994; French & Vince, 1999). Leaders who can sense and interpret these undercurrents are better equipped to manage ambiguity, foster trust, and guide adaptive responses. This calls for attentiveness to boundaries—across time, task, and role—as these offer containment, psychological safety, and the structure needed for productive functioning (Edmondson, 2018; Green & Molenkamp, 2005). Within such boundaries, interdependence must be actively nurtured, with strategic goals aligned across the system to prevent fragmentation (Senge, 2006).

Clarity around the organisational task cannot be underestimated—whether it's the primary task (core mission), the emergent task (arising from change), or the survival task (a defensive response) (Lawrence, 1977; Armstrong, 2005). Similarly, the type of leadership required must be aligned with context—be it strategic (Yap & Peveto, 2020), clinical

(Rao, Cate & Pote, 2023; NHS, 2019), operational (Swiderski & Winter, 2021), or professional (Rao et al., 2023; Koocher & Keith-Spiegel, 2016; BPS, 2008). Ambiguity across roles and tasks can derail collective efforts and heighten anxiety, often triggering institutional defences (Menzies, 1960).

As highlighted earlier, the relational element of leadership is crucial. Leadership does not emerge from position alone but through dynamic interactions between leaders, teams, and systems. Authority is fluid—granted from above (hierarchy), below (team expectations), and within (personal values and identity)—and must be continuously earned through trust, consistent presence, and alignment with shared goals (Reed, 2001; Heifetz et al., 2009). To lead effectively, one must understand how power is exercised, how influence flows, and how to mobilise collective energy toward a shared purpose (Kets de Vries, 2006; Antonakis & Day, 2017; Zhang et al., 2023). Crucially, unconscious dynamics—such as fear, group anxiety, and defensiveness—exert a subtle yet powerful influence on behaviour. Leaders who are attuned to these forces can identify and address them proactively, fostering open dialogue and ensuring adaptability during times of disruption.

Ultimately, leadership transcends decision-making; it involves reading the system, grasping its deeper context, and responding with awareness, courage, and integrity. By embracing this approach, leaders do more than navigate complexity—they transform organisations, guiding them to not only survive but to thrive.

Evolving Perspectives in Leadership: Leadership is often defined as the process of influencing others towards shared goals (Stogdill, 1974). However, as leadership challenges become more complex, Grint (2005) urges us to broaden our perspective by asking not only *who leads*, but *what they do*, *how they act*, and *where they lead*. This shift highlights that leadership is not static—it is multifaceted, relational, and shaped by context, power, and systemic dynamics explored throughout this book.

Leadership and management frequently overlap in organisational life and are required for the effective functioning of systems but differ in focus. While managers concentrate on operational *know-how*, leaders are more concerned with the '*know-why*'—navigating ambiguity, purpose, and transformation (Bennis & Nanus, 1985; Kotter, 2001). Leaders are required to integrate the strategic operational thinking of a manager and the inspirational qualities of a leader. Hickman (1992) emphasised the need for individuals to have the 'mind of a manager and the soul of a leader.' Leadership, after all, is not merely about achieving results; it involves navigating influence, resistance, and power dynamics within social and organisational systems (Foucault, 1977). To do this well, leaders must foster learning, enable innovation, and build collective adaptability (Senge, 1990).

Take the example of a senior leader in an organisation facing financial pressures while needing to update ageing technology and protect staffing levels. The leader must balance cost-saving decisions with preserving human capital. While managing operational concerns like technology upgrades, leadership involves addressing employees' job security, engaging them in the change process, and maintaining the organisation's values. This requires both the 'mind of a manager' for operational decisions and the 'soul of a leader' to communicate the vision, provide emotional support, and ensure the workforce feels valued during a challenging transition.

There is extensive literature on leadership theories and models. In contrast to traditional, hierarchical views, contemporary thinking reframes leadership as a co-produced, dynamic, and relational process. The concept of 'leaderhood' (Raelin, 2003) emphasises that leadership emerges through interaction, shared meaning-making, and mutual influence, positioning leadership as less of a top-down directive and more of a collaborative endeavour. The key question is: What kind of leadership is best suited to meet the organisational challenges a leader faces in their specific context? Is it the right style at the right time? Appelo (2025) notes that in a world shaped by distributed authority, agility, and collaboration, leadership depends less on formal position and more on presence, participation, and context.

No single discipline can fully capture the complexity of leadership. While traditional psychological and organisational frameworks offer foundational insights, they often overlook how leadership is embedded within broader social, cultural, and institutional systems (Meyer & Rowan, 1977; Bourdieu, 1986). Through my journey—spanning leadership, coaching, teaching, and reflective practice—I have witnessed firsthand how leadership is enriched by perspectives drawn from various disciplines and backgrounds. This diversity of thought not only unlocks new insights but fosters a more comprehensive understanding of leadership.

For psychologists in leadership roles, integrating diverse perspectives is crucial. They must navigate not only organisational structures and performance targets but also ethical dilemmas, unconscious group dynamics, and the broader societal context. Given the complexity and breadth of the challenges psychologists face, which extend beyond institutional boundaries into social, political, ecological, and global domains—leadership is required to be dynamic, adaptive, and socially responsible (Avolio & Gardner, 2005; Bass & Riggio, 2006).

The chapters ahead explore how adopting a multidimensional approach to leadership can cultivate more inclusive, psychologically safe, and resilient workplaces. By doing so, professionals can lead with greater integrity, purpose, and lasting impact.

Can Leadership Truly Be Impactful Without a Deep Understanding of the Self Behind the Role? As Aristotle wisely stated, 'Knowing yourself is the beginning of all wisdom.' This timeless insight sits at the heart of impactful leadership. Self-awareness—recognising one's values, emotions, motivations, and behavioural patterns—is essential for leaders navigating complex systems, building trust, and fostering collaboration (Goleman, 1995; Avolio & Gardner, 2005; Dweck, 2006). Self-awareness directly impacts leadership effectiveness by enabling leaders to make more informed decisions, manage conflict, and engage authentically with others.

For instance, a senior healthcare leader navigating service redesign during a period of acute staff burnout drew on their self-awareness to acknowledge their own limits and fears. By openly naming their concerns and inviting staff dialogue, they not only built trust but also diffused rising anxiety, enabling collective problem-solving to emerge.

Emotionally intelligent leaders demonstrate the attributes of self-awareness, regulation, motivation, empathy, and social skills that are associated with resilience and adaptability (Goleman, 1995; Cherniss, 2010). Integrating this with psychological and organisational knowledge—and insights into the importance of identity, power, marginalisation, and inclusion (Burnham, 1993; Buchanan, 2020)—enhances leadership impact in today's diverse workplace contexts. Goleman's (2013) Triad of Awareness extends this further, urging leaders to balance self-awareness with cognitive empathy, emotional empathy, and empathic concern. This layered awareness is vital to address inequities, discrimination, and privilege—issues explored further by several contributors in this book. It also equips leaders to recognise when they may be operating from unexamined biases or emotional triggers, thereby enhancing their capacity to lead more inclusively.

Leadership style plays a critical role in shaping team dynamics and responding to organisational anxieties. Whether authoritarian, transformational, servant, or participative, a leader's approach is shaped by both personality and context (Goleman, 1998; Greenleaf, 1977; Bass & Avolio, 1994). While emotionally attuned and connected leaders tend to cultivate trust, creativity, and openness, more authoritarian styles may heighten anxiety and limit adaptability (Cherniss, 2010). Beyond styles, unconscious processes such as groupthink, splitting, and projection can subtly destabilise leadership unless consciously managed (Hinshelwood, 2007; Krantz, 1998). Leaders attuned to these undercurrents are better equipped to provide psychological containment during uncertainty (Menzies, 1970). Emotionally intelligent leaders, with a deep understanding of their inner world, can sense when these dynamics emerge and intervene before they escalate, thus promoting a healthier, more adaptive organisational environment.

Take the case of a project lead in a global firm who noticed escalating tension between remote teams. Rather than imposing a directive, she used reflective listening and emotional awareness to unpack underlying group anxieties, rooted in job security concerns, loss of human connection due to online work, and perceptions about who can meet in person. By co-designing a more transparent communication structure and establishing discussion forums, she not only reduced interpersonal friction but also re-established psychological safety across the team.

Critically, leaders must understand the 'self-in-role'—how personal identity interfaces with role, authority, and task (Newton, Long & Sievers, 2006). Tools like the Johari Window (Luft & Ingham, 1955) and the Conscious-Unconscious Competence model (Noel, 2006) support deeper reflection and help expose blind spots. Leadership development, then, is not simply about acquiring new skills but expanding capacity across both horizontal (knowledge, skills) and vertical (mindset, values) dimensions (Kuipers & Murphy, 2023). This approach to leadership development encourages ongoing reflection and growth, both on a personal level and within the organisational context. Throughout this book, you'll encounter case examples of such developmental journeys, where leaders grow by navigating inner and outer complexities simultaneously.

Reimagining Leadership for the Future

The complexities of the 21st century compel us to rethink, redefine, and reimagine leadership through open dialogue and reflective conversation. This book invites psychologists to critically reassess the nature of leadership and consider what forms of leadership are most needed in today's rapidly changing world.

It examines leadership across a series of interwoven themes, offering multiple entry points into the evolving landscape of leadership: the contextual groundwork; rising with the tide by harnessing influence; cultivating phoenix leadership to navigate cycles of change and renewal; developing healthy hives for collective wellbeing; breaking the mould—identity around race, culture, and personal narrative; and embracing the Tao of leadership to orient ourselves in precarious times and shape future horizons.

As Heifetz et al. (2009) argue, leadership that fails to adapt risks becoming disconnected—or even harmful. Psychologists, with their deep understanding of human behaviour, are well placed to lead with empathy, insight, and influence. Yet today's context demands more: strategic thinking, cultural literacy, self-awareness, openness to learning, and confidence in navigating uncertainty. It calls for stepping into what we describe as *Living Leadership*—a practice-based approach that fosters learning, creativity, innovation, and growth through real-world experience rather than abstract theory. This is especially vital amid the pressures of a post-pandemic, cost-conscious, and often depleted environment (Binney, Wilke, & Williams, 2005).

This book aims to expand on what psychology has to offer to leadership, explore what it can learn from other disciplines, and show how leadership can be celebrated and embraced, regardless of role, to contribute to a thriving workplace. It distils insights from a range of leaders and experts across disciplines, offering reflective tools, real-world examples, and theoretical models. While it is not an exhaustive leadership compendium, it serves as a springboard for further exploration.

Contributors to this book come from diverse fields, reflecting the belief that leadership, especially in today's global context, benefits from multiple perspectives. In our interconnected world, where problems are increasingly complex and interdependent, cross-disciplinary dialogue provides a deeper understanding of leadership's evolving nature. Throughout, readers will encounter an exploration of leadership frameworks and actionable insights grounded in evidence and enriched by the lived experiences of professionals across sectors. Through diverse voices and perspectives, the book encourages exploration of leadership not as a fixed trait but as a dynamic, evolving process. It bridges theory and practice, offering insight into how leadership is experienced, developed, and transformed in real-world contexts. Though primarily aimed at psychologists, the book's insights are broadly applicable. Whether managing teams, leading transformation, or supporting workplace wellbeing, the principles here can guide effective leadership across various sectors and geographies.

The following section provides an overview of the chapters, organised around key themes. The journey towards impactful leadership begins with a deep understanding of yourself, your role, your context, and the changes on the horizon. As you move through this book, take time to reflect on how its insights resonate with your own leadership experience and context. Consider your experiences of being led and leading others, and how you view your role and key tasks. Reflect on whether your understanding aligns with others' expectations of you. Think about your identities, biases, blind spots, and leadership style, and how you can lead with authenticity and integrity. Identify the challenges you face in your leadership journey and contemplate how you might evolve to meet the demands of this complex, ever-changing world, making work a meaningful experience.

Part One: Building the Groundwork: Understanding Leadership and Its Context

Grounded in the understanding that leadership is a dynamic and multifaceted process—shaped by environmental conditions, role expectations, and the continuous interplay between leaders, followers, and systems—this section explores the foundational dimensions of leadership. It challenges reductive, one-size-fits-all models by foregrounding the significance of context, complexity, and the diversity of leadership expressions across cultural and organisational settings (Gibson et al., 2020).

The section begins by defining core leadership concepts and revisiting foundational theories, alongside organisational systems that illuminate the inherently complex and relational nature of leadership (Heifetz et al., 2009; Edmondson, 2018). Emphasis is placed on how leadership is shaped through ongoing interaction with its environment, highlighting the importance of agility, mutual co-production, and the ability to foster meaningful connections (Grint, 2017). Drawing on perspectives such as adult developmental theory, eco-leadership, and systems psychodynamics, the chapters deepen our understanding of leadership as a socially constructed, psychologically informed, and systemically enacted process. By situating leadership within both workplace dynamics and broader societal frameworks, the section reveals the nuanced, context-sensitive approaches necessary for navigating complexity and managing performance effectively (Day et al., 2014). These foundational insights lay the groundwork for the examination of more advanced leadership practices in the subsequent sections.

Chapter 1, 'Leadership in a VUCA | BANI World' by Stephen Murgatroyd, explores leadership in the context of VUCA (Volatility, Uncertainty, Complexity, Ambiguity) and BANI (Brittle, Anxious, Nonlinear, Incomprehensible) environments. It argues for a shift towards Agile, Adaptive, and Compassionate Leadership, moving away from rigid performance-based models toward approaches grounded in engagement, courage, and emotional intelligence. Rooted in the African philosophy of Ubuntu—'I am because we are'—the chapter promotes a relational, collective ethos of leadership. It emphasises building anti-fragile organisations that become stronger under stress (Taleb, 2012) and encourages leaders to act from a place of deep purpose, drawing on developmental models such as Kegan's stages of adult development. The focus is on cultivating leadership that can thrive in, and respond meaningfully to, complexity and change.

Chapter 2, 'Eco-Leadership: Leading clinical change' by Dr Simon Western, explores leadership as a psycho-social influencing dynamic, proposing Eco-Leadership as a framework for systemic change. Emphasising decentralisation, collaboration, and adaptability, Eco-Leadership offers a model for fostering inclusive leadership that integrates diverse perspectives and promotes the collective good. This approach is particularly vital in the face of global interdependence and environmental challenges, ensuring that leadership remains sustainable and people-centred.

Chapter 3, 'Theoretical perspectives and practical approaches to leadership' by Ian MacRae, examines why leadership theories exist and how they address the inherent complexity of organisational life. He discusses the overlap between leadership and management, stressing the importance of balancing strategic vision with operational delivery. Understanding these complexities helps psychologists bridge theory and practice.

Chapter 4, 'System psychodynamics of leadership roles: Understanding systems and Organisations' by Dr David Lawlor, introduces the Systems Psychodynamics framework that combines psychoanalysis, group relations, and open systems theory to uncover unconscious processes in leadership. This chapter reveals how anxieties, power dynamics, and systemic tensions shape organisational behaviour and leadership effectiveness. Using reflective examples, it offers practical strategies for leaders and practitioners to address these challenges, fostering healthier, more resilient organisations capable of navigating change.

Part Two: Rising with the Tide: Harnessing Influence for Impact and Transformation

Leadership in applied psychology transcends technical expertise, demanding not only the ability to inspire change and motivate others but also the capacity to facilitate transformation within organisations and communities. This section critically examines how leaders can foster change and collaboration while addressing emotional challenges and overcoming systemic barriers. The integration of trauma-informed leadership principles and systems thinking (Goleman et al., 2013; Senge, 1990) is explored, demonstrating their contributions to fostering sustainable change in healthcare and other settings. By leveraging their unique skills, psychologists have the potential to influence both individual lives and organisational systems, thereby driving lasting and meaningful transformation (Northouse, 2018).

Chapter 5, 'Political skills in everyday leadership—What you need to know, but might be hesitant to ask?' by Dr Ashley Weinberg, considers the professional and ethical pressures on practitioners and researchers to promote change for the public good and argues that political skills are ways of facilitating positive change. Readers are invited to consider how to build political will for positive change in their contexts and to reflect on the qualities of their leadership styles and use of power. A proposal is made for recognising the strategic need for relevant training that makes political skills essential prerequisites for enabling progress.

Chapter 6, 'Responding to challenges and opportunities when "the only constant is change"' by Dr Esther Cohen-Tovée, addresses how to navigate organisational change by finding anchor points. The chapter outlines how health leaders can identify drivers of change and foster collaboration for service improvement, ensuring that change leads to meaningful outcomes.

Chapter 7, 'Strategic leadership—translating vision into reality' by Dr Lynne Taylor, discusses strategic leadership within clinical and healthcare systems, illustrating how leaders can transform a vision into reality. Using a case study from the Scottish Government, the chapter highlights the role of strategic thinking, collaboration, and data-driven decision-making in driving successful organisational change. The chapter puts forward insights into how applied psychologists have unique skills as strategic leaders and how these skills could be applied within government to influence policy.

Chapter 8, 'Clinical leadership within systems: Integrating theory into practice and building relationships to enable change' by Dr Rachel Bradley and Dr Andrew Roberts, examines clinical leadership and how it is relevant for psychologists at different career stages, from direct work up to working strategically. The theory is brought to life through examples of clinical leadership practice from the authors' experiences, and to illustrate the importance of collaboration with stakeholders as a key part of success.

Chapter 9, 'Fostering transactional business skills, creativity and psychological principles to lead well' by Professor Aimée Aubeeluck, explores how integrating business skills with psychological principles can lead to more nuanced leadership. By leveraging transactional business skills, leaders can enhance team dynamics and organisational effectiveness, ultimately supporting better patient outcomes.

Chapter 10, 'How business skills can strengthen effective and impactful leadership' by Dr Rosie Gilderthorpe and Dr. Amra Saleem Rao, builds on this foundation by further examining the intersection of business and psychology. The chapter demonstrates how the synergy between these two areas empowers leadership, drives professional growth, and strengthens organisational impact. It highlights how integrating psychological expertise with business acumen can enhance leadership effectiveness, enabling the creation of value-driven, inclusive organisations that foster diversity, design impactful services, and transform lives.

Chapter 11, 'What does good leadership look like?' by Professor Aimée Aubeeluck, follows up on the ideas of rising with the tide for influence. It explores the common themes of leadership journeys, offering insights into the personal and professional growth necessary to become a transformative leader through a conversation with an experienced Health Psychologist and academic leader. It draws on insights to show that while each leadership journey is unique, many share common themes.

Part Three: Phoenix Leadership: Navigating through Change, Renewal, and Transformation

Phoenix leadership embodies the concept of transformation through adversity, drawing on the mythological idea of the phoenix rising from its ashes. In this section, we explore how healthcare leaders can navigate complex organisational changes while fostering resilience, innovation, and renewal. The chapters that follow examine various models and frameworks of change, illustrating their application in fostering sustainable transformations within healthcare and other settings. By understanding these processes, leaders can better equip themselves to guide organisations through challenges, ensuring long-term success and organisational renewal (Cameron, Dutton, & Quinn, 2003).

Chapter 12, 'A model for understanding organisational leadership and change and its application in health and social care' by Professor (Emirtus) Tony Lavender, opens the section by acknowledging the importance of work and organisations in our lives, impacting our wellbeing, sense of purpose and belonging. It discusses organisational leadership and management models for understanding change. Professor Lavender focuses on the need for adaptability and resilience in healthcare systems, using the NHS as a case study to distinguish between organisational leadership and managerial functions. The chapter offers practical frameworks for managing both transformational and transactional change.

Chapter 13, 'A view from the inside: Leading as a psychologist in times of conflict' by Dr Adrian Neal and Dr Kathryn Walters, brings a personal and professional perspective on leading in times of conflict. Through a case study, they explore the psychological contract between individuals and organisations, and how managing both interpersonal and organisational conflict is central to effective leadership. The work of moving forward is examined to consider restoration and rebuilding.

Chapter 14, 'Large scale change and communities of practice: development of the psychological professions network' by Gita Bhutani, Liz Kell, and Clare Baguley, discusses the importance of networks in leadership. The chapter highlights key principles of large-scale change: inform, enable, and influence, which can help with renewal and transformation to navigate complex organisational changes.

Part Four: A Healthy Hive: Fostering Thriving Culture and Sustainability through the Tempest

A caring work culture is essential for quality and sustainability, necessitating a systemic focus (Rao et al., 2021). In healthcare and wider settings, however, leaders and the workforce are increasingly confronted with challenges such as mental health issues, organisational stress, and workforce burnout. The complexity of modern work environments calls for organisational strategies that not only destigmatise mental health at work but also foster psychological safety, relational resilience, and systemic change (Edmondson, 1999; Masten, 2001).

This section of the book explores the importance of cultivating a 'healthy hive'—a thriving organisational culture where wellbeing is prioritised, and workplace relationships form the foundation for achievement and purpose. The chapters in this section examine how leaders can create supportive, innovative, and resilient teams, with approaches ranging from trauma-informed leadership to political office wellbeing. In this context, psychologists are urged to prioritise their wellbeing while supporting clients and organisations, recognising that their mental health is integral to their effectiveness as leaders and caregivers (Maslach & Leiter, 2016; Acker, 2013).

Chapter 15, 'Wellbeing as leadership: From paradox to collective practice' by Dr Amra Saleem Rao, Gita Bhutani, Dr Adrian Neal, and Professor (Emeritus) Tony Lavender, explores how workforce wellbeing can be understood and practised as a core leadership responsibility, rather than a peripheral concern. Focusing on psychological professionals, it argues that their wellbeing is essential not only for ethical reasons but also for sustaining organisational performance, staff retention, and long-term resilience. The chapter critiques individualised approaches and highlights the limitations of agendas that overlook systemic pressures. It calls for a shift towards collective, systems-based leadership practices that embed collaboration, shared responsibility, and structural care. By doing so, wellbeing becomes an integrated and generative force, supporting healthier organisations and more sustainable professional practice.

Chapter 16, 'The composition and wellbeing of the psychological professions in the UK (2014 to 2021)' by Professor (Emeritus) Reg Morris, Gita Bhutani, Dr Amra Saleem Rao, Jeremy C. Clarke, and Professor (Emeritus) Tony Lavender, draws on national surveys to explore their composition and wellbeing. Across 6,871 responses—mostly NHS-employed, female clinical psychologists—wellbeing was consistently lower than NHS and general population norms. Ethnic diversity improved over time, but disabled professionals remained underrepresented and reported significantly poorer workplace experiences. The findings highlight systemic challenges within the psychological workforce, particularly for disabled staff, and draw attention to the need for more equitable, inclusive, and sustainable organisational practices.

Chapter 17, 'Workforce wellbeing across healthcare partnerships: A systemic and relational approach' by Dr Kerry Hinsby and Dr Rajinder Dhanjal, considers the application of psychological models to workplace wellbeing. The authors argue that sustainable workforce wellbeing cannot be achieved through quick fixes but must involve systemic, multi-level changes that foster trust, respect, and curiosity. Leaders are encouraged to focus on relationships, collaboration, and investment in relational change to ensure sustainable improvements in workforce wellbeing.

Chapter 18, 'Connections' by Kalpita Kunde and Lawrence Welch, explores the power of building authentic, deep connections in leadership. It highlights the transformative potential of trauma-informed leadership, which goes beyond managing tasks to fostering human connections through empathy, trust, and inclusivity. It argues that leaders who understand the impact of trauma on employees create workplaces that are more than just productive—they foster spaces where individuals feel safe, respected, and seen. The chapter encourages leaders to embrace vulnerability, engage in self-reflection, and resist quick fixes, instead prioritising open dialogue and emotional safety to build cultures of mutual respect and compassion.

Chapter 19, 'Leading wellbeing practices in Prime Ministers' Offices' by Jennifer Lees-Marshment, sheds light on the often-overlooked aspects of wellbeing within political offices, where high-pressure environments contribute to stress and burnout among advisers. Drawing on interviews with political advisers from several countries, Jennifer Lees-Marshment identifies key strategies for supporting mental health in these high-stakes roles, including strategies on acknowledging pressures, fostering a culture of care, normalising self-care, and supporting resting spaces. The chapter argues that prioritising the wellbeing of political advisers is not just an ethical imperative but also a strategic necessity to ensure effective governance. It also underscores the role of psychologists and organisational experts in supporting sustainable wellbeing practices within these environments.

The concluding chapters of Part Four offer a critical appraisal of leadership through conversations with two leading figures in the field. Their insights provide valuable reflections on how to foster a thriving culture and sustainability in the face of ongoing challenges through the tempest.

Chapter 20, 'Hope in the dark: Compassionate leadership for high-quality care'—interview with Michael West, advocates for compassionate leadership in healthcare, where burnout and workforce shortages are critical challenges. Michael West highlights the vital role of psychological safety, teamwork, and a non-hierarchical, appreciative culture in fostering an environment where staff feel valued and engaged. Compassionate leadership—embodying 'attending, understanding, empathising, acting'—is put forward as promoting high-quality care. Michael West underscores the importance of humility, active listening, and inclusive leadership to drive innovation, reflection, and the overall wellbeing of healthcare teams and organisations.

Chapter 21, 'Psychological safety and leadership—a conversation with Amy Edmondson' by Dr Amra Saleem Rao, delves into the essence of leadership as a skill rooted in humility, curiosity, and empathy. Amy Edmondson argues that true leadership isn't about having all the answers but creating environments where collaboration, learning, and innovation can flourish. Leaders who prioritise psychological safety encourage open dialogue, the sharing of mistakes, and experimentation without fear of blame. By embracing failure as a tool for growth, leaders can cultivate high-performing organisations where continuous learning and innovation thrive. Amy Edmondson emphasises that leadership is not a fixed trait but a skill that must be intentionally developed to foster fearless, resilient teams.

Part Five: Breaking the Mould: Race, Culture, and Identity Can Leadership Truly Transform without Confronting Power Dynamics?

Leadership cannot be fully understood without addressing identity, power dynamics, and authority. Although these themes are explored elsewhere, this part of the book offers a focused examination of the tensions and dilemmas in creating empowering environments, particularly within healthcare and social care contexts (Kellerman, 2008; Long, 2018). It highlights the urgent need for leadership that actively dismantles systemic racism and bridges cultural divides. Emphasising antiracist practice and cultural competence, it explores both the challenges and opportunities involved and calls for cross-cultural leadership and community-based solutions to address structural inequities (Zhang et al., 2023). By exploring the intersections of leadership, identity, race, and culture, this section challenges conventional models that ignore systemic inequality and calls for a more equitable, sustainable approach to organisational and societal change.

Chapter 22, 'How can psychologists lead well? Anti-oppressive leadership principles and practices for practitioner psychologists' by Dr Charlotte O'Brien, King-Yin Chan, and Dr Laura Anne Winter, advocates for integrating anti-oppressive leadership into psychological practice. It highlights the challenges and opportunities of this approach, calling for collaborative efforts to promote social justice and accessible, anti-oppressive leadership practices. The authors emphasise that this ongoing work requires creativity, community, and collective action, themes further explored in Section Five and several other contributions.

Chapter 23, 'Identity and leadership—Understanding the meaning for clinical psychologists' by Professor Jan Hughes and Professor Gary Latchford, examines the evolving role of leadership for clinical psychologists, highlighting the growing recognition of clinical psychology's importance within the NHS. The chapter urges clinical psychologists to overcome reluctance to take on leadership roles, emphasising the potential for significant impact. Leadership may present challenges related to personal identity and recognition, but it also offers the opportunity to align professional identity with broader systemic change.

Chapter 24, 'Leading antiracism in health and care systems' by Dr Lorraine Gordon, focuses on the urgent need for antiracist leadership within health and care systems, particularly regarding mental health inequalities that disproportionately affect Black communities. It emphasises the need for psychologists to challenge historical and structural racism in the NHS and adopt co-production with communities to develop culturally competent care models and address deeply rooted inequities.

Part Six: The Tao of Leaderhood in Precarious Times: Towards Future Horizons

In an era of rapid change and uncertainty, leadership must continuously evolve. Drawing on foundational works by Schein (2010), Weick & Sutcliffe (2007), Huang (2017), and Friedman (2006), this section explores leadership models that prioritise flexibility, resilience, and forward-thinking strategies. These models equip leaders to navigate challenges such as technological disruption, societal instability, and the increasing demand for inclusivity while fostering innovation, collaboration, and resilience in times of crisis. Chapters in this section examine the emotional labour and risk inherent in leadership, the importance of cultural humility and community-centred leadership, as well as the need to anticipate future challenges such as technological change, inequalities, and social justice. These insights help ensure that both individuals and organisations can not only survive but thrive amidst uncertainty, with a focus on long-term sustainability, systemic reform, and empowering diverse voices.

Chapter 25, 'A relational model of leadership and its risks' by Dr Anton Obholzer, delves into the emotional labour and risk associated with leadership, particularly in high-pressure settings such as healthcare.

Dr Anton Obholzer argues that leadership should be grounded in humility, risk awareness, an inquiring mindset and managing internal and external anxieties. He encourages leaders to reflect on their state of mind, be open to multiple perspectives to unblock blockages and foster thoughtful engagement, avoiding the temptation to conform to one-dimensional solutions. By investing in alignment with the human relational core of their work, cultivating sources of support and reflection, foreseeing and managing risks, leaders can mitigate the pressures of their roles and enhance fulfilment at work.

Chapter 26, 'Centring leadership around the communities we serve: Truth, hearing, and ceding power', by Joanne Hemmingfield advocates for a leadership approach that emphasises cultural humility, co-production, and listening to the lived experiences of marginalised communities. Leaders are urged to move away from traditional authority-based models and embrace collaboration and human partnership, ensuring that diverse voices are heard and that community engagement is genuine and meaningful. Fostering inclusive, power-sharing leadership can feel challenging. The chapter calls for leaders to admit their limitations and to take responsibility for fostering systems that learn and evolve together, ensuring that service redesign is meaningful and reflective of the community's needs.

Chapter 27, 'Leadership for an anxious future: Leading in a technological age', by Stephen Murgatroyd examines rapid technological change in sectors like healthcare. He encourages leaders to embrace uncertainty and anticipate the future, particularly as AI and other technologies reshape work environments. An invitation is set out to embrace 'The future isn't what it used to be', as the change and uncertainty about 'what's next' are constant, requiring leadership to be focused on both courage and anticipation. He advocates for leadership that cultivates resilience, agility, and innovation, and that integrates technology into organisational culture in a way that empowers staff and enhances outcomes.

Chapter 28, 'Why we need a paradigm shift: Thoughts from young leaders' by Dr Olga Luzón, Dr Hannah Shaw, Dr Sarina Afzali Shamsabad, Charlotte Baribeau, Dr Arshia Amin Choudhury, Dr Maryam Haghiran and Dr Saim Kirhan, calls for a shift towards human-rights-based leadership and systemic reform to address mental health disparities rooted in inequality, racism, and socio-economic factors. It amplifies the voices of emerging leaders, urging psychologists to move beyond neutrality and engage in social justice through policy advocacy and culturally responsive, decolonised practices. Emphasising diverse, community-led leadership, the chapter highlights the need for inclusive, transformative approaches to dismantle structural barriers and promote equitable mental health care. It ultimately calls on psychologists to champion a holistic view of mental health that supports both individual and collective wellbeing.

Part Seven: Epilogue

The Leadership Odyssey—Key Insights and Reflecting Forward

The final section reflects on the journey of leadership, drawing insights from the chapters and looking toward the future. It emphasises the importance of adaptability, generativity, humility, and inclusivity in leadership, while acknowledging the challenges and complexities that lie ahead. It concludes with a call to action for today's and tomorrow's leaders to rethink what leadership means in times of complexity and change, fostering thriving workplaces grounded in integrity, compassion, and shared purpose.

References

Acker, J. (2013). Inequality regimes: Gender, class, and race in organizations. *Gender & Society, 20*(4), 441–464. https://doi.org/10.1177/0891243205278638

Antonakis, J., & Day, D. V. (2017). *The nature of leadership* (3rd ed.). SAGE Publications.

Appelo, J. (2025). *Human robot agent: New fundamentals for AI-driven leadership with algorithmic management*. Jojo Ventures.

Armstrong, D. (2005). *Organization in the mind: Psychoanalysis, group relations, and organizational consultancy: Occasional papers 1989–2003*. Karnac Books.

Avolio, B. J., & Gardner, W. L. (2005). Authentic leadership development: Getting to the root of positive forms of leadership. *The Leadership Quarterly, 16*(3), 315–338. https://doi.org/10.1016/j.leaqua.2005.03.001

Bass, B. M., & Avolio, B. J. (1994). *Improving organizational effectiveness through transformational leadership*. Sage Publications.

Bass, B. M., & Riggio, R. E. (2006). *Transformational leadership* (2nd ed.). Psychology Press.

Bennis, W., & Nanus, B. (1985). *Leaders: Strategies for taking charge*. Harper & Row.

Binney, G., Wilke, J., & Williams, B. (2005). *Living leadership: A practical guide for ordinary heroes*. The Spencer Foundation.

Bourdieu, P. (1986). The forms of capital. In J. G. Richardson (Ed.), *Handbook of theory and research for the sociology of education* (pp. 241–258). Greenwood Press.

Bourke, J., & Dillon, B. (2018). The diversity and inclusion revolution: Eight powerful truths. *Deloitte Insights*. https://www2.deloitte.com/insights/us/en/deloitte-review/issue-22/diversity-and-inclusion-at-work-eight-powerful-truths.html

British Psychological Society. (2008). *Professional practice guidelines: Division of Clinical Psychology*. BPS.

Buchanan, D. (2020). *Power, politics, and organizational change: Winning the turf game* (3rd ed.). Sage Publications.

Burnham, J. (1993). *Group relations, management, and organization*. Oxford University Press.

Cameron, K. S., Dutton, J. E., & Quinn, R. E. (Eds.). (2003). *Positive organizational scholarship: Foundations of a new discipline*. Berrett-Koehler.

Cherniss, C. (2010). Emotional intelligence: Toward clarification of a concept. *Industrial and Organizational Psychology, 3*(2), 110–126. https://doi.org/10.1111/j.1754-9434.2010.01231.x

Day, D. V., Fleenor, J. W., Atwater, L. E., Sturm, R. E., & McKee, R. A. (2014). Advances in leader and leadership development: A review of 25 years of research and theory. *The Leadership Quarterly, 25*(1), 63–82. https://doi.org/10.1016/j.leaqua.2013.11.004

Dweck, C. S. (2006). *Mindset: The new psychology of success*. Random House.

Eagly, A. H., & Carli, L. L. (2007). *Through the labyrinth: The truth about how women become leaders*. Harvard Business Review Press.

Edmondson, A. (1999). Psychological safety and learning behavior in work teams. *Administrative Science Quarterly, 44*(2), 350–383. https://doi.org/10.2307/2666999

Edmondson, A. C. (2018). *The fearless organization: Creating psychological safety in the workplace for learning, innovation, and growth*. Wiley.

Foucault, M. (1977). *Discipline and punish: The birth of the prison* (A. Sheridan, Trans.). Pantheon Books (Original work published 1975).

French, R., & Vince, R. (Eds.). (1999). *Group relations, management, and organization*. Oxford University Press.

Friedman, T. L. (2006). *The world is flat: A brief history of the twenty-first century* (Updated and expanded ed.). Farrar, Straus and Giroux.

Gibson, C. B., Gibbs, J. L., Stanko, T. L., Tesluk, P. E., & Cohen, S. G. (2020). Including the "I" in virtuality and modern job design: Extending the job characteristics model to include the moderating effect of individual experiences of electronic dependence and copresence. *Organization Science, 31*(6), 1400–1424. https://doi.org/10.1287/orsc.2020.1361

Goleman, D. (1995). *Emotional intelligence: Why it can matter more than IQ*. Bantam Books.

Goleman, D. (1998). What makes a leader? *Harvard Business Review, 76*(6), 93–102.

Goleman, D. (2013). The focused leader. *Harvard Business Review, 91*(12), 50–60.

Goleman, D., Boyatzis, R., & McKee, A. (2013) *Primal leadership: Unleashing the power of emotional intelligence* (10th anniversary ed.). Harvard Business Review Press.

Green, Z., & Molenkamp, R. J. (2005). *The BART system of group and organizational analysis: Boundary, authority, role and task*. Group Relations International.

Greenleaf, R. K. (1977). *Servant leadership: A journey into the nature of legitimate power and greatness*. Paulist Press.

Grint, K. (2005). *Leadership: Limits and possibilities*. Palgrave Macmillan.

Grint, K. (2017). *Leadership: A very short introduction* (2nd ed.). Oxford University Press.

Heifetz, R., Grashow, A., & Linsky, M. (2009). *The practice of adaptive leadership: Tools and tactics for changing your organization and the world*. Harvard Business Press.

Hickman, G. R. (1992). Ethics in leadership: The 1990s and beyond. In G. R. Hickman (Ed.), *Ethics and leadership: Putting theory into practice* (pp. 1–24). Greenwood Publishing Group.

Hinshelwood, R. D. (2007). *Therapeutic action in groups and organisations: Psychoanalytic approaches*. Routledge.

Huang, P. Y. (2017). A framework for research and practice: Relationship among authentic leadership, employee well-being, organizational innovative climate, and innovative behavior. *Open Journal of Leadership, 6*(3), 126–134. https://doi.org/10.4236/ojl.2017.63009

Kellerman, B. (2008). *Followership: How followers are creating change and changing leaders*. Harvard Business Review Press.

Kets de Vries, M. F. R. (2006). *The leadership mystique: Leading behavior in the human enterprise* (2nd ed.). Prentice Hall/Financial Times.

Koocher, G. P., & Keith-Spiegel, P. (2016). *Ethics in psychology and the mental health professions: Standards and cases* (4th ed.). Oxford University Press.

Kotter, J. P. (2001). What leaders really do. *Harvard Business Review, 79*(11), 85–96.

Krantz, J. (1998). The unconscious in organizations: Group dynamics and psychodynamics. In J. R. Meisler (Ed.), *Handbook of organizational consulting psychology* (pp. 113–132). Jossey-Bass.

Kuipers, B., & Murphy, C. (2023). Vertical and horizontal development for leaders: Expanding capacity for complexity. *Journal of Leadership Studies, 17*(1), 23–38. https://doi.org/10.1002/jls.21752

Lawrence, W. G. (1977). *Management development: Some ideals, images and realities*. Grubb Institute.

Long, S. (2018). *Leadership in healthcare: Essential values and skills* (3rd ed.). Routledge.

Luft, J., & Ingham, H. (1955). The Johari window: A graphic model of interpersonal awareness. *Proceedings of the Western Training Laboratory in Group Development*. University of California, Los Angeles.

Maslach, C., & Leiter, M. P. (2016). *Burnout: A multidimensional perspective*. In G. Fink (Ed.), *Stress: Concepts, cognition, emotion, and behavior* (Vol. 1, pp. 351–357). Academic Press. https://doi.org/10.1016/B978-0-12-800951–2.00027-9

Masten, A. S. (2001). Ordinary magic: Resilience processes in development. *American Psychologist, 56*(3), 227–238. https://doi.org/10.1037/0003-066X.56.3.227

Menzies, I. E. P. (1960). Nurses under stress. *International Nursing Review, 7*(2), 9–16.

Menzies, I. E. P. (1970). The functioning of social systems as a defense against anxiety: A report on a study of the nursing service of a general hospital. *Human Relations, 23*(4), 95–121. https://doi.org/10.1177/001872677002300404

Meyer, J. W., & Rowan, B. (1977). Institutionalized organizations: Formal structure as myth and ceremony. *American Journal of Sociology, 83*(2), 340–363. https://doi.org/10.1086/226550

Newton, B., Long, S., & Sievers, B. (2006). *Leadership, identity and power: Using psychoanalytic ideas in the workplace*. Karnac Books.

NHS. (2019). *Interim NHS people plan*. NHS England. https://www.longtermplan.nhs.uk/publication/interim-nhs-people-plan/

Noel, J. (2006). The conscious-competence learning model. *Journal of Continuing Education in Nursing, 37*(6), 257. https://doi.org/10.3928/00220124-20061101-03

Northouse, P. G. (2018). *Leadership: Theory and practice* (8th ed.). Sage Publications.

Obholzer, A., & Roberts, V. Z. (Eds.). (1994). *The unconscious at work: Individual and organizational stress in the human services*. Routledge.

Raelin, J. A. (2003). *Creating leaderful organizations: How to bring out leadership in everyone*. Berrett-Koehler.

Raelin, J. A. (2011). From leadership-as-practice to leaderful practice. *Leadership, 7*(2), 195–211. https://doi.org/10.1177/1742715010394808

Rao, A., Kemp, N., Bhutani, G., Morris, R. C., Summers, E. M., Brown, K., Clarke, J. C., & Neal, A. (2021). *Building a caring work culture – What good looks like.* British Psychological Society.

Rao, A. S., Cate, T., & Pote, H. (2023). Supporting leadership development through mentoring. Clinical Psychology Forum, 363, 58–62. https://doi.org/10.53841/bpscpf.2023.1.363.58.

Reed, B. (2001). An exploration of role. In J. Neumann, T. Kellner, & A. Dawson-Shepherd (Eds.), *Developing organizational consultancy* (pp. 19–30). Routledge.

Samma, A. (2025). Organisation and organising from structure to flex. In B. Huppertz (Ed.), *The psychology of organizations and workplace issues: Resolving everyday conflicts* (pp. 37–51). Lexington Books.

Schein, E. H. (2010). *Organizational culture and leadership* (4th ed.). Jossey-Bass.

Senge, P. M. (2006). The Fifth Discipline: The Art and Practice of the Learning Organization (Revised ed.). Doubleday.

Snowden, D. J., & Boone, M. E. (2007). A leader's framework for decision making. *Harvard Business Review, 85*(11), 68–76.

Stacey, R. D. (2012). *Tools and techniques of leadership and management: Meeting the challenge of complexity.* Routledge.

Stogdill, R. M. (1974). *Handbook of leadership: A survey of theory and research* (2nd ed.). Free Press.

Swiderski, M., & Winter, L. A. (2021). Operational leadership in applied psychology: Lessons from practice. *The Psychologist, 34*, 44–47.

Taleb, N. N. (2012). *Antifragile: Things that gain from disorder.* Random House.

Uhl-Bien, M. (2006). Relational leadership theory: Exploring the social processes of leadership and organizing. *The Leadership Quarterly, 17*(6), 654–676. https://doi.org/10.1016/j.leaqua.2006.10.007

Weick, K. E., & Sutcliffe, K. M. (2007). *Managing the unexpected: Resilient performance in an age of uncertainty* (2nd ed.). Jossey-Bass.

Yap, J., & Peveto, M. (2020). Strategic leadership in complex adaptive systems: Navigating healthcare's uncertainty. *Healthcare Management Forum, 33*(2), 93–96. https://doi.org/10.1177/0840470419893791

Zhang, Y., Waldman, D. A., Han, Y. L., & Li, X. (2023). Paradoxical leadership and team innovation: The role of team perspective taking and team reflexivity. *Journal of Organizational Behavior, 44*(1), 1–16. https://doi.org/10.1002/job.2690

PART ONE

BUILDING THE GROUNDWORK

UNDERSTANDING LEADERSHIP AND ITS CONTEXT

Leadership in a VUCA | BANI World 1

Stephen Murgatroyd

Introduction

Leadership is about becoming, personal mastery, and being more of yourself. It is, as Bennis (2009) observed, "as simple as that, and it is also that difficult." It is about courage, determination, compassion, care, and connection. It is increasingly about living and working with uncertainty, ambiguity, and paradox. Today, leaders need to be champions of their organisation's purpose – what the organisation stands for and what impact it seeks to have. They need to show courage in enabling all in the organisation to deliver that purpose and their potential every day. They need to show skill in enabling this to happen. They have to "muddle through" complex, demanding, and strange times to make happen what needs to happen (Rodgers, 2021).

This *work of leadership*, which has always been demanding, is becoming more difficult and challenging no matter what kind of organisation one works in (Zhang et al., 2020). Complexity and ambiguities grow as change accelerates (Alimardanian & Heffernan, 2024). Not only is the world VUCA (volatile, uncertain, complex and ambiguous), but it is also BANI (brittle, anxiety-making, non-linear, and, for many, incomprehensible), with new fractures and discontents occurring almost daily (Cascio, 2020).

As society becomes more complex, more multicultural, more divided socially and economically, and increasingly captured by technology, it becomes more fractured and complex. With AI technologies displacing jobs (Susskind, 2021) and governments struggling with mounting

DOI: 10.4324/9781003492399-3

debts (Graeber, 2021), many individuals feel anxious, vulnerable, and unheard (Haidt, 2024). Health professionals, in general, and psychologists and psychotherapists, in particular, are at the "sharp end" of what our volatile, uncertain, complex, ambiguous, brittle, anxiety-making, non-linear, and (for many) incomprehensible world is like. The psychological (and therefore psycho-physical and psycho-social) well-being of individuals, communities, and organisations is deeply impacted by the speed and range of change. The change also seems to be accelerating (Jacobson & Ferguson, 2023). Health systems suddenly seem vulnerable and have yet to reset after the pandemic.

In healthcare and clinical settings, whether public or private, leaders and their teams face growing challenges of a rapidly increasing demand for service, especially in relation to the core presenting conditions of stress, anxiety, depression, suicidal thoughts, bipolar disorder, schizophrenia, and children with exceptionalities, but also newer conditions such as climate eco-anxiety and solastalgia (Upward et al., 2024), prolonged grief disorder (Shear et al., 2022) and, in North America at least, a growing number presenting with "delusion-like beliefs" (DLBs) – culturally sanctioned and shared beliefs based on conspiracy and lies resulting in psychological distress (Sullivan-Bissett, 2024).

As demand increases, available resources to support this work in most jurisdictions – skilled and effective clinicians, administrative staff, and finance – are getting scarcer. Leaders are under tremendous pressure, resulting in less satisfying engagement levels between leaders and clinicians, amongst clinicians, and between clinicians and their clients, as well as increased pressure on all to "perform." Other stakeholders – commissioners, community leaders, patient leaders – feel increasingly disengaged, and there is palpable political tension within the health care ecosystem. These also create complex relationship issues within the team and challenges of moral distress (Lamoureux, 2024). Coupled with growing levels of bureaucracy and accountability (Bolton, Willis & Byrne, 2020) and the growing complexity within health and care systems caused by mass immigration, leadership is becoming more complex and challenging.

On top of all this, healthcare organisations in Canada, the UK, the USA, and many other countries are constantly reorganising, rightsizing, reshaping, and redefining what they do, how they are organised, and adding new public assurance and certification requirements to already complex systems. In the UK's NHS, the reforms recommended by Sir Gordon Messenger and Dame Linda Pollard[1] created a climate of competition in what used to be a much more collaborative environment, which has negatively impacted staff morale and increased inefficiencies, repeating the mistakes made by the USA in the 1970s. These kinds of reforms focused on process and competition rather than supporting professional judgement and practise, together with others introduced as part of the Deliverology® strategy of Sir Michael Barber (2017) and the new public management (Lane, 2020) and neo-liberalism (Giddens, 2013) rampant since the Blair administration, all undermine the very ideology of the NHS as envisaged by Nye Bevan, the founder of the NHS, in 1948. With a new government, a return to Blairite delivery strategies seems inevitable.

In Canada, public health care struggles with rising costs and rising demand as the population ages and staff shortages become acute. Sweden is in the midst of yet another reform of its healthcare system aimed at creating a more "person-centred" and integrated approach – exactly the opposite of what some Canadian provinces are doing. Some of the complexities faced by leaders of service organisations that deal directly with people in need are caused by the self-inflicted volatile and uncertain change management activities of health executives and political entities, most of which fail (Milella et al., 2021). It is not surprising, therefore, that it is increasingly difficult to recruit and retain courageous, innovative leaders (Zhang et al., 2020; Shaw, 2016).

Becoming a Leader as a Developmental Challenge

Robert Kegan is insightful about the relationship between leadership, self, situation, and society. In a series of books (Kegan, 1982, 1998; Kegan & Lahey, 2009, 2016), he and his colleagues have offered a deep understanding of the challenge of leading in a VUCA | BANI world. Leveraging the theory of constructive development (Kegan, 1982), built on the ideas of Piaget and a number of philosophers, Kegan sees leaders as "meaning-seekers" and "meaning makers" – always seeking to deepen their understanding of the present moment and anticipating the future. In this never-ending work, Kegan (1998) suggests that an individual has the possibility of moving through a series of five stages. Here, we focus on the three most often seen in those in leadership roles – the first two stages being more concerned with child and adolescent development:[2]

> **Socialised Mind (Stage 3):** The leader's vision of the future is shaped by the values and beliefs of important others in their lives and the roles one is expected to fulfill. The future is not yet a distinct

object that can be reflected upon and authored independently. As individuals develop to later stages, the future increasingly becomes an object that can be considered from a self-authored perspective. Their preoccupations are with the present and overcoming the past. Their mantra might be, "I am my relationships – I follow the rules."

Self-Authoring Mind (Stage 4): leaders construct a personal vision of the future of their organisation based on their values, goals and ideologies. The future is acted upon and shaped through their own agency and choices. They lead towards a different future and are not just preoccupied with the present. Their mantra might be "I have an identity, I make choices."

Self-Transforming Mind (Stage 5): Leaders can hold multiple possibilities for the future as objects of reflection. They are less identified with any single vision or strategy, recognising the partial nature of any one perspective or ideology (Kegan, R., 1994). This allows for more fluid and adaptive thinking about the future in the face of complexity and uncertainty.[3] They lead agile and adaptive organisations by thinking back at the future (Murgatroyd & Simpson, 2010). Their mantra might be, "I hold many identities – I embrace paradox."

In systematic studies of these stages of development, Kegan (1998) suggests that the majority are at Stage 3 (58%), Stage 4 finds many stuck between trying to change their organisation and resistance from both above and below (35%), and only a fraction of leaders (1%) operate at Stage 5. This is hardly surprising since hierarchy and risk avoidance are dominant leadership frames in many organisations (especially publicly funded organisations) despite the clear and present need to shift the mindset to agile and adaptive leadership. The VUCA | BANI world needs more leaders in Stages 4 and 5. Coaching and mentoring may help (Aris et al., 2024), but so would engagement and empowerment of teams. The less centralised the health system is, the more agile it can be.

Leaders only function and perform to the degree that their followers permit. What followers look for is a relentless focus on purpose achieved through engagement and empowerment. Command and control leadership, especially for millennials and Generation Z colleagues, produces resistance and higher staff turnover rates (Liborius & Kiewitz, 2022).

"Big Time Bad's" and Resistance to Change: Leadership Challenge

For health system leaders, understanding and anticipating how their staff colleagues think about and anticipate the future and the imperative of frequent change, one of the important ideas embedded in Kegan's work is that of "Big Time Bads" (BTBs): change which induces resistance and helps to develop immunity to change amongst staff colleagues (Lu, Loeb & Waymack, 2025.). A "Big Time Bad," in Kegan's thinking, represents the seemingly devastating consequences of an unconscious belief that something bad will occur if they violate their hidden assumptions and competing commitments – workplace engagement rules (Mills & Murgatroyd, 1991). Key characteristics of BTBs are typically a threat response that grows over time and is characterised by the following:

- "**Big assumptions**" are the unconscious beliefs and worldviews that drive their behaviours and competing commitments, as well as the tacit understanding of organisational rules coupled with the dynamics of interaction (Mills & Murgatroyd, 1991).
- **Big assumptions always have a "Big Time Bad" conclusion** – people believe something significant will happen to them or their organisations if they violate these assumptions, so they resist or behave in ways which minimise the change and subvert the intentions of leadership. Many are very enterprising about being seemingly supportive, but are actually subverting the proposed change. They become "contrapreneurs" (Mills & Murgatroyd, 1991).
- **BTBs represent a limit or boundary that people feel they cannot cross without severe consequences**. They make the competing commitments feel necessary.

Big Time Bads are expressions of anticipation that frame the VACU BANI ecosystem of healthcare and psychological services in ways that limit the potential for agile, adaptive leadership. As Rousseau (2020) observes, this risk-avoidance and BTB fear get in the way of leaders doing the right thing. These ideas also confirm Peter Drucker's remark that "culture eats strategy for breakfast" (Campbell et al., 2011).

Some examples of BTBs in health and psychological services include:

- Clinicians resist adopting new digital health technologies because they fear they will be held liable if something goes wrong, leading to patient harm. The BTB is a malpractice lawsuit (Mela et al., 2016) or exposure on social media. They also fear that, if the technology is successful – e.g., AI-enabled therapy – it may result in job loss.

- Mental health professionals are reluctant to discuss their own mental health challenges and seek support, fearing it will be seen as a weakness and negatively impact their credibility and career prospects. The BTB here is a loss of professional standing and (potentially) employment.
- Healthcare organisations avoid transparently sharing data on errors, mistakes and near misses, believing it will irreparably damage their reputation and lead to a catastrophic loss of public trust. The BTB is the collapse of public trust in the organisation, as occurred over gender identity treatments and support at the Tavistock Clinic[4] and from the continuing challenges to secure transparent reporting of failures and iatrogenesis in health systems (Wood et al., 2023).
- Physicians are hesitant to challenge the status quo and advocate for major reforms in care delivery models, worried they will be labelled as troublemakers and ostracised by their peers. The BTB here is the fear of ejection from the profession and job loss. Rufus May was disciplined by the NHS in 2012 for publicly criticising it for the over-reliance on psychiatric medications and coercive practices in the UK mental health system.[5] Canadian psychologist Brent Macdonald spoke out in 2017 about the need to expand public funding for psychotherapy and reduce wait times in Alberta. His criticism of government policy led to tensions with his health authority employer and colleagues, who felt he was overstepping his role[6].
- In a period of major cuts to healthcare funding, managers resort to short-term cost-cutting rather than innovative solutions, fearing that failed initiatives will be a stain on their leadership and perhaps lead to be fired. The BTB is career ruin and exposure through the press and social media.

In the volatile, uncertain, complex, and ambiguous landscape of modern healthcare, these hidden assumptions and worst-case fears can powerfully constrain leadership behaviours and organisational adaptability. Uncovering and confronting BTBs is crucial for fostering the psychological safety and bold vision needed to transform health systems and secure followership.

Agile, Adaptive, Compassion Leaders – The Renaissance Way

What is a leader to do when faced with increasing and constant pressure to improve performance, lower costs, increase impact, and manage the dynamics of a healthcare team? Given the complex, volatile, brittle, and anxiety-inducing nature of the world in which they have to operate, what can leaders do to better equip themselves for the rapidly changing world of health systems and care? How can leaders build a more agile, anti-fragile (Taleb, 2012) organisation?

Despite pressure to adopt national guidelines, "best practices," and protocols, leaders of front-line teams need to be agile, adaptive, and responsive to local conditions and circumstances. Being agile and responsive is the key to improving performance and surviving in an uncertain, brittle, and ambiguous world. This requires leaders to show:

- **Compassion and Empathy** – agile leaders exhibit compassion by acknowledging other people's perspectives, giving them the care they need to meet their work and personal goals, involving them in decisions where appropriate, and building a sense of partnership and community within their teams. This compassion leads to higher engagement, more trust, and stronger relationships with team members and stakeholders.
- **Transparency and Openness** – agile leaders foster a culture of transparency by being emotionally transparent themselves – they practise personal mastery (Murgatroyd & Simpson, 2010). This creates environments of trust where team members feel empowered to share more of themselves, leading to deeper trust and more empathetic, compassionate leader-team relationships. Transparency also helps mitigate the perception of ambiguity as threatening and prevents team members from interpreting a lack of full disclosure as "social rejection."
- **Empowerment and Autonomy** – agile leaders recognise that people work best when they are enabled, engaged, and energised. Empowering individuals is a key skill of the agile leader, as is protecting staff from interference by executives and commissioners so as to enable them to work without excessive micro-managed oversight. Agile workplaces thrive when individuals and teams are empowered to own their work. Leaders should offer a powerful statement of the purpose of the work and the organisation, create a framework

for them to operate within, and then let their people decide how to achieve those outcomes. Too much "command and control" produces too few outstanding outcomes.

- **Adaptability and Flexibility** – agile leaders must be adaptable and flexible and adjust their actions and behaviours as circumstances change. Among the most important elements for success is their desire and ability to learn from experience paired with changes in the environment and then use that learning to perform well in new situations (Akkaya et al., 2022). Agile leaders encourage teams to experiment with new ways of working, quickly test new ideas, and refine them over time. In this work, they strive to move from Stage 4 in Kegan's developmental stage to Stage 5.
- **Continuous Learning and Improvement** – agile leaders have a strong focus on developing people and a passion for learning. They encourage regular feedback loops, emphasise the importance of data-driven decision-making and experimentation, and foster a culture of continuous learning through training, workshops, and knowledge-sharing. Providing learning opportunities helps sustain team motivation while encouraging open discussion of important issues. They also practise cross-boundary learning by exploring ideas, practices, and research in fields other than their own.
- **Courage and Passion** – Courage enables leaders to take calculated risks, challenge the status quo, and make difficult decisions when necessary. It allows them to stand up for their beliefs and values, even in the face of adversity or uncertainty. Conversely, passion fuels the leader's drive and commitment to their work and the people they serve. It inspires and motivates team members to strive for excellence and fosters a sense of purpose and meaning in their work (Murgatroyd, 2023).

These six characteristics, in turn, require the leader to be a systems thinker – to understand systems dynamics and interaction so as to better anticipate consequences and challenges. It also requires them to connect and understand what is happening in other parts of the world and the way in which their peers in Canada, Australia, New Zealand, the USA, and elsewhere have tackled the issues they find challenging. Thinking globally so as to strengthen actions locally (thinking "glocal") is a strong capability that is evident in agile leaders in health systems. It reinforces our global interdependence and can accelerate innovation, especially through intelligent technologies for sharing, coaching, exploring, and innovation. To move beyond "best practices" to "next practices" demands collaboration across boundaries.

The underlying principle of this view of leadership in a VUCA | BANI world is that leaders should practise what Africans call "Ubuntu": "I am because *we* are" as opposed to "I think. Therefore, I am!" The term reminds us of our shared humanity and the importance of treating mental health issues not as individual failings but as part of the broader human experience that we must face together with compassion. It also reminds leaders that there is no leadership without followership, which ultimately depends on purpose, passion, courage, trust, and compassion. Taken together, this section of this chapter has described a new renaissance in leadership (Murgatroyd & Simpson, 2010), which is practised by leaders all over the world in health, business, arts, and non-profit organisations.[7]

Leadership Development Programs and Coaching for Success

This approach to leadership requires rethinking many of the current leadership development practices, which give too much emphasis to accountability, business processes, and performance, and do not sufficiently focus on the idea of leadership as becoming (Bennis, 2009) or of leadership as the practise of engagement, encouragement, and courage. Leaders in development need to embark on a journey to move from Kegan's Stage 3 to 4 and lead from a strong, deeply ingrained sense of purpose with courage and skill.

They also require mentoring for their growth and coaching for their interactions with followers and stakeholders. The intention is to significantly improve performance through the process of engagement and becoming. A strong focus on coaching for success needs to be balanced with mentoring for growth and development, including the task of helping leaders find the balance between work, wellbeing, and reflection.

At a brittle, vulnerable time when social media and technologies challenge the work health providers do and foster a climate of mistrust, health system leaders need to be amongst the most trusted leaders in the community (Edelman, 2024) – a position currently held by business leaders and academics.

Conclusion

Many believe the speed of change is accelerating, especially in technology-enabled healthcare (Werner, 2023; Hallett et al., 2024) and mental health services. Improving quality, costs, and access requires innovations in care delivery, and many health systems often lack the full capabilities to rapidly design, implement, and scale care delivery innovations (Sandhu et al., 2023). This suggests an urgent need to *reimagine* the ways in which change in health systems occurs, and leaders are selected, developed, and supported. More devolution to teams, more empowerment, more courage, and risk-taking focused on improving outcomes and increasing trust are needed. To enable this, leaders need mentorship focused on helping them to become more effective and coaching focused on day-to-day practise and performance (Aris et al., 2024; Murgatroyd, 2024a, 2024b).

They also need to develop an innovation-risk mindset – a strong sense of anticipation of "what's next?" (Couture & Murgatroyd, 2024). With AI technologies rapidly transforming diagnostics, patient care, and therapy – with much more to come – leaders need to overcome anxiety and fear of "the next thing" and be the ones who lead the "next thing," overcoming the Big Time Bads many of their colleagues and peers may experience. Leadership is more than the mastery of process and procedure and being able to enforce the "rules" – it is about being the person you need to become to lead a high-performing team to success.

Ideas in Brief

- Embrace agile and renaissance leadership to navigate volatility, uncertainty, complexity, and ambiguity with purpose and adaptability.
- Anticipate disruption and develop an innovation-risk mindset to lead through rapid technological, systemic, and cultural change.
- Support psychological wellbeing by recognising and responding to resistance, fear, and "Big Time Bads" in self and others.
- Foster empowered, high-performing teams by modelling courage, learning, and reflective practise – leading not just through strategy, but through who you become.

Notes

1 For more information, see https://www.gov.uk/government/news/biggest-shake-up-in-health-and-social-care-leadership-in-a-generation-to-improve-patient-care
2 They are Stage 1: Incorporative – managing impulses and learning to be; and Stage 2: Impulsive but developing self-sovereignty and finding the line between selfishness and social engagement.
3 See Kegan's commentary at https://books.byui.edu/Adult_development/meaning_making_model
4 See https://www.tortoisemedia.com/2024/04/02/tavistock-britains-biggest-gender-identity-clinic-has-closed/ for a commentary about the Tavistock Clinic.
5 The case is explored in depth at https://pure.manchester.ac.uk/ws/portalfiles/portal/54542630/FULL_TEXT.PDF
6 See https://theconversation.com/in-canadas-two-tiered-mental-health-system-access-to-care-is-especially-challenging-in-rural-areas-202121
7 For more information, see https://donaldsimpson.ca/

References

Akkaya, B., Panait, M., Apostu, S. A., & Kaya, Y. (2022). Agile leadership and perceived career success: The mediating role of job embeddedness. *International Journal of Environmental Research and Public Health, 19*(8), 4834. https://doi.org/10.3390/ijerph19084834

Alimardanian, M., & Heffernan, T. (2024). *The anthropology of ambiguity.* Manchester University Press.

Aris, S., Rao, A., Roycroft, P., & Clutterbuck, D. (Eds.). (2024). *Mentoring in health, social care and beyond: Handbook for practice, training and research.* Pavilion.

Barber, M. (2017). *How to run a government: So that citizens benefit and taxpayers don't go crazy.* Penguin.

Bennis, W. (2009). *On becoming a leader.* Basic Books.

Bolton. S., Willis, E. & Byrne, A-E. (2025). The role of leadership in supporting and mitigating moral distress in nursing: A scoping review. Journal of Nursing Management, 2025(1), https://doi.org/10.1155/jonm/5443770

Campbell, D., Edgar, D., & Stonehouse, G. (2011). *Business strategy – An introduction.* Palgrave Macmillan.

Cascio, J. (2020, April 29). *Facing the age of chaos.* Medium. https://medium.com/@cascio/facing-the-age-of-chaos-b00687b1f51d

Couture, J-C., & Murgatroyd, S. (2024). *Education futures for school leadership – Evidence-informed strategies for managing change*. Routledge.

Edelman. (2024). *The 2024 Edelman trust barometer – European region report.* https://www.edelman.com/sites/g/files/aatuss191/files/2024-05/2024%20Edelman%20Trust%20Barometer_Europe%20Report.pdf

Giddens, A. (2013). *The third way.* Polity.

Graeber, D. (2021). *Debt: The first 5,000 years [updated and expanded].* Melville House.

Haidt, J. (2024). *The anxious generation: How the great rewriting of childhood is causing an epidemic of mental illness.* Penguin.

Hallett, E., Simeon, E., Amba, V., McConnell, K. J., & Zhu, J. M. (2024). Factors influencing turnover and attrition in the public behavioral health system workforce: Qualitative study. *Psychiatric Services, 75*(1), 55–63. https://doi.org/10.1176/appi.ps.20220516

Jacobson, L., & Ferguson, S. (2023). Improving change management by quantifying the relationships between margins and design variable flexibility. In *49th Design Automation Conference (DAC).* https://api.semanticscholar.org/CorpusID:265377663

Kegan, R. (1982). *The evolving self – Problem and process in human development.* Harvard University Press.

Kegan, R. (1994). In Over Our Heads: The Mental Demands of Modern Life. : Harvard University Press

Kegan, R. (1998). *In over our heads – The mental demands of modern life.* Harvard University Press.

Kegan, R., & Lahey, L. L. (2009). *Immunity to change: Overcoming it and unlocking the potential in yourself and your organization.* Harvard Business Review Press.

Kegan, R., & Lahey, L. L. (2016). *An everyone culture: Becoming a deliberately developmental organization.* Harvard Business Review Press.

Lamoureux, S., Mitchell, A. E., & Forster, E. M. (2024). Moral distress among acute mental health nurses: A systematic review. *Nursing Ethics.* https://doi.org/10.1177/09697330241238337

Lane, J-E. (2020). *New public management – An introduction.* Routledge.

Liborius, P., & Kiewitz, C. (2022). When leader humility meets follower competitiveness: Relationships with follower affective trust, intended and voluntary turnover. *Journal of Vocational Behavior, 135,* Article 103719. https://doi.org/10.1016/j.jvb.2022.103719

Lu, A., Loeb, S., & Waymack, N. (2025). Business Not as Usual: Understanding Factors for Organizational Change after a Crisis. Teachers College Record, 0(0). https://doi.org/10.1177/01614681251368631

Mela, M., Luther, G., & Gutheil, T. G. (2016). Forty-five years of civil litigation against Canadian psychiatrists: An empirical pilot study. *The Canadian Journal of Psychiatry, 61*(2), 112–118. https://doi.org/10.1177/0706743715625943

Millella, F., Minelli, E. A., Strozzi, F., & Croce, D. (2021). Change and innovation in healthcare: Findings from the literature. *Clinical Economics and Outcomes Research, 13*, 395–408. https://doi.org/10.2147/CEOR.S301169

Murgatroyd, S. (2023). *Becoming courageous – The skills of courage.* Lulu Press.

Mills, A., & Murgatroyd, S. (1991). *Organizational rules – A framework for understanding organizational action.* The Open University Press.

Murgatroyd, S. (2024a). Mentoring leaders for courage. In S. Aris, A. Rao, P. Roycroft, & D. Clutterbuck (Eds.), *Mentoring in health, social care and beyond: Handbook for practice, training and research.* Pavilion. 137–146

Murgatroyd, S. (2024b). Changing minds through futures-focused mentoring. In S. Aris, A. Rao, P. Roycroft, & D. Clutterbuck (Eds.), *Mentoring in health, social care and beyond: Handbook for practice, training and research.* Pavilion. 173–183

Murgatroyd, S., & Simpson, D. G. (2010). *Renaissance leadership – Rethinking the future.* Lulu Press.

Rodgers, C. (2021). *The wiggly world of organizations – Muddling through with purpose, courage and skill.* Routledge.

Rousseau, D. M. (2020). Making evidence-based organizational decisions in an uncertain world. *Organizational Dynamics, 49*(9), 1–12. Available at https://www.researchgate.net/publication/339463933_Making_Evidence-Based_Organizational_Decisions_in_an_Uncertain_World

Sandhu, S., Sendak, M. P., Ratliff, W., Knechtle, W., Fulkerson, W. J., & Balu, S. (2023). Accelerating health system innovation: Principles and practices from the Duke Institute for Health Innovation *Patterns, 4*(1), Article 100710. https://doi.org/10.1016/j.patter.2023.100710

Shaw, P. (2016). *The reluctant leader.* Canterbury Press.

Shear, M. K., Skritskaya, N., & Bloom, C. (2022). Prolonged grief disorder therapy (PGDT). In U. Schnyder & M. Cloitre (Eds.), *Evidence-based treatments for trauma-related psychological disorders* (pp. 309–326). Springer. https://doi.org/10.1007/978-3-030-97802-0_15

Sparks, D. (2002). Inner conflicts, inner strengths – Interview with Robert Kegan and Lisa Lahey. *Journal of Staff Development, 23*(3), 66–71.

Susskind, D. (2021). A world without work: Technology, automation, and how we should respond. Picador.

Sullivan-Bissett, E. (Ed.). (2024). *Belief, imagination, delusion.* Oxford University Press. https://doi.org/10.1093/oso/9780198872221.001.0001

Taleb, N. N. (2012). *Antifragile – Things that gain from disorder.* Random House.

Upwards, K., Usher, K., Saunders, V., & Maple, M. (2024). Understanding solastalgia from a decolonised, indigenist lens: A scoping review. *Frontiers in Public Health, 11*, Article 1261247. https://doi.org/10.3389/fpubh.2023.1261247

Werner, L., Puta, C., Chilalika, T., Walker Hyde, S., Cooper, H., Goertz, H., Rivera Hildebrand, M., Bernadotte, C., & Kapnick, V. (2023). How digital transformation can accelerate data use in health systems. *Frontiers of Public Health, 11*, Article 1106548. https://doi.org/10.3389/fpubh.2023.1106548

Wood, D., Robinson, C., Nathan, R., & McPhillips, R. (2023). The practice of incident reporting and management: Current challenges and opportunities for mental health trusts in England. *The Journal of Mental Health Training, Education and Practice, 18*(3), 248–260. https://doi.org/10.1108/JMHTEP-05-2022-0038

Zhang, C., Nahrgang, J. D., Ashford, S., & DeRue, S. (2020, December 17). Why capable people are reluctant to lead. *Harvard Business Review*. https://hbr.org/2020/12/why-capable-people-are-reluctant-to-lead

Eco-Leadership

Leading Clinical Change

2

Dr Simon Western

Introduction

This chapter explores leadership within clinical and therapeutic settings from a diverse vantage point. Throughout my career, I have worked as a clinician and leader in the healthcare sector and as an organisational consultant in many other sectors. My work has given me a unique perspective on how leadership, and in particular Eco-Leadership, can bring about the radical change that is urgently needed in the healthcare sector today.

During the first half of my career, I worked as a general nurse, psychiatric nurse, family therapist, and clinical manager in the health sector. This gave me an embodied experience of leadership in mental health and general medicine settings. I worked in community care and with the elderly and dying. I experienced excellent, mediocre, and very poor individual leadership, but more importantly, I took a real interest in observing how systemic leadership patterns and organisational cultures informed individual and team practice.

Following this, I studied psychoanalysis, leadership, and organisational culture, utilising critical theory and systems thinking to gain a PhD in Leadership and publish academic papers and books on this research. I then worked in executive education at a leading university business school, became their Director of Executive Coaching, and in the past decade have worked with senior leaders in companies across the globe and in diverse sectors such as finance, manufacturing, technology, and education. I have also revisited the health sector, coaching

DOI: 10.4324/9781003492399-4

CEOs in the NHS, and most recently working with international NGOs to deliver Eco-Leadership in the humanitarian sector. As a psychoanalytically informed coach, I work intimately with leaders, which gives me unique insights into the emotions, dilemmas, and challenges they face.

This diverse experience enables me to cross-fertilise my learning and apply it to the healthcare sector I know so well. What is most striking is recognising how entrapped most clinical and healthcare leadership is, entrapped in modernist mindsets and outdated leadership practices and theories. Whilst innovative individuals and teams do amazing work bucking the system, the general trends are biased towards hierarchy and top-down, "expert or manager knows best" practices. There is an urgent need to re-think clinical leadership approaches within the sector. Specifically, clinical settings require an Eco-Leadership approach, one that shifts leadership thinking from transactional approaches to ecosystemic approaches that can deliver a mutualistic co-production of healthcare and well-being. This paradigm shift calls for the adoption of Eco-Leadership principles. The following chapter will share what this means, but will first offer a definition of leadership.

Defining Leadership

Clinical and therapeutic leadership can mean different things to different people, and an important starting point is to define what we mean by leadership. Leadership studies encompass a broad interdisciplinary field. As Stodgill (1974) noted, "There are almost as many different definitions of leadership as there are persons who have attempted to define the concept." Hollander (1978) characterised leadership as a process of influence between leaders and followers, a definition that often privileges the leader and casts followers as passive participants.

However, leadership is a nuanced and complex phenomenon. It encompasses influence not just from individuals but also from groups and wider collectives. Increasingly, it is recognised that leadership can manifest through informal networks, demanding a broader definition to acknowledge this complexity (Heifetz, 2009; Western, 2014; Laloux, 2014). Leadership is not just the property of an individual; it can be enacted by individuals, but it also transcends individuals. It is relational and can be collective and dispersed.

A Comprehensive Definition of Leadership

"Leadership is a psycho-social influencing dynamic" (Western, 2019, p. 36). This definition can be dissected into four key components:

- **Psycho:** Leadership exists within and between individuals, stimulating emotional and unconscious responses as well as relational dynamics.
- **Social:** It is also a product of social constructs and dynamics, involving power, authority, and resource control. The social context—shaped by discourse, history, culture, and politics—must be considered.
- **Influencing:** Leadership denotes agency aimed at influencing others, but this influence is reciprocal; followers can and do influence leaders.
- **Dynamic:** Leadership is fluid, not fixed; it is a dynamic process, one that evolves rather than being a defined set of skills or competencies.

Four Dominant Discourses of Leadership

These four discourses emerged from my PhD and post-doctoral research (Figure 2.1) (Western, 2005). Over the last century, four dominant leadership discourses have shaped the perceptions and practices of leadership in the West. Further research found that these four leadership discourses were also present in different international regions, albeit in specific cultural ways (Western & Garcia, 2018). All of these discourses are relevant and useful; they coexist, but typically, one or two dominate in each specific context and setting. The aim is to get the right balance of

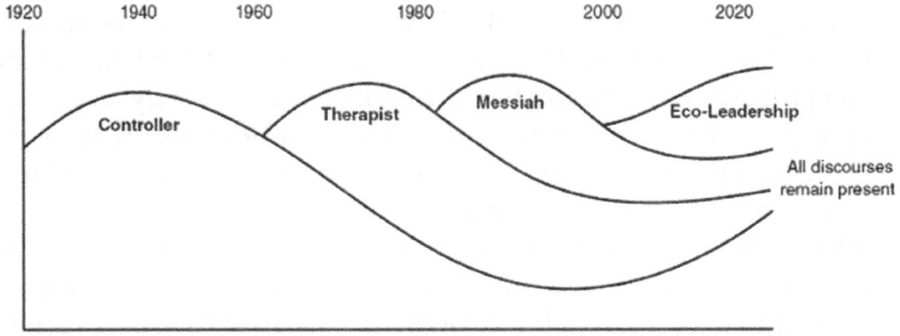

Figure 2.1 Illustration from (Western 2019).

these discourses within an organisation. To do this, it is necessary to utilise Eco-Leadership approaches to observe the local ecosystem and identify which balance of leadership discourses is required to deliver success.

1. **Controller Leadership Discourse:** Originating during industrialisation, this approach emphasises efficiency through strict control of resources and personnel, utilising science and rationality to deliver success. Frederick Taylor's scientific management (1997) and Fordist production lines epitomised this approach that dominated manufacturing, and these methods were later transmitted to the bureaucratic office. Controller Leadership remains present in today's digital age—evidenced by algorithmic management—it is often criticised for being dehumanising and overly focused on short-term productivity, lacking strategic thinking, and being unable to realise employees' potential. Maximising efficiency, careful control of resources, and focusing on tasks are important in all organisations, but when too much Controller Leadership is exercised and not balanced with other leadership approaches, it can be very dysfunctional and demoralising to workforces.

   In clinical settings, Controller Leadership can be very dominant. It aligns with ideas of maximising service efficiency, and clinical managers are often faced with the pressure of delivering to targets, which leads them to adopt Controller Leadership approaches. Additionally, healthcare and medicine are underpinned by the discourse of science, which produces ideas including evidence-based practice. This also leans into the Controller Leadership discourse, which draws on the same scientific discourse. However, the scientific discourse is a reductionist discourse. The reductionist approach in science involves breaking complex systems into their simpler components to better understand how they work. This method has led to significant advancements in fields like biology, chemistry, and physics. However, it is also important to recognise the limitations of reductionism. Complex systems often exhibit behaviours and properties that cannot be fully understood by merely analysing their parts. Balancing reductionism with holistic and systemic perspectives can provide a more comprehensive understanding, which comes from the Eco-Leadership discourse.
2. **Therapist Leadership Discourse:** Emerging from post-1960s counter-cultural movements, this approach centres on individual motivation and personal development. Therapist Leaders nurture

employee potential through emotional intelligence and supportive relationships. "Happy workers are productive workers" is the underlying premise of this approach. Therapist leadership focuses on getting the best from individuals and teams utilising psychometric tests, investing in coaching, training and development, and understanding team dynamics to maximise human potential. However, Therapist leaders often overlook broader strategic goals. Therapist Leadership can foster dependency, as their followers feel cared for by a "parental" leader figure. In clinical, and particularly in therapeutic settings, the therapist discourse can be very popular, as it aligns closely with the work. It sometimes clashes with the medical model and hierarchical managerial approaches, which lean more towards scientific expertise and Controller/Messiah Leadership. In many clinical settings, defence mechanisms against working with trauma create a taboo on emotional sharing, which can also undermine Therapist Leadership approaches.

3. **Messiah Leadership Discourse:** Gaining traction in the 1980s, this discourse highlights charismatic leadership and the cultivation of strong organisational cultures. While Messiah Leaders can inspire loyalty and commitment, they can also polarise employees—some love the leader, others dislike them intensely. Messiah Leaders create conformist environments that marginalise dissent and stifle creativity. Any critique of the leadership, however well-meaning, is seen as disloyalty. This creates "silent cultures" which close down dissent and limit creativity and innovation.

When I was a nurse 30 years ago, the consultant doctors were totalising Messiah Leaders who would lead either benevolently and with kindness (whilst retaining total power) or with fear, and often with a mixture of both. In more recent years, Messiah Leaders have been appointed as CEOs of healthcare organisations, transferring leadership approaches from corporate life to healthcare with the aim of mobilising their organisations to meet demanding targets and to drive organisational culture change. In clinical settings, Messiah Leadership is hugely problematic, mainly because it creates dependent followers who won't speak up. Clinical leadership relies on each actor in the system being able to speak up, both to prevent harm and to enable learning. Messiah Leadership undermines this capacity. Occasionally, a Messiah leader in healthcare will lead a breakthrough in how to deliver change; i.e., they will create a dynamic clinical team that pioneers a breakthrough in the delivery of care. In this scenario, the Messiah leadership mobilises the strength of the team and creates a culture of can-do and a team spirit that drives change. However, this is an unusual scenario!

4. **Eco-Leadership Discourse:** In response to the complexities of a globalised society, Eco-Leadership advocates for a decentralised, participatory approach that maximises the potential of the workforce. Eco-Leadership distributes and disperses leadership; i.e., leaders are everywhere in the organisation, and informal leadership is encouraged. Leadership is not seen as fixed to positional power, but something that is fluid and can be taken up by individuals and teams when the need arises.

   Eco-Leaders think of their organisations as "ecosystems within ecosystems." Organisations are ecosystems; they are connected and interdependent webs of life. Organisations also exist within wider ecosystems, and Eco-Leaders look externally to see potential collaborations and to look for disruptions that offer opportunities or dangers.

   For years, healthcare and clinical settings have lacked this ecosystemic leadership perspective, focusing more on an industrial healthcare model that relies on Controller/Messiah approaches, balanced by Therapist Leadership. Eco-Leadership is centred on creating shared value, ensuring that patients, their families, the community, and all stakeholders and participants are engaged and have agency in their clinical care. It emphasises prevention and public health, rather than waiting for crisis intervention. Eco-Leadership also takes an ethical stance, focusing on social purpose, environmental issues, and adaptability in a rapidly changing landscape.

These discourses reflect evolving views on leadership, from hierarchical control to collaborative and adaptive approaches. In clinical settings, each discourse has its strengths, but gaining a good balance across the four discourses is vital.

Shifting Clinical Mindsets: From Controller Leadership to Eco-Leadership

To navigate the challenges in clinical settings, there is an urgent need to transition from the dominance of the Controller Leadership discourse to an Eco-Leadership framework. The traditional Controller mindset leads to a transactional view of care, with too much focus on operational efficiency and resource management rather than on strategic engagement and systemic change. In old-school language, there is too much bureaucratic management and not enough adaptive and systemic leadership. Eco-Leadership maximises the potential of the resources, human and non-human, in the ecosystem. This means utilising technology with strategic precision. Eco-Leadership emphasises collaboration and mutual benefit. It fosters environments where all stakeholders—clinicians, patients, families, and communities—are engaged in co-producing their care and well-being. This shift not only enhances the quality of care but also delivers economic value as it cultivates better uses of resources, improved engagement of employees, and resilience and adaptability within healthcare systems.

Eco-Leadership, Healthcare, and Well-being

Eco-Leadership approaches lead to a new ethos of healthcare and well-being, one that advocates for participatory ethics that challenge traditional power dynamics. Key elements include:

- **Mutualist Cultures:** Promoting shared benefits and equitable power dynamics. Patients' families and communities become active mutual participants in ecosystems of provision and prevention.
- **The Citizen Turn:** Encouraging individuals to move from dependency to interdependency, fully engaging in their care.
- **Ecosystems:** Clinical Eco-Leadership means mapping ecosystems to seek resources, engagement, and connections. It fosters diverse collaborations that blur the lines between healthcare and social care, and between private, public, and non-profit organisations (Mintzberg, 2015).

The world is transitioning from the concept of stable, growth-driven economies to an era characterised by Precarious Interdependence (Western, 2020). This new age is shaped by the environmental crisis, technological advancements, and hyper-globalisation, all intertwined with rapid social and political changes. These factors influence one another, creating a precarious, interdependent reality that will likely persist for the foreseeable future.

In this context, Eco-Leadership approaches are emerging as crucial frameworks. By conceptualising health, social, and well-being ecosystems, we can envision pathways to a sustainable future. The current paradigm of healthcare is primarily transactional. The aim on a micro level is that experts provide care to passive patients, while on a macro level, the aim is to create an efficient system to deliver scaled care to populations. This transactional approach is reactionary rather than preventative, and it works within a vertical understanding of healthcare.

In contrast, health, social, and well-being ecosystems advocate for a more horizontal and mutualist collaboration that integrates people, technology, and the environment. To make this shift, we must establish a clear vision of our destination and the reasons behind it. Currently, there is a lack of clarity, resulting in a fragmented landscape of ideas—some promising, others merely functional, and many conflicting or distorted by political dynamics and power struggles. Eco-Leadership, grounded in the ethos of mutual ecosystems, offers a coherent vision and a leadership framework that can be applied and developed to achieve the necessary paradigm shift.

A Case Study of Eco-Leadership in a Clinical Setting

Hospice Care—Turning a Hospice Inside Out

Introduction

I was engaged as an external organisational consultant to apply an Eco-Leadership perspective for further improvement at an award-winning hospice facility that provided excellent care services. After discussions with the CEO, we identified two main challenges: first, despite delivering outstanding care, the hospice served only a small number of patients due to limited bed availability; second, care was primarily top-down, with minimal involvement from families or the community.

The normative way of approaching this challenge would be to seek greater improvements in existing services. The Eco-Leadership approach focuses on looking at the ecosystem of hospice care, both internally and externally, and taking a much more strategic and radical approach.

We decided to adopt an Eco-Leadership approach focused on two key objectives:

1. Transforming the hospice model of care
2. Reconnecting life and death by returning the dying to the living community

Instead of merely improving existing services, we aimed to re-imagine hospice care as a community-centred initiative. Our goals included:

- **Creating ecosystems of care** to significantly increase patient engagement with the community.
- **Leveraging community resources**—patients, families, and local organisations—to deliver care collaboratively.
- **Reconnecting life and death** by engaging families and neighbours in the dying process, moving away from the professionalisation of death.
- **Extending hospice care** to marginalised groups such as the homeless and ethnically diverse populations.

An excerpt of a reflection note written to hospice staff following months of consultation with them reads:

> The vision is to turn the hospice "inside out" by adopting a social model of hospice care that involves family, friends, neighbours, local charities, professionals, and volunteers. The aim is to redefine hospice from being just a physical space for dying to a model that "mobilises hospitality" within the community. Care will be returned to those best positioned to provide it—family and friends—while professionals support when needed.

Key Advantages of This Model

1. The Moral Case: Expanding Access
   - Currently, only 4% of those dying have access to hospice care. By empowering the community to provide care, we can significantly increase this percentage, maximising benefits from existing resources.
   - Engaging diverse populations by including marginalised groups, such as the homeless and racially excluded communities, to improve accessibility to hospice care.
2. The Quality Case: "Light Touch" Interventions
   - Community engagement allows for personalised, home-based care that addresses holistic needs rather than just medical interventions. A "better death" is achieved by incorporating support from family, friends, and familiar surroundings.

3. The Social Case: Reconnecting Life and Death
   - By integrating dying back into the community, we can reclaim the collective wisdom and experience surrounding death, moving away from an expert-dominated model. Hospice facilities play a role but should not be the central focus of care.

Eco-Leadership Challenges

The Eco-Leadership challenges for the hospice were fourfold:

1. **Gain critical mass support:** Share the vision with stakeholders—including staff, the board, and funding bodies—to gain widespread support and influence the broader community.
2. **Construct a new business model:** Adapt the existing model to support social hospice care, moving beyond the "patients in beds" paradigm and exploring new funding avenues.
3. **Develop internal structures and culture:** Foster generative leadership that encourages fluid collaboration and learning from the community.
4. **Transform professional identities:** Rethink the roles and identities of professionals to allow for a more adaptable approach that values non-expert carers.

Outcomes and Impact

Over four years, the Eco-Leadership consultation process achieved significant outcomes:

- Increased community and volunteer engagement.
- Over 100 "hospice neighbours" were recruited and trained to provide non-expert support, alleviating pressure on professional staff.
- Community "walk-in hubs" made hospice resources more accessible, particularly in underserved areas.
- Greater integration and understanding among hospice and community staff, promoting holistic care.
- Enhanced collaboration between public, not-for-profit, and private organisations to deliver networks of care.
- Increased involvement of service users and their families in care decisions.

The internal culture shift posed challenges; while some staff found it liberating, others struggled with the changes, particularly regarding their professional identities. However, the process ultimately led to a more inclusive, community-centred model of hospice care.

Conclusion: Four Key Tasks in Delivering Eco-Leadership Approaches

Infusing Mutualism in Health and Social Care

The primary goal of Eco-Leadership in clinical settings is to embed the principle of mutualism as the foundational social purpose within health and social care ecosystems. This ethos should guide all teamwork, departments, and projects, encouraging everyone—from clinicians to patients—to reflect on whether mutualism is truly being practised. Questions like "Are we integrating mutualism into our work?" and "Are we fostering inclusivity and diverse voices in the healthcare ecosystem?" should be commonplace. Eco-Leadership emphasises that small changes can lead to significant transformations, and social purpose is not merely a top-down mission statement; it is a lived experience that thrives on active engagement.

Fostering Participative Cultures

The second task is to cultivate participative cultures that break away from traditional top-down structures and the notion that "the doctor or manager knows best." This involves distributing leadership throughout the organisation and challenging the idea that only hierarchical power holds sway. Valuing diverse perspectives allows marginalised voices to be heard and ensures that specialised knowledge is integrated into broader discussions. Creating a participative culture requires both structural and cultural changes. Change often arises from the margins, and it is the potential that every individual—managers, professionals, citizen-patients, families, and communities—can actively participate and deliver this transformation.

Developing Eco-Mindsets

The third task is to cultivate eco-mindsets, shifting away from the factory-hospital model and re-envisioning health and social care as interconnected ecosystems and networks. This involves regular network mapping and moving beyond silos to identify patterns that perpetuate certain behaviours and outcomes. Ecosystemic thinking means recognising unintended consequences, such as how setting targets may resolve immediate issues but create new ones elsewhere. To foster eco-mindsets, healthcare professionals must engage with perspectives outside their usual realm.

Eco-Leadership is about initiating a process of change with a clear vision. Eco-Leadership does not wait for directives from above; instead, diverse actors engage, learn, and share within their communities, connecting their insights with others. Eco-Leadership means distributed leadership, not simply training a hierarchical leader with a new perspective. Leadership needs to be set free from positional power and unleashed across the organisation.

In summary, by shifting the ethos from a "professional or manager knows best" mentality to an Eco-Leadership perspective, individuals, families, and communities will become active participants in their care. Shifting from a Control Leadership to an Eco-Leadership approach unleashes the potential of the ecosystem. It changes the gaze from top-down to seeing what potential exists in the ecosystem and to harness the dormant resources that lie within. It leverages best practices through peer-to-peer learning, sharing best practices, breaking down silos, and, most of all, by thinking systemically and holistically about health and well-being.

This transformation unlocks vast resources, fostering a culture of mutual responsibility and care—an essential shift for the future of healthcare. To deliver this approach, Eco-Leadership is the required skill set within clinical and therapeutic settings

Ideas in Brief

- Shift from top-down control to distributed leadership rooted in mutualism, participation, and interconnectedness.
- Infuse mutualism as the foundational social purpose within health and social care ecosystems.

- Foster participative cultures by engaging patients, professionals, and communities as co-leaders in care, valuing diverse voices and systemic insight over positional authority.
- Develop eco-mindsets and think beyond silos using networked, systemic awareness to identify unintended consequences and unlock dormant resources within the system.
- Drive transformation through lived purpose. Embed mutualism and shared responsibility into the everyday fabric of clinical work—moving from mission statements to meaningful, inclusive action.

References

Heifetz, R. A., Grashow, A., & Linsky, M. (2009). *The practice of adaptive leadership: Tools and tactics for changing your organization and the world*. Harvard business press.

Hollander, E. P. (1978). *Leadership dynamics: A practical guide to effective relationships*. Free Press.

Laloux, F. (2014). *Reinventing organizations* (Vol. 58). Nelson Parker.

Mintzberg, H. (2015). *Rebalancing society: Radical renewal beyond left, right, and center*. Barret-Koehler Publishers.

Stogdill, R. M. (1974). *Handbook of leadership: A survey of theory and research*. Free Press.

Taylor, F. ([1911] 1997). *The principles of scientific management*. Dover Publications.

Western, S. (2005). *PhD Thesis: A critical analysis of leadership: Overcoming fundamentalist tendencies*. Lancaster University Management School. [Unpublished].

Western S. (2012). *Coaching and mentoring: A critical text*. Sage.

Western, S. (2014). Autonomist leadership in leaderless movements: Anarchists leading the way. *Ephemera: Theory & politics in organization, 14*(4), 673–698.

Western S. (2019) *Leadership: A critical text* (3rd ed.). Sage.

Western, S. (2020). Covid-19: An intrusion of the real the unconscious unleashes its truth. *Journal of Social Work Practice, 34*(4), 445–451.

Western, S. (2023). From paternalism to mutualism Eco-Leadership: The cultural transformation of healthcare. In N. Chambers (Ed.), *Research handbook on leadership in healthcare* (pp. 793–817). Edward Elgar Publishing.

Western, S., & Garcia, E. J. (2018). *Global leadership perspectives: Insights and analysis*. Sage.

3 Theoretical Perspectives and Practical Approaches to Leadership

Identifying Potential, Organising Leadership Structures, and Managing Performance

Ian MacRae

What Is Leadership?

Leadership involves organising people, systems, or both at a strategic level, guiding them towards a shared objective or goal. It is fundamentally about influencing others to align their actions with a common purpose, where the leader sets out a vision, coordinating efforts to achieve a specified outcome. Effective leadership involves motivating others and mobilising resources, ensuring progress is made towards shared objectives.

Leadership can encompass a range of roles. Leadership is most often viewed as a workplace role, such as the role of a CEO or President of a company. Any role that involves moving people or systems towards a common objective can be considered leadership. This may not involve directly supervising or directing individuals to behave in a certain way. For example:

- Company/organisational leadership
- Political leadership
- Moral leadership

DOI: 10.4324/9781003492399-5

- Spiritual leadership
- Educational leadership
- Thought leadership

The chapter focuses on leadership within the context of the workplace.

What Isn't Leadership?

Leadership and management are often confused or used interchangeably, but they represent distinct functions. Leadership is about influence: guiding, inspiring, and aligning people or systems towards a common vision. Management is about direct oversight and involves organising, coordinating, and ensuring that systems or people follow a structured plan. Managers ensure tasks are completed as expected, whereas leaders prioritise long-term goals, innovation, and motivating others to push beyond the status quo. Leaders shape the systems while managers ensure people fulfil their roles within the system. A manager may oversee performance and workflows, but that does not necessarily make them a leader.

Most leadership roles involve a combination of leading people and managing people and their tasks. For example, a clinical leader might inspire a team to explore or adopt new treatment protocols (leadership) while also ensuring compliance with operational legal and ethical standards (management). Similarly, strategic leadership may set the vision for an organisation's future, while operational leadership focuses on ensuring day-to-day activities align with that vision.

Limitations of a Mechanistic Model of Leadership

We cannot yet fully explain what makes a good leader because leadership is complex and influenced by a vast number of contextual and relational factors. While many leadership theories and models provide useful insights, they remain highly debated and offer only partial explanations for the success of organisations and individuals.

This does not mean leadership is unknowable. Theories and models provide useful frameworks to clarify what leadership is and how it works. They help us identify potential in others, create organisational structures that work within complex interpersonal and cultural dynamics, and manage performance in high-pressure and ever-changing environments.

If we are to understand leadership, we need a shorthand to explain what it is and how it works. This is where theories, models, and effects come in.

Theoretical Approaches and Models

To better understand leadership, it is helpful to look at different theories of leadership and reflect on what a theory is and what it is supposed to do. This can help us choose the right tools and adopt practical perspectives. While there is no shortage of leadership models and theories, relying too heavily on just one can limit our understanding and effectiveness in practice.

Theories, models, effects, and how we get there

One of the challenges in psychology is that much of the work is atheoretical (Haines, 2019) and too many results are found by chance but do not add to our practical or theoretical understanding (Meehl, 1990; McPhetres et al., 2021). We often find a model that seems sensible, fits the data well enough, and may reflect our understanding or experience of the world, but has little relation to broader theories (Kline, 2011; Haines, 2019). This continuous development of isolated models often fails to advance or refine cumulative knowledge in the field.

So what is a theory, a model, and an effect, and what is the difference?

Theories are broad conceptual frameworks that help organise information into coherent bodies of knowledge (Fried, 2021) to explain robust phenomena in a way that accurately represents how the world works. Theories are supported by a body of evidence that has accumulated over time, based on multiple studies that have tested but not falsified it (See Figure 3.1).

Models explain more specific, focused, and limited phenomena or enhance our understanding within a certain context. While a single study only contributes in a small way to an overall theory, a model is often useful at the level of a single research study or practical application of a topic, highlighting precise mechanisms or effects.

Finally, an *effect* describes a specific relationship between two variables, but it does not explain why the outcome occurs. Effects are more straightforward and descriptive; they focus on what happens rather than providing a deeper understanding. For example, an effect might be that higher emotional intelligence in leaders is correlated with lower employee turnover (Jordan & Troth, 2011). The usefulness of effects is primarily in describing specific actions within models and broader theories.

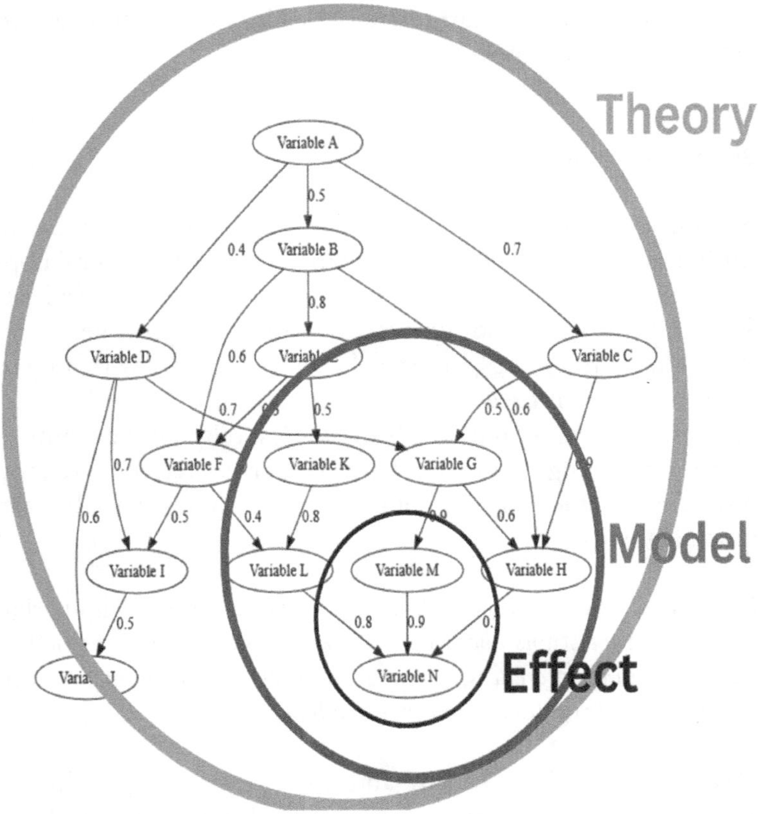

Figure 3.1 Theory, model, and effect.

A useful example from personality psychology illustrates this distinction. Trait *Theory* is a broad theoretical framework proposing that personality consists of stable traits that shape behaviour. The Five-Factor *Model* (FFM) builds on this theory by identifying five major personality traits (Openness, Conscientiousness, Extraversion, Agreeableness, Neuroticism) based on statistical patterns in personality data. From this, researchers have identified the specific *effect* of conscientiousness on job performance, showing that conscientious individuals consistently perform better at work.

Understanding the distinction between theories, models, and effects is essential in leadership studies. Many books and seminars promise "one simple solution" to revolutionise leadership, often describing an effect focused on a narrow relationship between specific variables. While effects may be based on empirical data, they offer limited insights and fail to capture the full complexity of leadership. Relying too heavily on overly simplistic solutions can restrict a leader's ability to adapt to different challenges and contexts.

Leadership Theories

There are numerous leadership theories. The chapter focuses on broad trends within theories and their central themes. It explores several popular contemporary models that align with these broader theoretical categories to provide some grounding in today's popular approaches.

The *Great Man Theory* suggests that leaders are born with innate qualities that make them exceptional. Historically, it explained leadership through the actions of individuals in politics, religion, or the military, credited with changing history. However, critics like Leo Tolstoy argued at the time that leaders are not inherently extraordinary but are shaped by social forces.

- *While outdated and controversial, this conceptualisation of leadership raises important questions about the nature of leadership and the importance of individual differences, personal attributes, and life histories in shaping the career trajectories of notable leaders.*

Zeitgeist Theory, favoured by Tolstoy and often resurfacing in discussions of leadership, argues that broader societal and cultural forces shape behaviour, while individuals merely ride the wave of change. This theory suggests that those credited with leadership are often just figureheads, with little real power to influence events. Zeitgeist Theory is not a *psychological* theory because it deliberately discounts psychological factors as predictors of leadership outcomes.

- *While it discounts individual traits or actions as predictors of outcomes, Zeitgeist Theory invites us to consider how much a leader's context limits or amplifies their power—an important factor in performance management.*

Trait Theory emphasises internal characteristics, such as intelligence, emotional intelligence, confidence, and personality, as key to leadership potential. It suggests that some individuals are predisposed to leadership but recognises that traits interact with situational factors to determine effectiveness.

- *Trait Theory helps in identifying potential leaders by focusing on personal characteristics that align with specific organisational needs, making it a useful tool for leadership selection and development.*

Situational or Contingency Theories propose that effective leadership depends on aligning a leader's behaviour with the demands of the situation. They highlight the importance of social context, task complexity, and the leader-follower relationship.

- *Emphasising adaptability, these theories are directly applicable to managing performance in dynamic environments.*

Relational Theory focuses on leadership as the process of building and maintaining relationships to drive change. *Transactional models* emphasise managing processes, structures, and performance through clear expectations and rewards, while *transformational models* highlight prosocial relationships, emotional connections, and ethical decision-making. What defines an effective relationship depends on the specific model.

- *Relational approaches highlight the importance of interpersonal relationships within the organisation, typically focusing on developing teams through strong, trust-based connections.*

Behavioural Theories focus on what leaders do, rather than who they are. These theories suggest that effective leadership is not necessarily about inherent traits but about the specific behaviours leaders display. This includes everything from decision-making and communication styles to how they interact with and motivate their teams. Behavioural theories range from *heroic leadership*, which emphasises bold, decisive action in difficult times, to *servant leadership*, which focuses on humility, empathy, and putting the needs of followers first.

- *These approaches are highly subjective and context-dependent. Yet they often provide specific guidelines on what is considered "optimal" or "ideal" behaviour, which vary based on differing views of leadership goals.*

Utility of Theories

Theories provide broad, general explanations that serve as conceptual frameworks to organise and interpret large bodies of knowledge. Psychological theories of leadership generally focus on individual differences and traits, situations, interpersonal relationships or behaviour. Within these types of theories, a huge number of different models suggest different lenses on what is optimal or effective in terms of leadership processes or outcomes.

The real challenge, in practice, is that workplaces are a lot more complex and nuanced than any of these theories. There are far more variables in any workplace or network of relationships than any theory can fully capture. Each theory and model has both benefits and significant criticisms; Northouse (2013) provides a very useful review.

In practice, we can use theories to make sense of our experiences and effects found in research, but we also need to adapt that to useful, practical tools that we can draw on in action. Over-reliance on a single theory can lead to ignoring other useful information. For example, a century of psychological research shows strong evidence for traits as a determinant of leadership success (Do & Minbashian, 2020). However, that does not diminish the importance of relationships, behaviour, or situational factors.

Leadership in Practice

In practice, leadership requires more than just inspiring others. It involves selecting the right people, developing potential into performance, and ensuring people's behaviour aligns with the organisation's objectives. Transforming organisations and structures is not just a matter of vision and communicating strategic objectives; translating goals into behaviour over the long term within any organisation requires managing performance effectively.

Most leaders must navigate both leadership and management, with the degree of overlap varying depending on the role. In health contexts, the two are often merged significantly, requiring leaders to juggle strategic vision with operational responsibilities. This overlap may also span diverse roles and responsibilities across different teams, organisations, workplaces, professional bodies, and advisory roles.

Identifying High Potential: Selecting Leaders

Potential refers to latent qualities or abilities that individuals may not yet have fully demonstrated but could develop under the right conditions (MacRae et al., 2018). Silzer and Church's (2009) model can be used by leaders to identify talent for any position, but it is useful for identifying and selecting leadership potential. Career Dimensions, would address leadership-specific skills and capabilities; Growth Dimensions, highlighting adaptability and motivation for development; and Foundational

Dimensions, such as intelligence and conscientiousness, which predict long-term performance (See Figure 3.2).

- *Career Dimensions* are specific skills essential for success in a job or field, such as technical expertise. These skills can be learnt and are context-dependent.
- *Growth Dimensions* enable learning and development over time. Growth depends on opportunities such as mentorship or training and thrives in supportive environments.
- *Foundational Dimensions* are stable traits like intelligence and conscientiousness that predict success across roles and environments (MacRae et al., 2018). These traits are key for identifying individuals with long-term leadership potential, even when they lack experience.

Silzer and Church's (2009) model can be used by leaders to identify talent for any position, but it is useful for identifying and selecting leadership potential. *Career Dimensions* would address leadership-specific skills and capabilities; *Growth Dimensions* highlight adaptability and motivation

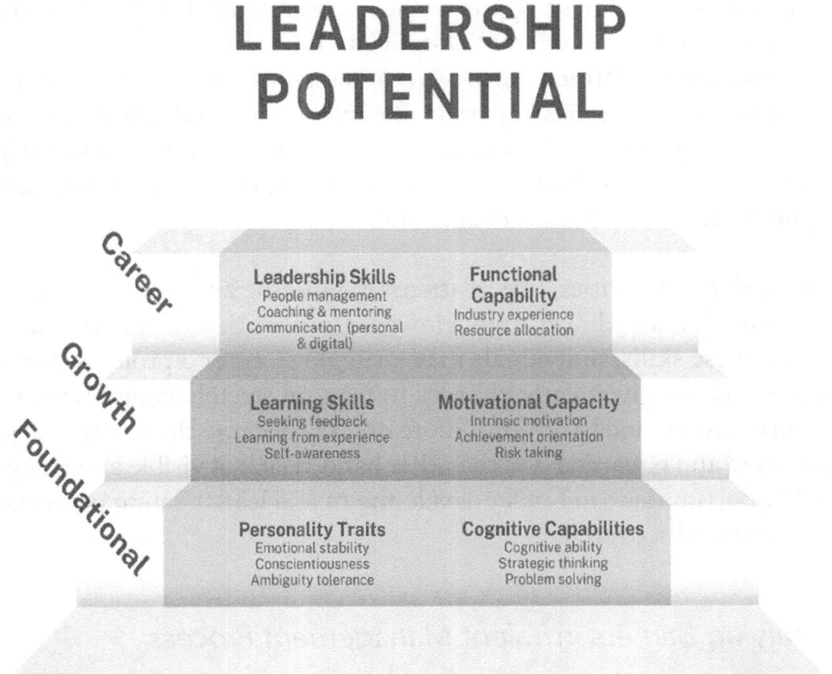
LEADERSHIP POTENTIAL
Career
Growth
Foundational
Leadership Skills
People management
Coaching & mentoring
Communication (personal & digital)
Functional Capability
Industry experience
Resource allocation
Learning Skills
Seeking feedback
Learning from experience
Self-awareness
Motivational Capacity
Intrinsic motivation
Achievement orientation
Risk taking
Personality Traits
Emotional stability
Conscientiousness
Ambiguity tolerance
Cognitive Capabilities
Cognitive ability
Strategic thinking
Problem solving

Figure 3.2 The three dimensions of leadership potential (Adapted from MacRae et al., 2018).

for development; and *Foundational Dimensions*, such as intelligence and conscientiousness, predict long-term performance.

This model helps identify both untapped potential and the barriers preventing it from being realised. It highlights opportunities to nurture high-potential individuals while also diagnosing obstacles that may be blocking their growth and development into leadership roles.

Barriers in the Potential Talent Pipeline

Shifting the lens from identifying individual potential across the above dimensions to looking at the development of high potential within an organisation, we can frame the question as "what are the systemic barriers to potential being realised"?

1. **Career Dimensions:** Limited access to training, biased recruitment, and role stereotyping restrict opportunities to build necessary expertise.
2. **Growth Dimensions:** Poor leadership, toxic cultures, and lack of trust or development opportunities hinder adaptability and learning, preventing high-potential individuals from thriving.
3. **Foundational Dimensions:** Over-reliance on unstructured interviews often overlooks key traits like intelligence and conscientiousness. A vague or subjective approach to hiring can fail to identify high-potential candidates, perpetuating inequity in talent management decisions (MacRae et al., 2018).

Many leadership abilities, like relationship-building and motivating others, can be developed over time. However, without early opportunities to build these skills, individuals may struggle to enter a profession and progress. Those given early chances to take on stretch assignments or mentoring roles tend to advance more quickly because their potential is recognised and rewarded. On the other hand, a lack of visible and recognised opportunities can hinder development and lead to latent potential remaining undiscovered.

Identifying Barriers in Talent Management Process

Organisations can use this model to identify barriers in **selecting**, **developing**, and **retaining high potential individuals** by asking key questions.

- **Selecting**: Are we missing potential by focusing only on immediate skills or the wrong attributes that ignore some aspects of potential?
- **Developing**: Do people have the opportunities, recognition, and support to develop and grow into their potential? Do we have the capacity to spot high potential across the organisation?
- **Retaining**: Are high-potential individuals leaving because they lack opportunities to grow or be recognised? Are there structural problems that make this career inaccessible to some groups or people with certain attributes?

Organising Leadership Structures

One of the key debates in leadership and organisational design is the balance between centralisation and decentralisation. This debate directly impacts leadership by shaping how power, authority, and decision-making are distributed within an organisation. Should leadership concentrate authority at the top for consistency and control, or delegate it broadly to enhance adaptability and innovation?

Proponents of centralisation argue that concentrating authority in a single leader or small group ensures consistent decision-making, strengthens control, and unifies organisational vision. Centralised leadership is often preferred in highly regulated industries, large bureaucracies, or crisis scenarios where quick, decisive action is essential. It minimises conflicting decisions across departments and establishes clear accountability.

The case for decentralisation emphasises resilience and individual autonomy (MacRae, 2024). Decentralised systems are intended to empower those closest to the problem, leveraging their local knowledge to respond quickly and effectively to dynamic and complex situations. This idea, central to leadership and the distribution or concentration of power, has changed little over the past 200 years, as Alexis de Tocqueville noted: "Decentralisation has not only an administrative value but also a civic dimension since it increases the opportunities for citizens to take interest in public affairs; it makes them accustomed to using freedom" (Schmidt, 1991).

Decentralised networks encourage individual autonomy and decision-making, aiming to enhance innovation, flexibility, and responsiveness by allowing decisions to be made closer to the specific role and context. This approach assumes that employees are skilled and knowledgeable enough to make informed judgements about their work. Extensive research indicates that decentralisation boosts job satisfaction and engagement, with autonomy being a key factor in work engagement (Decuypere & Schaufeli, 2020). Furthermore, decentralisation is essential for creativity and adaptability, particularly in fast-changing industries or geographically dispersed organisations.

While teams operate independently, coordination through communication, shared goals, and performance management ensures alignment. Collaboration is often delegated to individuals rather than management structures, making communication breakdowns a matter of interpersonal relationships.

While decentralised leadership enhances resilience, engagement, and innovation, it requires careful structuring and communication to ensure that autonomy is balanced with overall organisational coherence and accountability.

A key risk is fragmented information flow, where teams operate independently, limiting communication and collaboration. This can result in high-potential employees being overlooked, remaining isolated without recognition or development by talent management.

Decentralised systems face challenges when performance standards are inconsistent or unequally applied. Without formal structures, organisations may struggle to identify talent and ensure equitable development pathways. Overly centralised structures create over-reliance on a few decision-makers who may overlook diverse talent.

Organisations need a context-specific, balanced approach. But the key is aligning both accountability and responsibility at the same level. Centralising decision-making while decentralising accountability creates chaos; the reverse leads to gridlock. Imbalances cause the biggest problems.

Continuous Performance Management

A comprehensive discussion of performance management is beyond the scope of this chapter. Instead, this section will introduce the concept of **continuous performance management,** which aligns with Silzer and Church's (2009) model of potential and complements a decentralised leadership structure.

Continuous performance management is an ongoing process of providing frequent, real-time feedback and maintaining regular conversations between employees and their managers. Unlike traditional annual appraisals, which focus on one-off evaluations, continuous performance management adds short-term goals and immediate feedback. This is intended to be complementary, not a replacement.

In decentralised leadership structures, where decision-making is distributed across various levels, continuous performance management is essential for maintaining alignment and accountability. This isn't about constant direct communication, but rather ensuring useful information flows freely and can be measured and evaluated effectively. Regular feedback and review help keep teams and individuals on track, provide a clear structure and framework for evaluating performance across different roles.

Continuous performance management typically involves:

- **Regular check-ins**: Short, informal meetings that focus on immediate feedback, addressing short-term goals, and adjusting behaviour. These allow for quick corrections, identifying successes and offering opportunities to raise issues.
- **Annual or biannual formal reviews**: More formalised evaluations of long-term performance, development, and strategic goals. These reviews are less frequent but focus on broader objectives and the overall contribution to the organisation.

Effective leadership isn't just about inspiring people; it's about strategically designing and managing and may involve management to ensure they function as intended. That requires identifying and developing high-potential talent within a clear framework. Leadership structures must balance centralisation and decentralisation to maintain accountability and adaptability based on the requirements of the situation and context. Without clear performance management processes, both talent identification and organisational strategy flounder.

Ultimately, leadership is about designing systems that align individual development with organisational goals. A well-structured leadership framework ensures that talent is nurtured, decision-making is effective, and strategic goals translate into action. Leaders who prioritise organising systems, balancing autonomy with accountability, are better positioned to create high-functioning teams and effective organisations.

Ideas in Brief

Leadership

- Leadership and management are often confused; leadership is about influence, while management is about oversight.

- Many leadership roles, especially in clinical, counselling and health settings, require both leadership and management in the same role. This involves balancing long-term planning with immediate priorities and delegating responsibilities. Practical managerial tasks such as performance management and employee selection and development can directly enhance or hinder leadership objectives.

Theoretical Approaches and Models

- Leadership theories provide frameworks to understand and apply different perspectives in practice.
- While theories can overlap and remain contested, they offer valuable tools for addressing the complexity of leadership in real-world settings.
- Effective leadership requires synthesising these theoretical ideas to suit specific organisational challenges, ensuring they translate into realistic, measurable, and practical strategies.

Leadership in Practice

- Identifying and nurturing potential requires creating conditions that allow individuals to grow into leadership roles through structured opportunities and support.
- Centralised and decentralised leadership each has trade-offs: centralised structures offer control and consistency, while decentralisation enhances autonomy and responsiveness. Leaders must evaluate which approach suits their objectives and adapt accordingly.
- Continuous performance management, with regular feedback and goal-setting, is essential for maintaining alignment and accountability. This is particularly important in decentralised systems where flexibility in methods and approaches supports clear objectives and measurable outcomes.
- Leaders must focus on linking these elements: selecting and developing potential; choosing structural approaches; and maintaining performance management systems to support their overall leadership vision and objectives.

References

Decuypere, A., & Schaufeli, W. (2020). Leadership and work engagement: Exploring explanatory mechanisms. *German Journal of Human Resource Management, 34*(1), 69–95.

Do, M. H., & Minbashian, A. (2020). Higher-order personality factors and leadership outcomes: A meta-analysis. *Personality and Individual Differences, 163*, 110058.

Fried, E. I. (2021). Theories and models: What they are, what they are for, and what they are about. *An International Journal for the Advancement of Psychological Theory, 31*(4). https://doi.org/10.1080/1047840X.2020.1854011

Haines, N. (2019). *Thinking generatively: Why do we use atheoretical statistical models to test substantive psychological theories?* Computational Psychology.

Jordan, P. J., & Troth, A. (2011). Emotional intelligence and leader member exchange: The relationship with employee turnover intentions and job satisfaction. *Leadership & Organization Development Journal, 32*(3), 260–280.

Kline, R. B. (2011). *Principles and practice of structural equation modeling* (3rd ed.). The Guilford Press.

MacRae, I. (2024). *Web of value: Web of value: Understanding blockchain and web3's intersection of technology, psychology and business*. Alexandria Books.

MacRae, I., Furnham A., & Reed, M. (2018). *High potential: How to spot, manage and develop talented people at work* (2nd ed.). Bloomsbury Business.

McPhetres, J., Albayrak-Aydemir, N., Barbosa Mendes, A., Chow, E. C., Gonzalez-Marquez, P., Loukras, E., et al. (2021). A decade of theory as reflected in *Psychological Science* (2009–2019). *PLoS ONE, 16*(3), e0247986. https://doi.org/10.1371/journal.pone.0247986

Meehl, P. E. (1990). Appraising and amending theories: The strategy of Lakatosian defense and two principles that warrant it. *Psychological Inquiry, 1*(2), 108–141.

Northouse, P. G. (2013). *Leadership: Theory and practice* (6th ed.). Sage Publications.

Schmidt, V. A. (1991). *Democratizing France: The political and administrative history of decentralization*. Cambridge University Press.

Silzer, R., & Church, A. (2009). The pearls and perils of identifying potential. *Industrial and Organizational Psychology, 2*, 377–412. https://doi.org/10.1111/j.1754-9434.2009.01163.x

System Psychodynamics of Leadership Roles 4

Understanding Systems and Organisations

Dr David Lawlor

Key Concepts of Systems Psychodynamics

Gould et al. (2001, pp. 2–15) show that the field of systems psychodynamics had its birth with the publication of Miller and Rice's seminal volume *Systems of Organisation* (1967). The "systems" designation refers to open systems concepts that frame the understanding of organisational structures, including design, division of labour, authority levels, reporting relationships, tasks, processes, mission, the nature and patterning of the organisation's task and sentient boundaries, and the transactions across them. They provide a perspective for understanding the structural aspects of an organisational system.

Psychodynamics studies the interplay between conscious and unconscious processes, emotions, motivations, and behaviours, focusing on how past experiences shape an individual's psychological state and influence their thoughts, feelings, and actions. The term psychodynamics refers to psychoanalytic perspectives on individual experiences and mental processes (e.g., transference, resistance, object relations, phantasy), as well as the experiences of unconscious group and social processes that are simultaneously both a source and a consequence of unresolved or unrecognised organisational difficulties (Freud, 1921; Jaques, 1955; Menzies, 1960).

The following are the core concepts of systems psychodynamics practice:

DOI: 10.4324/9781003492399-6

Mechanisms of defence: Kets de Vries (2006) and Gabriel (1999) highlight that unconscious motivations and defences significantly impact individual and group behaviour within organisations. These processes include repressed desires, fears, and unresolved conflicts that affect how leaders relate to their teams and their work.

Roles and boundaries: According to Hirschhorn (1997) and Gould, Stapley, and Stein (2001), roles provide a structure for individuals to understand their place within the organisation, while boundaries delineate the limits of roles, tasks, and responsibilities. This clarity is vital for effective leadership.

Group processes: Drawing on Group Relations Theory, Miller and Rice (1967), and Trist and Murray (1990) explore how individuals function within groups and how group dynamics influence individual behaviour. This theory emphasises the interplay between personal psychodynamics and group processes, providing insights into leadership dynamics and team interactions.

Social defences: Menzies Lyth (1988) and Jaques (1955) examined how social systems in organisations can act as defences against collective anxieties and uncertainties. These defences can manifest as rigid structures, rituals, or cultural norms that protect individuals from emotional discomfort but may also hinder organisational effectiveness and change.

Boundaries: The systems psychodynamic model emphasises the importance of boundaries as critical zones where internal and external systems meet—zones where anxieties and defences are projected and negotiated, and where organisational health and dysfunction often become most visible.

Systemic Systems Theory

Von Bertalanffy (1968) and Senge (1990) present organisations as interconnected wholes, focusing on the complex interrelations and interdependencies among their parts. This theory examines how organisational structures, cultures, and processes influence—and are influenced by—individual and group behaviour.

Organisation in the Mind

Armstrong (2005) refers to the mental representation of an organisation that individuals hold. This concept explores how these internal models shape individuals' behaviour and interactions within the organisation.

Armstrong emphasises the importance of understanding these representations to address organisational issues effectively.

Primary Task

Miller and Rice (1967) introduced the concept of the *primary task* as the core mission or purpose an organisation or group is designed to accomplish. It forms the foundation upon which organisational roles, boundaries, and leadership are constructed. The primary task defines the business objective, clarifies responsibilities, and mediates the relationship between task-related and emotional dynamics—making it essential for achieving organisational success. Alignment with the primary task ensures smoother operations, while misalignment can result in inefficiency and conflict. Balancing task boundaries (related to work duties) and sentient boundaries (related to emotional dynamics) is vital for productivity and well-being.

The BART (Boundary, Authority, Role, and Task) Model

Molenkamp and De Beer (2000) summarised the BART model, which invites leaders to reflect on how these four elements interact within an organisation. By examining issues such as unclear roles, misaligned authority, or fuzzy boundaries, leaders can uncover systemic tensions and enhance organisational effectiveness.

Boundary: Defines limits such as time, space, tasks, and membership, which determine who is included or excluded. Boundaries are essential for maintaining structure and function.

Authority: Refers to both formal and informal power dynamics that influence decision-making and control. It can be based on roles or personal traits such as expertise.

Role: Involves the expectations and responsibilities tied to a position within the organisation. Clear roles ensure duties and decision-making authority are well understood.

Task: The primary mission or objective of a group. Task clarity helps align efforts and avoid confusion.

Complexities of Authority, Authorisation, Power, and the Leadership Politics

Authority, power, and politics are central to leadership. Leadership is not just a function of individual traits or behaviours but is deeply intertwined with the unconscious processes and emotional undercurrents that shape organisational life.

Authority and Power

In organisational dynamics, leadership is entwined with authority, power, and the politics of leadership. Power is not just about formal authority; it also involves emotional and psychological undercurrents, such as dependency, rivalry, and fear. Leaders who are aware of these unconscious power dynamics are better equipped to manage authority ethically and effectively.

Armstrong (2005) suggests that leadership requires *discernment*. This involves bringing into view and articulating the often-tacit aspects within an organisation, particularly how it embodies meaning in its work.

French and Raven (1959) identified six power sources: legitimate (formal authority), reward (compensating compliance), expert (skills and knowledge), referent (respect), coercive (ability to punish), and informational (control of information). Understanding these dynamics helps leaders navigate complexities, build trust, and drive success.

Leadership and Followership

Leadership and followership are co-created processes, where both leaders and followers influence each other in unconscious ways. Leaders often project their desires, fears, and anxieties onto followers, while followers, in turn, transfer their hopes, needs, and expectations onto the leader. This unconscious interplay forms the foundation of the leadership-followership dynamic.

System psychodynamics focuses on how authority, power, and political dynamics unfold. Authority refers to the right to make decisions, while power is the ability to influence others, shaped by unconscious motivations like repressed desires and fears. Leaders must manage their own and their followers' unconscious motivations, which impact how authority is perceived and exercised.

Authority is not only granted by position but also by the group's ongoing authorisation, influenced by competence, integrity, and emotional intelligence. Psychological safety is key to effective followership, allowing followers to express concerns without fear. Leaders who foster this environment build trust and maintain their authority.

Leadership and followership are interdependent, with followers seeking guidance and leaders relying on their support. This relationship is shaped by unconscious processes like dependency and idealisation. Trust, built through empathy and transparency, is essential. Leaders must also manage projections from followers, such as unrealistic expectations, using emotional intelligence to navigate these dynamics and create a supportive work environment.

Politics of Leadership

Leadership politics is not merely about organisational strategy or external influence but about managing the hidden emotional tensions within the group. Power struggles are played out in subtle ways, with unconscious competition, loyalty shifts, or hidden resentments influencing organisational outcomes. Leaders must navigate these dynamics, balancing their own psychological needs with the organisational goals and managing the emotions that arise within their teams.

Understanding the unconscious drivers behind organisational politics allows leaders to better manage conflicts, alliances, and power plays within the organisation. By being attuned to these deeper dynamics, leaders promote healthier power relations, foster balanced, ethical, and productive collaborative environments, and avoid the pitfalls of unchecked power, such as authoritarianism or disengaged followership.

How Can a System Psychodynamic Approach Help with Taking Up the Leadership

Systems psychodynamics offers insights into how leaders exercise authority and how followers respond to it. The unconscious dynamics of power, control, and dependency shape leadership behaviour and organisational outcomes. Leaders who understand these underlying processes wield their authority more effectively and ethically, fostering a balanced and productive organisational climate.

> **Question to Consider:** What are your observations of how power, control, and dependency are exercised in your team/organisation? How do you see it impacting the way you take leadership?

Change management is an area where systems psychodynamics prove invaluable insights. Organisational change triggers unconscious fears and anxieties that hinder transformation efforts. Leaders who are attuned to these dynamics design interventions that address the root causes of resistance, facilitating smoother and more successful transitions. This approach helps in mitigating the emotional and psychological barriers that obstruct change initiatives.

> **Question to Consider:** What unconscious fears and anxieties might have been triggered during organisational change? What can be done to reduce resistance and facilitate a more successful transformation?

Effective leadership involves enhancing team dynamics by addressing unconscious processes within teams. Leaders improve team cohesion, communication, and collaboration by identifying and managing hidden conflicts, rivalries, and alliances. This proactive approach to team dynamics boosts team performance but also fosters a more collaborative and supportive work environment.

> **Question to Consider:** What do you see are the unconscious conflicts, rivalries, and alliances within your team? What resources do you need to identify and manage them to foster greater cohesion and improved team performance?

The Use of Consultation to Enhance Service Effectiveness

A systems psychodynamics consultant plays a vital role in helping organisations navigate the complexities of leadership, authority, and power dynamics. An external consultant can facilitate conversations that enable leaders and teams to explore underlying issues that may be hindering organisational effectiveness. By creating a safe and reflective space, the consultant helps the organisation examine unconscious processes—such as projections, anxieties, and power struggles—that are often difficult to address internally.

Miller and Rice (1967), Hirschhorn (1997), and French and Vince (1999) describe role analysis and boundary management as strategies that enhance organisational effectiveness by helping leaders understand how unconscious processes influence role perceptions and enactments. This understanding aids in identifying role conflicts and ambiguities. Managing and clarifying boundaries within organisations reduces uncertainty and anxiety, creating a stable environment for confident operation.

The consultant's role is to guide the organisation through questions and areas that require exploration, including:

Leadership and Followership Dynamics: Consultants encourage leaders and teams to reflect on how unconscious expectations, dependencies, and projections influence their relationships. Are leaders being idealised or feared? How is this affecting their decision-making and team dynamics?

Power and Authority: By helping the organisation explore how power is distributed and exercised, consultants assist in identifying imbalances or unspoken power struggles. This might involve asking, "How is authority being used, and how are followers responding to it?" or "Are there unacknowledged sources of power influencing the organisational culture?"

Boundary Management: Consultants help examine the boundaries within the organisation—such as roles, responsibilities, and control over resources—and how these boundaries might contribute to conflict or inefficiency.

Team Dynamics: Consultants ask questions that lead teams to explore hidden alliances, rivalries, or unresolved conflicts that could be impacting collaboration and productivity.

Obholzer and Roberts (1994), Hirschhorn (1997), Miller and Rice (1967), and Kets de Vries (2006) highlight that the benefits of systems psychodynamics for leadership are substantial. Through facilitated conversations, a systems psychodynamics consultant enables organisations to uncover and address the deeper emotional and psychological dynamics at play—ultimately fostering healthier, more effective leadership and team functioning. Systems psychodynamics interventions contribute to sustainable change by addressing root causes, ensuring lasting improvements in organisational health and effectiveness.

Application of Systems Psychodynamics Approach

This section provides examples of the application of the systems psychodynamic approach through a case study. Reflective questions and exercises are offered for readers to explore the areas discussed earlier.

A Case Study

A psychological service had significant challenges such as high employee turnover, low morale, and leadership conflicts. Despite its innovative practice, these internal issues threatened its success. The Head of Service invited a systems psychodynamics consultant to help navigate these complex dynamics.

The consultant began by conducting in-depth interviews and facilitating group discussions at various levels. This revealed several critical issues: unconscious competition and power struggles among the leadership team, hidden fears of failure and self-doubt regarding intellect, skills, or accomplishments among individuals, affecting decision-making, and underlying anxieties about rapid changes and job security.

The consultant organised workshops to surface hidden emotions and conflicts through role-playing and reflective exercises, fostering a safe space for open dialogue. Senior leaders received one-on-one coaching sessions focused on self-awareness and emotional intelligence. The Head of Services, for example, realised that her fear of failure led to micromanagement and mistrust of her team. Team-building activities were introduced to improve organisational health, aiming to build trust and improve communication across departments. Staff engaged in collaborative problem-solving tasks requiring open communication and mutual support. Additionally, a structured, anonymous feedback system was implemented to gather insights from staff about the organisational climate, allowing the consultant to tailor interventions more precisely and address specific concerns as they arose.

As a result of these interventions, leaders gained a deeper understanding of the unconscious factors influencing their behaviour, leading to more empathetic and effective interactions within the team. Through coaching, leaders developed greater self-awareness, with the Head of Services becoming more mindful of her tendencies and starting to delegate more, which improved trust and collaboration. Addressing underlying psychological issues improved the overall organisational climate, making employees feel more secure and valued, leading to increased morale and reduced turnover. A culture of innovation was fostered by encouraging risk-taking without fear of negative repercussions. The improved trust and collaboration translated into a more resilient and adaptive organisation.

Exploring Authority, Authorisation, Power

Leaders can reflect on how traits like confidence, empathy, and assertiveness affect power dynamics and decision-making, ensuring alignment with organisational values. Expertise influences authority, and knowledge-sharing impacts collaboration. Fair resource distribution and access to opportunities promote inclusiveness and balance.

Leaders can consider how organisational structure shapes their authority and balance personal agency with system constraints. Understanding unconscious power dynamics, managing resistance, and balancing formal authority with personal influence are crucial for mindful leadership. Reflecting on unconscious power use, power distribution within teams, and responses to resistance helps leaders foster a more equitable, supportive environment.

Reflective Question

How do you navigate power dynamics in your organisation while balancing your political skills with ethical considerations to build trust and legitimacy?

A power mapping exercise is illustrated below.

Power Mapping Exercise

1. Identify Key Areas of Power
   Create a diagram of power sources in your organisation, including personal power (e.g., expertise, charisma), formal power (e.g., authority), and control of resources (e.g., budgets, knowledge).
2. Reflect on Your Position
   Place yourself in the power map. Reflect on how you influence others and which power sources you rely on in your leadership role.
3. Analyse Power Dynamics
   Examine power distribution among team members. Who controls key resources? Who is excluded from decisions? Consider any unconscious biases affecting these dynamics.
4. Discuss with a Colleague
   Share your power map with a trusted peer. Discuss where power is effective and where it could be more equitably distributed.

Reflective Areas and Questions for Leadership and Followership Dynamics

1. Projections and Transference:
   - Reflection: How do unconscious projections from followers shape your leadership?
   - Question: Do you feel idealised or overly relied on, and how do you manage this?
2. Authority and Power:
   - Reflection: How do authority and power manifest in your leadership?
   - Question: Is your authority based on position, or earned through actions and emotional intelligence?
3. Mutual Dependence:
   - Reflection: How do you and your followers rely on each other for support and direction?
   - Question: How does this dependency influence team interactions, and are unconscious dynamics at play?

4. Psychological Safety:
   - Reflection: How do you create psychological safety for open communication?
   - Question: Do followers feel safe expressing concerns, and how can you improve this?
5. Emotional Intelligence:
   - Reflection: How do you use emotional intelligence to meet your team's emotional needs?
   - Question: Are you missing emotional cues, and how can you enhance your awareness?
6. Unconscious Motivations:
   - Reflection: How do your unconscious motivations affect your leadership?
   - Question: Are unresolved personal experiences influencing your approach to power and authority?

Exercise: Exploring Leadership and Followership Dynamics

Step 1: Leadership and Followership Mapping

Instructions: Draw a map that highlights the relationships between you and your followers. On this map, identify key individuals or groups and reflect on the emotional and relational dynamics at play. Consider areas such as:

- How do different followers respond to your leadership style?
- What projections or expectations do they place on you?
- How do you feel towards certain followers (e.g., over-protection, frustration, dependency)?

Step 2: Identify Projections and Transference

Instructions: For each key relationship on your map, note any unconscious projections or transference that may be occurring (both from followers towards you and from you towards them). Examples may include feelings of dependency, idealisation, or unrealistic expectations.

- **Reflection**: How might these unconscious processes be influencing your leadership style and decision-making? How do they impact the group dynamics?

Step 3: Take Action to Manage Dynamics

Instructions: Choose one relationship or dynamic from your map that requires attention. Reflect on how you can address this dynamic to improve communication, trust, or emotional engagement.

- **Reflection**: What practical steps can you take to manage these projections and build a more balanced, transparent relationship? What role does emotional intelligence play in this process?

Political and Conflict Resolution Skills

Leaders need political skills such as social astuteness, networking, influence, and sincerity to manage relationships, resolve conflicts, and drive change. Conflict, often arising from competition or personality clashes, is natural. Ethical leadership builds trust and legitimacy, requiring integrity and transparency in the use of power.

Exercise: Conflict Resolution Analysis

Step 1: Identify a Current Conflict

- Reflect on a conflict within your organisation that involves competition for resources, differences in values, or power struggles.
- Identify the key individuals involved and consider the underlying dynamics at play.

Step 2: Analyse Power Dynamics and Political Skills

- Reflect on how power is distributed among the parties involved. Are there hidden alliances or unconscious motivations influencing the conflict?
- Consider your own political skills (e.g., networking, interpersonal influence) and how they can be applied to address the conflict.

Step 3: Develop a Conflict Resolution Strategy

- Using your analysis, create a strategy that balances assertiveness and empathy to manage the conflict constructively.
- Reflect on how you can use your political skills to influence a positive outcome while maintaining ethical integrity.

Step 4: Reflect on Organisational Culture

- Consider how your organisation's culture influences political behaviours. Does it encourage collaboration or competition?
- Think about ways you can contribute to fostering a more supportive environment that values openness and respect.

Fostering a Culture of Trust

The concept of *holding environment* helps to think about the work environment and the role of leaders in shaping employees' psychological experiences and their overall effectiveness in their roles (Kahn, 1992). By creating a safe environment, organisations can enhance engagement, productivity, and overall well-being. *Psychological presence* or *being fully there* at work is crucial for staff engagement and well-being (Kahn 2005).

Reflective Questions

- **Meaningfulness:** Where we are regarding our sense of purpose. What values do we hold as a team?
- **Safety:** Does my team feel safe to share their views without fear of negative consequences?
- **Availability:** Do we have physical, emotional, and psychological resources to allow people to be fully present at work?

Key Points

Creating a Supportive Environment: Leaders shape employees' psychological experiences by fostering a safe and supportive "holding environment" that enhances engagement, productivity, and well-being.

Promoting Psychological Presence: Encouraging employees to be "fully there" at work improves engagement and well-being. Leaders can cultivate connection, value, and focus.

Key Conditions for Psychological Presence

1. **Meaningfulness:** Aligning work with purpose and shared team values.
2. **Safety:** Ensuring team members feel secure to express themselves without fear.
3. **Availability:** Providing the necessary resources for employees to be engaged.

Facilitating Reflection: Open team discussions help identify enablers and barriers to trust and presence. Reflective questions guide these conversations.

Implementing Insights: Leaders should use feedback to develop actionable steps to address challenges, foster trust, and enhance the working environment.

Ideas in Brief

- Recognise how unconscious dynamics shape leadership roles, team behaviour, and organisational culture.
- Develop insight into patterns of anxiety, projection, and group defences that hinder effective leadership.
- Explore how authority, identity, and role are negotiated in systems often beneath conscious awareness.
- Use reflective and relational practices to surface hidden tensions and strengthen leadership impact.

References

Armstrong, D., & French, R. (Eds.). (2005). *Organisation in the mind: Psychoanalysis, group relations and organisational consultancy*. Karnac.

Bion, W. R. (1961). *Experiences in groups and other papers*. London: Tavistock Publications. [Reprinted London: Routledge, 1989; London: Brunner-Routledge, 2001.]

French, J. R. P., Jr., & Raven, B. (1959). The bases of social power. In D. Cartwright (Ed.), *Studies in social power* (pp. 150–167). University of Michigan.

French, R., & Vince, R. (1999). *Group relations, management, and organisation*. Oxford University Press.

Freud, S. (1921). *Group psychology and the analysis of the ego*. International Psycho-Analytical Press.

Gabriel, Y. (1999). *Organisations in depth: The psychoanalysis of organisations*. Sage.

Gould, L. J., Stapley, L. F., & Stein, M. (2001). *The systems psychodynamics of organisations: Integrating the group relations approach, psychoanalytic, and open systems perspectives*. Karnac Books.

Hirschhorn, L. (1997). *Reworking authority: Leading and following in the post-modern organisation*. MIT Press.

Jaques, E. (1955). Social systems as a defence against persecutory and depressive anxiety. In M. Klein, P. Heimann, & R. Money-Kyrle (Eds.), *New directions in psycho-analysis* (pp. 478–498). Tavistock.

Kahn, W. A. (1992). To be fully there: Psychological presence at work. *Human Relations, 45*(4), 321–349. https://doi.org/10.1177/001872679204500402

Kahn, W. A. (2001). Holding environments at work. *The Journal of Applied Behavioral Science, 37*(3), 260–279. https://doi.org/10.1177/0021886301373001

Kahn, W. A. (2005). *Holding fast: The struggle to create resilient caregiving organisations*. Routledge.

Kets de Vries, M. F. R. (2006). *The leader on the couch: A clinical approach to changing people and organisations*. John Wiley & Sons.

Lawlor, D., & Sher, M. (2022). *An introduction to systems psychodynamics* (Vol. I). Routledge.

Lawlor, D., & Sher, M. (2023a). *Systems psychodynamics: Innovative approaches to change, whole systems & complexity* (Vol. II). Routledge.

Lawlor, D., & Sher, M. (2023b). *Systems psychodynamics: Voices from the field* (Vol. III). Routledge.

Menzies, I. E. P. (1960). A Case-Study in the Functioning of Social Systems as a Defence against Anxiety: A Report on a Study of the Nursing Service of a General Hospital. Human Relations, 13(2), 95–121.

Menzies Lyth, I. (1988). *Containing anxiety in institutions: Selected essays volume 1*. Free Association Books.

Miller, E. J., & Rice, A. K. (1967). *Systems of organisation: The control of task and sentient boundaries*. Tavistock.

Molenkamp, R. J., & de Beer, M. J. (2000). *The BART system of group and organisational analysis: Boundary, authority, role and task (Workshop manual)*. Leadership & Management Learning Institute.

Obholzer, A., & Roberts, V. Z. (Eds.). (1994). *The unconscious at work: Individual and organisational stress in the human services*. Routledge.

Senge, P. M. (1990). *The fifth discipline: The art and practice of the learning organisation*. Doubleday/Currency.

Trist, E. L., & Murray, H. (1990). *The social engagement of social science: A Tavistock anthology. Volume I: The socio-psychological perspective*. University of Pennsylvania Press.

Von Bertalanffy, L. (1968). *General system theory: Foundations, development, applications*. George Braziller.

PART TWO

RISING WITH THE TIDE

HARNESSING INFLUENCE FOR IMPACT AND TRANSFORMATION

Political Skills in Everyday Leadership 5

What You Need to Know, but Might Be Hesitant to Ask?

Ashley Weinberg

Politics has acquired a reputation of its own that too often leaves it outside the topics of civilised conversation. Unfortunately, this also means politics and its associated skills are consigned to spaces beyond those in which we train as health-focused professionals. This chapter shuns such unhelpful conventions in the hope that, as a discipline, psychology can not only recognise the strategic need for relevant training but also become equipped with the tools that make political skills just one prerequisite for enabling progress in the workplace and life beyond. This is not to give sway to Machiavelli's purported dark side, but rather to encourage readers to consider the mechanics of envisioning and creating thriving cultures, introducing change successfully, engaging stakeholders and providing influence that together can support the improved well-being and functioning of psychologists as practitioners, students, teachers, and leaders.

Politics with a Small 'p'?

> *'I'm not political', she said. 'I mean, I would never invest time in promoting myself or what I do because that's the kind of thing those 'others' do... you know, the colleagues that nobody likes'. 'When did you last have a promotion?' the listener asked. 'Er, almost 25 years ago' she replied.*

DOI: 10.4324/9781003492399-8

Being political is part of everyday life and often in ways we would not credit. For psychologists, this includes communicating ideas, facilitating new ways of being and doing, championing healthier lifestyles and successful habits, and empowering others. However, the idea of bringing about positive change means that not only are political skills part of our work, but they are also expected by clients, students and workplaces (Weinberg, 2023). Furthermore, the suggestion that everything we do is 'political' can extend to our lives beyond the workplace – just ask any parent attempting to persuade their child of the merits of homework, or a friend who keeps telling you it might do you good to come out for an evening.

Politics with a small 'p' is often about these everyday exchanges and perhaps sounds rather familiar after all? The use of political skills is fundamental to changing behaviour and mindsets. The chapter encourages you to consider their use in your everyday life and increase the positive impact you are working to achieve. You may also reflect on whether political skills training is sufficiently present in the formal qualification routes of Psychology, or perhaps needs to be brought into the light!

We are far quicker at recognising politics with a big 'P' in media headlines about world leaders and Members of Parliament. As such, we may be inclined to feel less positively about such skills, especially where events have not gone to plan and a professional politician endeavours to explain things away, or too commonly ignores awkward questions altogether. Not surprisingly, citizens find this kind of political practice off-putting. However, the reality – for colleagues in the field of Psychology and outside it – is that politics actually can be 'a force for good'. If this sounds familiar, it is not just because the UK Prime Minister elected in 2024 used the phrase, but this mantra has been alive and well for many years in the Political Psychology Section of the British Psychological Society. Importantly, evidence of the truth of such a statement owes more to using political skills in the application of psychological knowledge in order to persuade, support, enhance and promote positive values than to employing negative political tactics to delay, disguise, undermine or oppress.

Few of us start out as leaders, so our route to developing such skills and the opportunities to display them may seem haphazard. Yet leadership behaviours are apparent in daily life, as a reflection of political skills and our values. In other words, evidence of how we conduct ourselves can be indicative of leadership, whether emerging or aspiring to more official 'leadership' roles. Therefore, it helps to recognise the political skills that support positive behaviour. The next section considers what is 'political'?

Using Political Skills to Be the Change You Wish to See

In the hustle and bustle and pressures of daily existence, it is tempting to become preoccupied with grinding challenges and how they make us feel rather than the grander schemes of human progress to which we aspire. Yet, the potential to play our part as psychologists, trainees and students, in everyday positive change is clear in our interactions with clients, organisations and through education. One limiting issue is that immediate pressures capture our focus and, without much encouragement, we are inclined to feel that achieving broader change is beyond our scope. Therefore, deciding on and then keeping our aims and goals in mind is perhaps the first step towards the progress we hope for. So how can this be achieved?

The British Psychological Society Code of Ethics and Conduct (BPS, 2021) encourages Respect, Competence, Responsibility and Integrity as a clear map for 'how' we behave. These incorporate clear political considerations which are highlighted as values, including 'issues of power', 'self-determination', 'caution in making knowledge claims', 'professional accountability', 'fairness' and 'addressing misconduct'. Combined with the stated aims of psychological training across sub-disciplines, such values give all concerned a clear idea of the positive influence Psychology can wield. However, an explanation of the associated political skills – the 'how to' that facilitates effecting change – is more rarely stated.

Ferris et al. (2005) define political skills in an occupational context as 'the ability to effectively understand others at work and to use such knowledge to influence others to act in ways that enhance one's personal and/or organisational objectives' (p. 127). Their focus on social astuteness, interpersonal influence, networking ability, and 'political savvy' relates to emotional competencies exercised in psychological practice. Notably, interacting with people to promote positive change means knowing how to connect (e.g. social antennae), engage successfully (e.g. likeability) and discern others' motivations (e.g. positive enquiry).

Admittedly, opportunities to deploy political savvy can be limited to thinking 'We can't do that because of a decision above our pay grade', but that is more of a reflection of formal power structures (see French and Raven, 1959). While politics is about power, it comes in many forms and expertise is one such source, reflecting the importance of

Table 5.1 Everyday political skills for psychologists

Leadership in action	Political actions	Everyday political skills
Controlling/shaping	Enacting change	Making key decisions
Envisioning	Influencing policy/change	Providing informed/expert opinion
Inspiring	Campaigning for change	Communicating with key decision-makers
Energising	Raising awareness of an issue	Sharing information
Demonstrating political skills	Advocating for others	Representing clients' views/gathering information
Sharing political skills	Empowering others	Providing support/mentorship
Enhancing self-efficacy	Developing our personal resources and capacity	Requesting training/funding/support
Self-awareness	Reflecting on our actions	Making time for self-development

information and credibility (Kovach, 2020) of psychologists as professionals or trainee professionals. Political savvy for psychologists points to making appropriate use of relevant and up-to-date knowledge to inform and influence the positive change we wish to see. Accordingly, political skills can support the efforts of individuals to progress in their careers as well as promote social progress. Indeed, Ferris et al. (2007) go further to identify political skills as 'a necessary competency to possess to be effective in organisations', so perhaps it is not surprising that a subsequent large-scale review of research has found political skills are positively linked to career success (Chen et al., 2021). Table 5.1 provides examples of these in action at varying levels of leadership.

Case Study Examples: The Power of Well-Aimed Research

Broadening the application of political skills to advance psychological progress can entail being the person who leads or encourages others to show leadership. This might start with conversations with affected individuals, groups or communities, and recognition of the need for gathering more detailed information. Co-creating data tools with employee groups is one way in which psychologists as researchers can facilitate this, employing appropriate statistical analyses and producing relevant and readily digestible outputs, such as a report or executive summary. Similarly, using psychological knowledge to provide accessible information to raise awareness can stimulate change. We can support the process of raising awareness and may find that, as professionals trained in the use of research, the onus can lie with us to present the findings to an audience of relevant decision-makers. In other words, understanding information may also mean raising awareness by disseminating the findings. In this way, research has the potential to be political (and in a good way). Here are two examples.

Psychology graduate and former teacher Rosamund Adoo-Kissi-Debrah (The Psychologist, 2024) has found her knowledge of research invaluable in raising awareness of the effect of pollutants on children's health. The tragic death of her daughter Ella from a fatal asthma attack triggered by air pollution in 2013 has led her to become a campaigner, not only for awareness of the effects of pollutants among medical practitioners and politicians but also for 'Ella's Law', to ensure access to clean air for children is a right.

After delivering a workshop on well-being to MPs' staff during the Covid-19 lockdown, the author of this chapter was invited to conduct a survey of their working conditions (Weinberg, 2024a). Surveys evidenced working practices in need of reform. Results were presented to a Speaker's Conference of MPs, who had been appointed to scrutinise the working experiences of staff. The opportunity to use psychological knowledge as a force for good became clear, and subsequently Parliament accepted recommendations for positive change.

Psychologists Demonstrating Political Skills in Knowledge and Practice

It is likely that psychologists underestimate the soft power used in the context of everyday practice and teaching. Choices of theoretical models and modes of practice are influenced and determined by training and experience, which in turn shape approaches to perceived needs, not least as every case has its own individual features. Equally, psychological training and commitment to continuing professional development mean contact with new scientific information and an occupational requirement to interrogate such findings for both ethics and suitability.

Such a process signifies the impact of decisions made for psychologists as well as by psychologists – and choices tend to be political, whether rooted in traditions and conventions or arising from more recent consensus. Conformity across an entire occupational group may appear a prerequisite for consistent standards, yet ongoing debate about 'best practice' is always needed in the interests of enlightened and progressive science. In other words, the act of questioning amounts to a political process for those who propose, support or oppose ideas, by weighing up matters and raising issues for debate.

The interface between a psychologist and their client(s) – however they are defined in any of the sub-disciplines of our field – is itself political and fraught with the potential for misunderstanding if psychologists are shortchanged in training in everyday political skills. Additionally, those engaged in practising psychology have the potential and responsibility to raise awareness beyond the profession of psychological issues that have implications for clients, workplaces and society. This underscores the need for healthcare professionals to engage in what may be deemed political action. Indeed, the review of professional standards by the UK Health and Care Professions Council is headed by the revised emphasis to, 'Promote and protect the interests of service users and carers', with this message to practitioners: 'You must empower and enable service users, where appropriate, to play a part in maintaining their own health and wellbeing and support them so they can make informed decisions' (HCPC, 2024).

Similarly, raising concerns 'regarding colleagues if you witness bullying, harassment or intimidation of a service user, carer or another colleague' (HCPC, 2024) represents overtly political behaviour. This is clearly significant and raises many questions about how. HCPC guidance suggests 'following the relevant procedures within your practice or organisation and maintaining the safety of all involved'. Herein lies a common challenge for individuals: i.e. questioning power structures via processes often defined by organisations. Perhaps it is not surprising that employees frustrated with the lack of a safe route to raise difficult issues seek the support of outsiders to the organisational context, either through their professional body or other trusted external agencies. This is no less the case outside the practice of Psychology; for example, hundreds of UK sub-postmasters who waited decades for justice after wrongful convictions for fraud due to malpractice by the Post Office.

Questions to consider:

- Do I need to consider myself political?
- How adept am I at recognising the 'political' in the actions of others?
- How should I become more political, and what would this look like?
- Is it ethical to be non-political?

Building the Will to Bring about Change

It is exciting to see movements growing to raise awareness of so many issues that society has hitherto neglected to focus on. Part of this increase is linked to the social levers that can help build 'political will', generating the energy for change to take place. Whether linked to neurodiversity in the workplace, the menopause, experiences of minoritised groups or sexual harassment, people are connected via social media in ways that have not been so readily available previously, making the political skill of networking almost universal.

Not surprisingly, progress relies on deploying a range of political skills to carve out the building blocks of change. In providing a framework for this, Raile et al. (2021) outline some key steps:

1. Identify the key political and public stakeholders.
2. Understand the perceptions held by these stakeholders of the problem and possible solutions.
3. Consider how stakeholders' views of problems and solutions might be aligned.
4. Facilitate shared commitments for change, which incorporate mutual accountability among stakeholders.

How might this work in practice, whether it is introducing a new way of doing things or trying to regain effective practices that perhaps have been overtaken by competing commitments?

The following example is taken from an initiative by staff working in a UK university, who met to discuss staff well-being (Weinberg, 2024b). This became a regular meeting chaired by a member of the human resources team and drew sponsorship from senior leaders as well as a modest budget. What began as a voluntary role by staff supporting their colleagues became an organisation-wide 'Staff Well-being Working Group' with recognised responsibilities. To underpin progress, a written Commitment to staff mental well-being, co-authored by frontline staff, was drafted and championed by group members and became University policy. Recognising that this is so often the end point for envisaged change in organisations, the Group launched the Commitment on World Mental Health Day, inviting colleagues, senior leaders, and interested parties from other universities. The positive energy from the event led to a subsequent online meeting of Staff Well-being Leads from 30 higher education institutions (HEIs), and a national network was born. As well as an annual conference, hosted in turn by a different HEI, quarterly online events share best practices and provide support and resources to members. Generating their own data on HEI provision for staff well-being has attracted interest from relevant employers, helping to join together stakeholders across the sector with the potential to stimulate even wider positive change.

As an application of Raile et al.'s (2021) framework on generating will, this example illustrates the actions the initiative incorporated and some of the political skills required (See Table 5.2).

Understandably, a role in bringing about change is a challenge not all of us relish. Indeed, the concept of demonstrating leadership may seem 'something for others', yet as Psychologists, the ball often comes to rest with us. Our training, ethical and practitioner requirements amount to a discipline that plays an essential role in creating thriving cultures in workplaces and communities, whether this is built on a clear vision of our own or one on which we are well-placed to advise. As Psychologists, we have access to individuals and organisations who are hoping for – and likely needing – successful change. This encompasses engagement with stakeholders and shaping influence at the level of individuals, teams and beyond. From the political skills of social astuteness, interpersonal and networking reach, as well as 'savvy' proposed by Ferris et al. (2007), to concrete actions in generating political will (Raile et al., 2021), it is clear there are levels of leadership in psychological practice. Recent changes in HCPC rules go further by demanding these.

The next section considers the 'how' in a little more detail and highlights some indicative features to which you may want to add.

Personal Reflections on Leading

'Do good things' were my Uncle Monty's last words to me. Naturally, such wisdom stays with you and I reflect on them often, asking, 'Am I doing something useful or positive?', 'Have I been fair with others?', 'Do I exercise a sense of responsibility?' Hopefully, I have opportunities

Table 5.2 Using political skills and associated actions to generate the 'will' for change: A colleague well-being initiative

Generating will (Raile et al., 2021)	Examples of actions to bring about change	Political skills involved (Ferris et al., 2005)
Identify stakeholders	Engaging Human Resource colleagues Creating role of Staff Well-being Leads Transfer learning from NICE guidelines Meeting with sector leadership	Networking ability
Understand perceptions of problems and possible solutions	Co-design a Staff Mental health and well-being commitment Invite colleagues to an in-person conference on World Mental Health Day Host online follow-up events	Social astuteness and Political savvy, e.g. sensitive to political steps, inclusive of all staff groups, maintaining momentum
Consider alignment of stakeholders' views of problems and solutions	Chaired network meetings become regular Invitations for network members to speak at sector-wide events Conduct survey to assess provision for staff well-being Share survey findings with stakeholders	Interpersonal influence
Facilitate shared commitment among stakeholders and mutual accountability	Build community of stakeholders Identify and agree common principles Encourage 'active' membership Keep Network informed Evaluate provision for staff well-being Share good practice	All of the above

Note: Ferris et al. (2005) identify political skills as: social astuteness, interpersonal influence, networking ability, and political savvy.

to answer 'Yes', and underpinning success in any of this is earning the trust of colleagues, clients, and students. Demonstrating you care has many components and is vital, from being accessible to actively listening and showing consideration. However, it is worth remembering that the ground one gains in the minds of others is as likely judged by the positive difference one makes and is not always determined by how well one is liked. After all, impact is what happens when you are not there.

Becoming Leaders by Example

Practice is important. The same is true of political skills in leadership and is salutary in reminding us that leadership is never 'over'; for example, continuous development via learning, reflecting on our intentions and actions, and maintaining a healthy self-awareness with a concern for the impact on others (See Table 5.3). All are reminders of the importance of being mindful of our behaviour, whether starting out on a journey that may be defined as 'leadership' or advancing well down the track. Lord Acton's adage that 'power tends to corrupt' still echoes and is no less true in today's organisations. Complacency is a potential enemy of effective functioning as demands on our time eat into good intentions to consider the impact we are having on colleagues and organisations; thus,

Table 5.3 Potential tips for modelling leadership

Look after yourself, so you can best help others
Maintain an optimistic outlook and generate positive energy
Be prepared to listen
Do your research
Take others with you
Earn trust
Show your care
Show tolerance and respect for others' views (including those you disagree with)
Maintain dignity in your communications
Play fair, or play for fairer rules
Invest time in your own development, e.g. Have a mentor/coach
What else you consider important:

ensuring leadership development time is 'booked in for us' is a must and can even maintain our well-being in challenging times (Weinberg, 2016).

As we reflect on our own psychological contract – or unwritten expectations – with our workplaces, the role of a coach or mentor is significant as sometimes our 'self-talk' is not always kind. There are considerable benefits in finding a psychological 'trainer' who can help you harness your enthusiasm and talents, helping to steer things back on course when distractions overtake you, as well as revitalising your potential should obstacles seem overwhelming. Sometimes, this person is a senior colleague, a respected professional in your field, a professional coach, or a significant other who not only encourages you to reflect but facilitates you in doing something positive about what you discover about yourself.

The need for, and role of, supervision is clearly recognised in psychological training routes. In other words, 'becoming' is not exclusively about outcomes, but just as focused on the process of 'getting there', however long the road ahead. In this way, how we might lead others necessitates thinking about our own approach for us to 'be the change we wish to see'. Indeed, when contemplating our own expectations of the potential improvements we desire, it helps to reflect on the lessons of history. Progress is slow, change is possible, persistence is the key!

Ideas in Brief

- Recognise, harness and develop political skills to achieve change.
- Encourage the realisation of your occupational and ethical purpose.
- Adopt ways in which this can be enhanced through acceptable political means.
- Consider how we might utilise sources of power and positive leadership strategies in applied contexts.

References

BPS (British Psychological Society) (2021). Code of conduct and ethics. Available at: https://explore.bps.org.uk/content/report-guideline/bpsrep.2021.inf94

Chen, H., Jiang, S., & Wu, M. (2021). How important are political skills for career success? A systematic review and meta-analysis. *The International Journal of Human Resource Management, 33*(19), 3942–3968. https://doi.org/10.1080/09585192.2021.1949626

Ferris, G. R., Treadway, D. C., Kolodinsky, R. W., Hochwarter, W. A., Kacmar, C. J., Douglas, C., & Frink, D. D. (2005). Development and validation of the Political Skill Inventory. *Journal of Management, 31*(1), 126–152. https://doi.org/10.1177/0149206304271386

Ferris, G. R., Treadway, D. C., Perrewé, P. L., Brouer, R. L., Douglas, C., & Lux, S. (2007). Political skill in organizations. *Journal of Management, 33*(3), 290–320. https://doi.org/10.1177/0149206307300813

French, J. R. P., Jr., & Raven, B. (1959). The bases of social power. In D. Cartwright (Ed.), *Studies in social power* (pp. 150–167). University of Michigan.

HCPC (Health and Care Professions Council) (2024). Details of the revisions compared to the current standards. Available at: https://www.hcpc-uk.org/standards/standards-of-conduct-performance-and-ethics/revised-standards/what-is-changing/

Kovach, M. (2020). Leader influence: A research review of French & Raven's (1959) Power Dynamics. *The Journal of Values-Based Leadership, 13*(2). Available at: https://doi.org/10.22543/0733.132.1312

Raile, A. N., Raile, E. D., & Post, L. A. (2021). Analysis and action: The political will and public will approach. *Action Research, 19*(2), 237–254. https://doi.org/10.1177/1476750318772662

The Psychologist. (2024). *When breathing clean air becomes political.* Interview with Rosamund Adoo-Kissi-Debrah, p. 40–43. Available at: https://www.bps.org.uk/psychologist/when-breathing-clean-air-becomes-political

Weinberg, A. (2016). The preventative impact of management coaching on psychological strain. *International Coaching Psychology Review, 11*(1), 93–105.

Weinberg A. (2023). Political considerations in implementing initiatives to improve the mental well-being of employees in the workplace. *Medical Research Archives, 11*(5). https://doi.org/10.18103/mra.v11i5.3725

Weinberg, A. (2024a). Just another day in politics? *The Psychologist, 37*, 52–54. Available at: https://www.bps.org.uk/psychologist/just-another-day-politics

Weinberg, A. (2024b). Why it's time to promote staff wellbeing in universities. *British Psychological Society*, 10th October. Available at: https://www.bps.org.uk/blog/why-its-time-promote-staff-wellbeing-universities

6 Responding to Challenges and Opportunities when "the Only Constant is Change"

Dr Esther Cohen-Tovée

Introduction

In UK Health and Social Care, change appears to be the only constant—whether in systems, priorities, culture, and prevailing climate (whether political, environmental or social). This is alongside smaller-scale, localised shifts in structure, leadership and organisational ethos. But some things do stay the same. How then can we navigate these constant changes to the status quo? This chapter will consider how understanding the context of structures and functions, drivers for change and mechanisms for improvement offers opportunities for leadership and influence. Although based on UK health and social care contexts and experiences, the principles, opportunities and challenges discussed are likely to have broader relevance.

Understanding the Whole System Context

Wherever one is practising, the context in which we work includes the political climate, the organisational structure and the dynamics of the health and social care system; as such, that context is always changing and developing.

However, there are observable repeating cycles of change: the purchaser-provider split versus co-production, competition versus

DOI: 10.4324/9781003492399-9

partnerships and collaboration, financial austerity versus investment, retraction versus re-establishment of corporate and infrastructure roles, integration versus separation of health and social care, restructuring focused on the benefits of small-local versus economies of scale and care consistency offered by large provider organisations.

Following the NHS England-commissioned review by Dalton (2014), which considered international evidence to develop proposals for service improvement through organisational form and system change, there has been an attempt in England to combine local (place-based) and large-scale efforts, and to achieve partnerships across health and social care through the ICS (Integrated Care System) model (NHS England, 2020). The outcome of this is not yet clear, but some of the difficulties that have emerged include tensions between place-based and ICS commissioners, financial pressures across the ICS and a series of ICS restructures aimed at achieving significant savings, which disrupt relationships and result in a loss of continuity. A more equitable distribution of power and resources, which might have been achieved through a whole-system approach, remains rare, particularly from the perspective of mental health and learning disability services. That said, there are notable examples of good practice, such as:

- Formulation-based and trauma-informed collaborations among local councils, local authorities and mental health providers, rather than diagnostically driven (e.g. Gateshead Council and CNTW NHSFT, 2024).
- Health and wellbeing hubs delivering mental wellbeing support across health and social care, jointly commissioned during the Covid-19 pandemic (e.g. British Psychological Society, 2023).

To develop influence and instigate positive change or to protect against emerging threats, we need to:

- Understand the whole system context
- Identify and understand the levers
- Understand how decisions are both ostensibly and actually made
- Develop relationships with those who make decisions directly or indirectly
- Establish formal roles within the decision-making structures

These aspects can be held in mind when considering the functions and structures operating within the system.

NHS and Social Care Functions and Structures

There are four central functions of the NHS and Social Care:

- Commissioning: Assessing healthcare needs and purchasing services to meet them.
- Providing: Delivering services as commissioned according to the standards set.
- Performance Management: Monitoring performance against standards and targets.
- Governance and assurance: Ensuring safe services and accountable organisational practice.

To navigate the complexities of the structures, it is helpful to examine the functions above and identify opportunities for influence, bearing in mind how quickly the landscape can change. For example, the UK government's sudden announcement in March 2025 that NHS England is to be abolished and its functions subsumed into the Department of Health and Social Care. See also Chapter 12, where NHS England structures are considered as a case study.

A key question to consider is, where is decision-making truly taking place? In England, the high-level decision-making structures currently include Integrated Care Boards (ICBs), Health and Wellbeing Boards (HWBs), Trust Boards, Local Authorities, Provider Collaboratives and Regional Combined Authorities.

> *The 2022 (Health and Social Care) Act...put integrated care systems on a statutory basis. This has the makings of a sensible management structure, consisting of a headquarters, seven regions and 42 integrated care boards (ICBs) whose strategy to tackle inequalities, and to improve population health, is set by an Integrated Care Partnership (ICP) that includes local government and the third sector alongside the NHS itself.*
>
> Darzi (2024).

However, it is equally important to understand where (and how) local decision-making takes place, and where influence can be sought. This may include place-based commissioning, primary care networks (PCNs), local councils, and provider trust sub-structures, e.g. directorates and business units. While decision-making ostensibly takes place formally, informal relationships and influence are essential. These may also be cultivated across the system e.g. within regional or devolved nations' organisational structures, strategic clinical networks, and education and training structures.

In Scotland and Wales, the Health Board structures provide greater continuity and reach across population areas. Scotland has fourteen Health Boards, seven national NHS Boards, and a public health body. In Wales, there are seven Local Health Boards, three NHS Trusts and two Special Health Authorities. For a comparison between the NHS in England and Wales with a focus on waiting times, see Baker (2024).

Influence and Impact

Many of us are passionate about how the knowledge, skills and expertise of Practitioner Psychologists could be more impactful. This might be through, for example, the adoption of new models of service delivery (e.g. trauma-informed, systemic), resources to address unmet needs (e.g. neurodivergence), or the implementation of existing evidence. However, to gain support for such developments or changes, we first need to identify what drives the decision-makers and influencers in the system. These can often be found in the domains of safety, quality, finance, reputation, and kudos. This is not to say that those things are not important to psychologists, but we may need to find a different way into the issues and use different language and processes. We also, above all, need to cultivate relationships with these decision-makers.

In order to maximise our influence, there is strength in numbers and in diversity of expertise. We can use professional bodies and networks to unite and drive change—e.g. the British Psychological Society (BPS) and divisional networks in the UK, and the regional/national Psychological Professions Networks in England. Could we go further and establish Psychological Professions Councils or Faculties, similar to AHP structures within ICSs?

We also need to understand the system we are working within. How does the whole system work? When teaching trainee clinical psychologists on this topic, I ask them to explore this by choosing a theme or metaphor and illustrating their ideas on whiteboards. We have had some amazingly creative illustrations, including a zoo, a rollercoaster, a tree of life, and a tea party (to which some groups are not invited…). Figures 6.1 and 6.2 show two examples from 2025.

In an organic conception of many parts making up one body, "The Octopus" highlights interdependencies and mutual benefit within the system. This harmonious conceptualisation is, however, marred by the

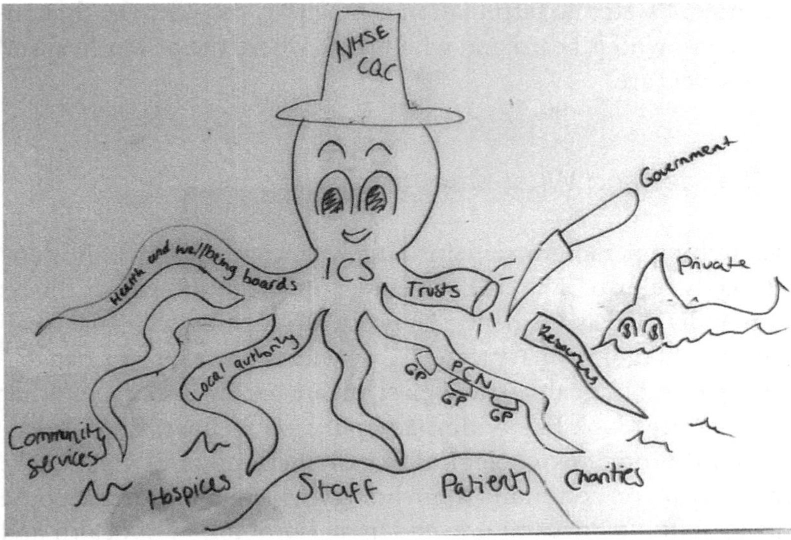

Figure 6.1 The Octopus.

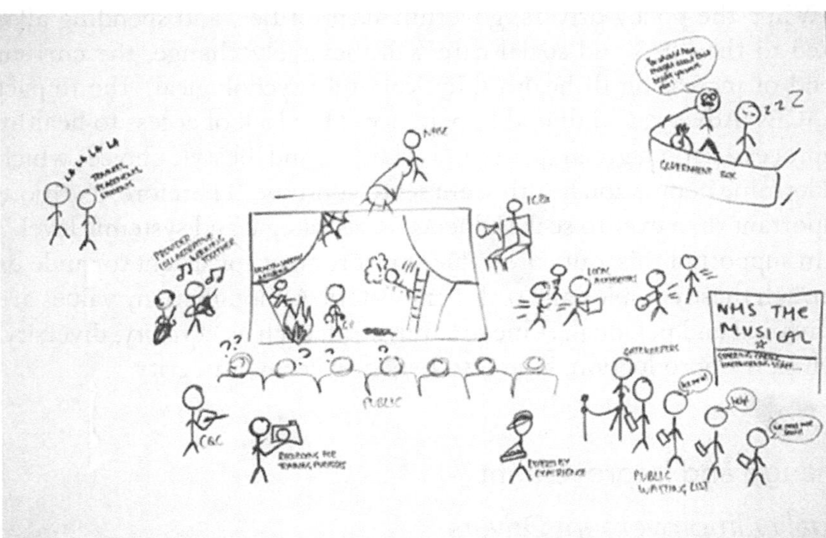

Figure 6.2 NHS The Musical.

threats of government action and the private sector conceived as a predator. "NHS The Musical" depicts chaotic illustrations of disconnected endeavour, with service users waiting in line, only able to observe, and contradictory drivers undermining the "performance".

Generating a systemic formulation can help us consider the dynamics of a system, who is heard and who is not, where the power lies, and where the levers are.

What Changes and What Stays the Same?

The overarching paradigm remains largely unchanged, though many agree it needs reform. The NHS operates under an individual illness paradigm: individual assessment, diagnosis/formulation, care and treatment and discharge. Primary care GP services, however, do not discharge people. Public health bodies exist but are poorly resourced. What could our services look like within a population wellness and wellbeing paradigm? From a psychological practitioner's point of view, there is a rich literature on community psychology which, if resourced, could allow us to shift our focus to prevention and promotion of health and wellbeing, in partnership with, and tailored to the needs and aspirations of, our communities.

While the policy drivers, government priorities, and spending allocated to the NHS and social care will inevitably change, the current trend of increasing ill health (physical and psychological); the impact of ACEs (Adverse Childhood Experiences); the lack of access to healthy unprocessed food, green spaces and clean air; and lifestyle choices which undermine population health seem set to continue. Therefore, it is more important than ever to seek influence at a strategic and systemic level.

In support of this, our core values must remain consistent to guide us through these complex and turbulent waters. Although many values are individual and personal, some are universal, such as equality, diversity, inclusion, coproduction, kindness, beneficence and integrity.

Change and Improvement

Quality Improvement Drivers

The evidence for the effectiveness of a wide range of psychological interventions and therapies is set out in NICE (National Institute for Health and Clinical Excellence) guidance and in the Matrix (NHS Education for Scotland, 2023). Professional body publications can bring wider perspectives, particularly in co-production with people with lived experience. For example, compare NICE guidance for Depression in Adults (2022) with the BPS Division of Clinical Psychology's *Understanding Depression* (2020).

Where there is also a policy driver such as the *Community Mental Health Framework for Adults and Older Adults* (National Collaborating Centre for Mental Health, 2019), which sets out the imperative of increasing access to evidence-based psychological interventions, there is a very strong argument to be made that a suitably trained, clinically supervised and professionally led workforce is required to deliver this. But to whom should this argument be made? This depends on where the decisions regarding this will be taken, which could be at the system commissioning level or place-based commissioning, but is likely to be a decision taken by the provider organisation itself. Hence the importance of understanding how the internal system operates, and whether a more strategic argument or a business case would be more effective.

Where there is a Chief Officer or equivalent role for psychological professions, there is not only a crucial influence at the national level but also the opportunity to develop policy, workforce and quality improvement guidance from the perspective of our professions. A good example is the Psychological Professions Network *National Vision for the Psychological Professions* (2021).

Quality drivers may also be found in relevant changes to legislation, such as the reforms to the UK Mental Health Act of 2007, which extended the role of Approved Clinician/Responsible Clinician to a wider range of registered professionals, including Clinical Psychologists, Nurses, Occupational Therapists and Social Workers. I have co-led a regional project aimed at increasing understanding and implementation of these roles (see CNTW NHS FT, accessed 30.5.25).

Performance Management, Regulation and Inspection

These are all drivers for change and hopefully improvement, though they can also have paradoxical impacts.

In England, health and social care services must register with the Care Quality Commission (CQC), which can inspect them at any time. The CQC sets standards across five domains: safety, effectiveness, caring, responsiveness and leadership (CQC, 2022). Services receive ratings within each domain and overall. Even "outstanding" services may receive "should do" or "must do" improvement actions, with the latter subject to ongoing review. The CQC also has the power to close a service or provider. Given all this, it is unsurprising that the prospect of

CQC inspection is a powerful driver, in addition to the actual ratings provided and the actions required of health and social care organisations. Practitioner psychologists may lead CQC improvement actions, helping overcome practical or cultural barriers—for example, in clinical supervision. The Health and Safety Executive (HSE), with broader regulatory powers than the CQC, may sometimes mandate changes that conflict with CQC expectations. While the CQC focuses on service user safety, outcomes, and experience, the HSE prioritises environmental safety and staff wellbeing.

In England, NHSE performance management is a key driver. NHS Talking Therapies data on access, waits, and outcomes are reported monthly, with underperformance triggering "deep dive" reviews. Commissioners monitor performance and may tender contracts, though recent years have seen a shift from competition to collaboration.

Accreditation schemes set standards and help drive quality and safety improvements. For example, APPTS (Accreditation of Psychological Therapies Services), a BPS and RCPsych partnership I co-founded and co-chaired, developed standards aligned with CQC domains (Jethwa, 2024). These have supported service improvement and showcased good practice across the UK (Rosario et al., 2024).

Policy drivers can enable change, but without mechanisms for outcome reporting or accountability, the impact is limited. The community mental health transformation framework for adults and older adults (National Collaborating Centre for Mental Health, 2019) metrics include access to a tightly defined set of evidence-based psychological therapies/interventions and require outcome measures to be used and reported. Data provided back to providers and commissioners highlight the scale of the problem. Average data for England in March 2024 showed that only 1.47% of adults and older adults with complex mental health problems in mainstream community mental health services (excluding early intervention in psychosis services) were accessing an evidence-based psychological therapy. By March 2025, this had only increased to 1.87% despite the above drivers. Despite decades of evidence supporting the effectiveness of psychological interventions, it is the above policy driver and the availability of provider trust-level, regional, and national data that have enabled me, in a Trust leadership role, to gain traction for community workforce development to increase provision for people with complex mental health needs.

Commissioning models continue to evolve in England. Integrating Care (NHS England, 2020) introduced Provider Collaboratives. For those working in these areas, decision-making may be more accessible to practitioner psychologists than the ICS/ICB structures. It may also be possible to influence the ways in which decisions are reached and the underpinning principles (e.g. trauma-informed care).

Anchor institutions have system-wide responsibilities, offering opportunities for influence and innovation. Practitioner psychologists often work in or with these institutions, such as NHS provider trusts, Health Boards, Local Authorities, and Universities. Public Health Scotland (2025) and Maguire (2021) outline the NHS's role as an anchor institution.

Data and Service Improvement/Redesign Methodology

Data can drive quality improvement, but it is not always accurate, meaningful, or well used. Where essential data is missing, we must explain its importance for addressing quality or safety concerns. Evidence-based redesign methods (e.g. Six Sigma, Lean) offer Practitioner Psychologists opportunities to lead impactful change, using psychological skills—such as engagement, problem definition, negotiation, and facilitation—in combination with these models.

The voice of experts by experience should be embedded across all of the above. In my national roles with the BPS, I have sought to promote coproduction by jointly highlighting the principles and benefits with experts by experience (e.g. Hemmingfield & Cohen-Tovée, 2018) and co-developing a governance framework. Over time, we would hope to see full coproduction and expert-by-experience-led research, service improvement and policy become the standard rather than the rarity. *People Power: lessons from the health care response to the Grenfell Tower fire* (Wellings, Ross & Chikwira, 2024) is an example of lived experience voices driving change and improvement.

The Wider Role of Psychological Practitioners

In addition to making use of the existing quality improvement drivers, Practitioner Psychologists can make a valuable contribution to the drivers themselves. This can include the generation of evidence through research and service evaluation (evidence-based practice and practice-based evidence), and/or participating in the review of evidence, e.g. for NICE. Professional bodies such as the BPS generate guidance to which members can contribute or on which they may take a lead. There is often an opportunity across provider organisations, members of professional bodies and the public to contribute to the shaping of policy drivers such as the NHS Long Term Plans. Practitioner Psychologists working in a relevant field can apply to become CQC reviewers and can contribute to the development of CQC standards, processes and methods. They can also contribute to the review and revision of HCPC standards. In England, the Provider Collaboratives have established Clinical Director posts which are open to Psychological Practitioners, enabling them to take on broader commissioning and clinical leadership roles.

Psychological Services-Specific Developments and Drivers

Practitioner Psychologists and the wider psychological professions in health and social care can instigate and develop psychological initiatives that benefit the communities we serve. Examples include the NHS Talking Therapies programme, innovations such as Virtual Reality interventions, psychologists taking up the Approved Clinician role, and leading on staff wellbeing during the Covid-19 pandemic. Trauma-informed approaches and community psychology could radically improve population wellbeing.

In summary, there is a wide variety of opportunities for change and improvement in the health and social care system, including the opportunity to shape the drivers themselves. However, although these drivers may be levers for change, the levers that influence decision-makers may be different, e.g., reputational and financial considerations. The most effective approach is to understand the relationship between these drivers and the system in which one is working, as well as the opportunities to build relationships and influence decision-making. The key may be in enabling the voice of experts by experience to be heard, the power of data to benchmark performance and highlight risk, and the role of regulatory bodies in holding to account.

Looking Ahead

Horizon Scanning

Today's horizon scanning is tomorrow's old news, but horizon scanning is a very helpful adjunct to everything in the preceding section, and some might say this should have been the first consideration. In the context of the health and social care system there are some important places to look for the priorities, developments and changes that are in the offing. For example, a government-commissioned review such as that of Darzi (2024), which sets out a well-informed agenda for change. External reviews of high-profile serious incidents and investigations can be drivers for change even when the failings uncovered represent well-known issues. New paradigms from the psychological literature can be proposed and piloted, making use of the innovation curve (Rogers, 2003) and an understanding of the local system levers and decision-making hierarchies.

Working with These Systems

As practitioner psychologists, we can often identify what seem to be obvious areas for change and improvement. But is the system ready for these changes? In instances where change is strongly resisted, it may be helpful to use the Prochaska and DiClemente (1983) model of change as a "diagnostic" tool to help direct our efforts. Is the problem we have identified not recognised as a problem at all (pre-contemplation)? Are some stakeholders considering the need for change (contemplation)? Have previous efforts to make a change/implement something new failed (relapse)?

If motivation among decision-makers is difficult to develop, a more fruitful approach may be to seek to support them with issues they do want to address.

For example:

- What do Executive and Non-Executive Directors see as the key problems?
- What's on the organisation's risk register?
- What are the strategic priorities or ambitions?
- What is the system's/organisation's risk appetite?
- Review the Joint Strategic Needs Assessment.
- Review information on the NHS Futures website and how your organisation compares with others.

It is also important to communicate our specialist abilities for driving change clearly, such as:

- Formulation of an organisation's problems using psychological models
- Promoting trauma-informed service improvement with users and carers
- Helping others reflect to deepen insight and improve solutions
- Supporting staff wellbeing through reflective practice, clinical supervision, and therapy
- Providing organisational feedback ("holding up a mirror")
- Collective, collaborative and compassionate leadership

Conclusion

The UK Health and Social Care systems are part of a complex organisational environment that is in continual flux, and which can change rapidly due to changes in the prevailing political context, financial considerations and evolution of evidence and ethos. This can feel destabilising and difficult to navigate. Understanding the functions and purposes of different components of the system, and developing a systemic understanding of how these inter-relate, helps to make sense of organisational structures and priorities, and where they can be influenced. An awareness of the drivers for quality improvement in the present and anticipating future priorities and innovations can provide a wide range of opportunities; however, the focus and timing of our efforts need to be informed by the cycles of change, risks, finance and the organisational state of motivation for change.

There will always be change, and the need to adapt to challenges and setbacks, as well as to seek new opportunities, but we can remain grounded in our values and principles.

Practitioner Psychologists can, and should, take opportunities to lead and influence using our distinctive skills, in partnership with multidisciplinary colleagues, system partners, service users and carers.

Ideas in Brief

- Grounding ourselves in what does not change—our values, principles and professional expertise—helps us navigate a system in constant change
- Change is cyclical; recognising the patterns helps us manage challenges and setbacks, and find new opportunities
- Psychologists' skills in formulation and understanding motivation for change can be usefully applied in the NHS and social care systems
- Quality and safety drivers can provide a wide range of opportunities to instigate and lead productive change and improvement

References

Baker, L. (2024). *Can we make direct comparisons between the NHS in England and Wales?* NHS Confederation.

British Psychological Society. (2023). *Learning from NHS staff wellbeing hubs. Principles for staff mental health provision.* https://tinyurl.com/yt8kxs7m

Care Quality Commission. (2022). *Our new single assessment framework.* Care Quality Commission.

CNTW NHS FT. *Multi-professional Approved Clinician (MPAC) Project.* Retrieved 31, 2025, from from Cumbria, Northumberland, Tyne and Wear NHS Foundation Trust.

Dalton, D. (2014). *Examining new options and opportunities for providers of NHS care.* UK Government. The Dalton Review (publishing.service.gov.uk).

Darzi, A. (2024). *Independent investigation of the NHS in England.* UK Government.

Division of Clinical Psychology. (2020). *Understanding depression. Why adults experience depression and what can help.* British Psychological Society.

Gateshead Council and CNTW NHS FT. (2024). *Integrated trauma informed care in Gateshead children's social care.* https://gateshead.moderngov.co.uk/documents/s40026/Item%206%20-%20THG%20Annual%20Report%202023-24%20final.pdf

Hemmingfield, J., & Cohen-Tovée, E. (2018, January 17–18). *Are we all together? How far have we travelled towards co-production with Experts by Experience in the DCP and the profession?* Paper Presentation, Division of Clinical Psychology Annual Conference, Cardiff. British Psychological Society.

Jethwa, J. (Ed.). (2024). *Quality standards for psychological therapies services* (6th ed.). Accreditation Programme for Psychological Therapies Services: Royal College of Psychiatrists and British Psychological Society.

Maguire, D. (2021). *Anchor institutions and how they can affect peoples' health*. The King's Fund.

National Collaborating Centre for Mental Health. (2019). *The community mental health framework for adults and older adults*. NHS England and NHS Improvement.

National Institute for Health and Care Excellence. (2022). *Depression in adults: Treatment and management*. https://www.nice.org.uk/guidance/ng222

NHS Education for Scotland. (2023). *Matrix – A guide to delivering evidence-based psychological therapies in Scotland*. NHS Education for Scotland.

NHS England. (2020). *Integrating care: Next steps to building strong and effective integrated care systems across England*. NHS England.

Prochaska, J. O., & DiClemente, C. C. (1983). Stages and processes of self-change of smoking: Toward an integrative model of change. *Journal of Consulting and Clinical Psychology, 51*(3), 390–395.

Psychological Professions Network. (2021). *National vision for psychological professions*. NHS Briefing template.

Public Health Scotland. (2025). *Community wealth building and anchor institutions*. Overview – Anchor institutions – Economy and poverty – Social and economic impacts on health – Population health – Public Health Scotland.

Rogers, E. (2003). *Diffusion of innovations* (5th ed.). Free Press.

Rosairo, M., Bean, M., Shepherd, M., Lucas-Motley, H., Farquharson, L., Thornton, G., & Cohen-Tovée, E. (2024). APPTS (Accreditation Programme for Psychological Therapies Services) – A quality improvement programme for psychological therapies services, bringing benefits to service users, services and the wider system. *Clinical Psychology Forum*, 372, 20–27. British Psychological Society.

Wellings, D., Ross, S., & Chikwira, L. (2024). *People power; Lessons from the health care response to the Grenfell Tower fire*. The King's Fund.

7 Strategic Leadership

Translating Vision into Reality

Dr Lynne Taylor

When working in large systems and organisations like Health and Social Care or Government, implementing positive change can be challenging due to organisational systemic dynamics and complex operational structures. Data and evidence that support the case for change are helpful, but that alone does not necessarily result in change. Human factors such as our motives, fears and beliefs also influence how we engage in change processes (Sharot T., 2017). Having a strategic vision is key. The most effective vision is one that takes account of the interests of stakeholders, is adaptable, and meets identified needs by facilitating innovations and decision-making.

Vision alone will also not get results. Translating a vision into action requires a set of fundamental strategic leadership skills. Leaders need to inspire others to own and share in that same vision. It requires leaders to engage with others on an emotional level, provide the evidence, and use skills of influence to help others commit to a course of action. A good leader acknowledges that inspiring others is not a solo undertaking. It requires a vision to be widely shared and viewed as adding value to overall organisational aims. It should inspire confidence, provide direction, motivate others, and align efforts for a shared endeavour to make a difference to the people it aims to help. This is only possible through collective endeavour and jointly agreed priorities.

A core responsibility of the Principal Psychology Officer in the Scottish Government is advising, providing leadership, facilitating, and supporting change linked to policy objectives and improved clinical delivery. As stated in an interview with the British Psychological Society in 2025 the

DOI: 10.4324/9781003492399-10

role it is "about harnessing ideas and aspirations and thinking about how you make that tangible. I occupy that space in the middle between government and clinical systems, and advise, facilitate and influence to initiate change, where possible, in that space". Like any leader, this requires harnessing ideas and aspirations that are tangible through action, strategy, and collaboration. This chapter provides examples of strategic leadership by describing how a vision for a Scottish Government national specification for the delivery of psychological therapies and interventions was turned into reality by using skills of strategic leadership.

The Unique Skills of Applied Psychologists as Leaders

Psychologists have the unique skills to be effective strategic leaders, as the core training of any applied psychologist is about how to influence and change systems to help improve the lives of others. Applied psychologists intuitively understand relationships and systems. As stated by Lavander and Hope (2007, p. 41) psychologists, "by virtue of their training, competencies and experience, can lead and teams". They are also scientist-practitioners who can use data to support improvement. Applied psychologists are doing what they are trained to do – help others see a vision for positive change through our relationships with them (Taylor, 2023). This skill set to influence change can be just as effectively applied in systemic work environments as well as in people's personal lives.

Managers are also an important part of any organisation, but there is a fundamental difference between a manager and a leader. The most cited definition is from John Kotter (1996) who described how management helps systems function, whereas leadership roles are about building systems or transforming old ones. This is also further outlined in an article by the Kinds fund by Allen (2020) who shared that leadership skills involve establishing direction, aligning people, motivating, and inspiring others. There will always be a place for leadership and management at all levels, as health and social care systems cannot function without this.

There is also a subtle difference between leaders and strategic leadership. Strategic thinking can be defined as the process that determines the way people consider, assess, view, and create a vision for the future for others. Strategic planning is about identifying future opportunities, anticipating challenges, and creating a path to achieve both desired outcomes. High-quality, accountable collaborative strategic leadership should be linked to comprehensive planning, be adaptable, needs-led, and data-driven. As stated in a blog article by IMD business school (2025) "strategic leadership is the ability to guide an organisation toward long-term success while focusing on short-term goals. It involves setting a vision, making decisions that align with the organisation's objectives, and ensuring adaptability in an ever-changing environment". Leadership can also be challenging and isolating as leaders can become public figures where people project things, and leaders can be burdened by unrealistic expectations (Hulk, 2020).

Strategic leadership requires an ability to see the bigger picture, a mandate and support for change, adaptability, confidence in the face of competing views, and strong stakeholder relationships. Strategic leaders therefore need to be visionaries, have an approach of curiosity, practise accountability, create transparency, be innovative in uncertain situations, balance objectives with realistic outcomes, and always listen to feedback. The most common factor in strategic leadership is the need to inspire and build confidence in others and develop a culture that fosters change aligned to the values of the organisation and long-term goals. Leadership clarity is also crucial as it is associated with better outcomes and support for innovation (West et al., 2003). Strong strategic leadership can help others to engage collectively and courageously in a vision that is value and evidence-based, adaptable, emotionally understood, and people-focused (Bailey & West, 2022).

Every Change Starts with a Vision – Nothing Changes If Nothing Changes

A vision for change does not necessarily have to be bold or revolutionary. A vision is usually something that has not been accomplished, helps staff and stakeholders align, supports decision-making, and helps services manage inevitable challenges. It needs to be ambitious but also achievable. A vision can be about any possibility that can become a reality.

A strategic vision can often be more complex as it needs to align with the systems and structures of large organisations, whilst holding a common understanding of the aims they want to achieve and how. This is different from business planning, which focuses on short-term goals. Strategic planning is about achieving longer-term visions for systems to work towards. They help motivate systems to make positive differences to the people they aim to help. Developing a strategic vision into strategy is a core aspect of work within government.

In Scotland, the recently published Mental Health and Wellbeing Strategy (2023) sets out the strategic vision of a Scotland which recognises that it is essential that the services and support that people need should be built around clear national frameworks and high-quality evidence-based care to improve outcomes. This strategy, together with the identified gap in describing outcomes for people and services, helped support the emerging vision that the quality of delivery of services should be described to help improve the outcomes and experiences for the people of Scotland. As stated in the joint foreword by Ms Todd (Former Minister for Social Care, Mental Wellbeing and Sport) and Councillor Paul Kelly (COSLA Spokesperson for Health and Social Care), "we acknowledge that all areas of Government will need to work together to achieve our shared vision and to make progress towards our outcomes….we want this strategy to serve as a blueprint for what a high-functioning whole mental health system looks like".

Hitting the Target and Not Missing the Point

Targets and strategy are common aspects of service delivery and government objectives. Having a strategic vision and working with targets and the boundaries of published policy can present challenges. Targets often divide opinion, but they are a reality of many public sector environments. Equality and access matter in public services. When targets do not function well, they can pull services in different directions, provide the wrong incentives, and operate as a blunt tool. However, when they work well, they help focus resources and time to deliver key priorities; they can act as performance indicators, grow the workforce, promote accountability, and increase access. It is often said that what gets measured gets done, but the flip side is also true. It is therefore important that any target does not cause any unintended unhelpful consequences. Although the benefits and challenges of targets continue to generate debate, targets do serve an important function in public sector environments – especially when they both hit the target and do not miss the point.

One such target is the revised waiting times standard published by Public Health Scotland (2023) which clearly sets out the number of people who are being seen for psychological treatment within 18 weeks of a referral. There is also an important national framework developed and regularly updated by NHS Education for Scotland (NES), which sets out best practice in relation to the delivery of evidence-based psychological treatments (The Matrix, 2023). However, there was no national framework regarding what people should expect in relation to the quality of care they receive when accessing psychological treatments, or how services are expected to deliver these high-quality services. Engagement with stakeholders, policy officials, and those with lived experience indicated that a quality framework that supports effective psychological service delivery would be helpful. Further engagement with senior leaders, policy officials, and Ministers, therefore, agreed that this vision should be delivered, which provided a clear mandate to develop this strategic work.

The key overall aim of this strategic vision was that **irrespective of age or ability, people should be entitled to access high-quality psychological treatments that meet their needs**. Gilian Paton, the **Senior Policy Officer** for psychological therapies in the Scottish Government at that time, set out how her policy role supported the development of the specification:

> *I worked with the national psychology officer, other policy officials, and key partners to develop the new National Specification setting out clear expectations for what services will look like as they provide high-quality care. My role was to work with partners across government and within operational delivery, as well as those with lived experience to gather their important contributions together, working towards the same vision of setting outcomes that would improve equity and quality of psychological therapies. My policy role was important in setting the direction of the consultation prior to publication and the narrative around expectations on delivery of the Specification outcomes post publication. This was done collaboratively by working closely with services, senior civil servants, the Minister, and the national advisor to ensure successful implementation and improved access and quality of psychological services for all.*

Linking Vision to Goals

Having goals linked to a strategic vision and a mandate increases clarity and focus. It allows systems and teams to identify what matters and how they can use their time well. Decision-making is also easier when people have shared achievable goals and know the direction of travel. It can also enhance motivation, as any accomplished goal, no matter how small, supports a sense of achievement. The SMART objectives framework (2011) from the Chartered Management Institute was used to help drive the vision for a specification:

- **Specific:** small defined goals were set out nationally which were linked to the vision of stakeholders, policy officials and Ministers.
- **Measurable:** ways to track progress were agreed upon with internal policy teams and Board-wide Directors and Leads of Psychology.
- **Achievable:** realistic and attainable goals were agreed upon, which were challenging and ambitious yet possible.
- **Relevant:** tasks were aligned with larger relevant objectives of improved delivery of psychological services, which supported the value of the task.
- **Time-bound:** clear deadlines that motivated action while explaining extensions required to policy officials and Ministers were adaptable.

In government, any goals for change need to be aligned with wider policy objectives and stakeholders' broader objectives. This was set within the Scottish context of effective policy making as set out by Cairney (2020) where there should be an outcomes-based measure of policy success that is linked to greater local authority discretion in the delivery of national objectives. It notes that governance principles should be built on localism and the further inclusion of service users in the design of public policy. This alignment ensures that the product being developed not only solves a real problem for the public but also does have unintended negative consequences.

Underlying any policy development or change linked to a vision needs to consider the important question of what positive impact it can it make. Developing staffing and improving workplace culture are important for the success of any longer-term strategic aims. As set out by Ms Todd (Former Minister for Social Care, Mental Wellbeing and Sport) in the foreword of the Specification, "we acknowledge that the workforce plays a crucial part in how we provide, safe, effective, timely, trauma informed, and compassionate based service delivery.. . we also recognise that some of these outcomes may take longer for services to fully deliver in the face on ongoing systems pressures."

Systems pressures and work cultures are a crucial ingredient to the success of any strategic vision. We know that employees who are satisfied with their work environment and feel their wellbeing is supported are more productive and effective than those who aren't. This is especially true in health and social care where staff want to make a difference in the lives of those they serve. A gap in strategy and delivery is often impacted by culture and resources – and ultimately any effective strategic vision and leadership should seek to reduce this gap and ensure good line management is in place. An additional aim of the specification was therefore to set out nationally what good looks like for local resources, governance, and leadership.

Effective Collaboration and Communication

Turning a strategic vision into reality is not a solo endeavour. It requires buy-in from key stakeholders across all organisations. A vision is something that cannot be accomplished without enrolling others to participate in achieving shared goals. As indicated by Haslam et al. (2020) leadership is not just about leaders; it is also about followers who develop a shared sense of social identity to achieve shared aims. There were therefore three key aspects that were crucial to aiding the shared aims of the specification:

1. **Communication and engagement through local and national meetings, networking, and online communications:** The vision was shared widely with all stakeholders (including those with lived experience) to explain how it aligned with their hopes and objectives.
2. **Gathering feedback and views through national consensus meetings, surveys, and local engagement:** Regular stakeholder feedback provided valuable insights and helped refine content and shape the key areas of focus.
3. **Building consensus and agreements through a process of redrafting and engagement:** This ensured that everyone involved understood their role in bringing the specification to life and was aligned with the overall national strategy.

Repeated engagement during the development of the specification was crucial and can be seen as in Figure 7.1.

This process took an approach of constant collaboration, refinement, evaluation, curiosity, redrafting, and analysis to ensure the vision and content were relevant, achievable, and ambitious enough to make a difference to the people of Scotland. This also helped the Scottish Government be aware of any risks, how to mitigate these, and how to

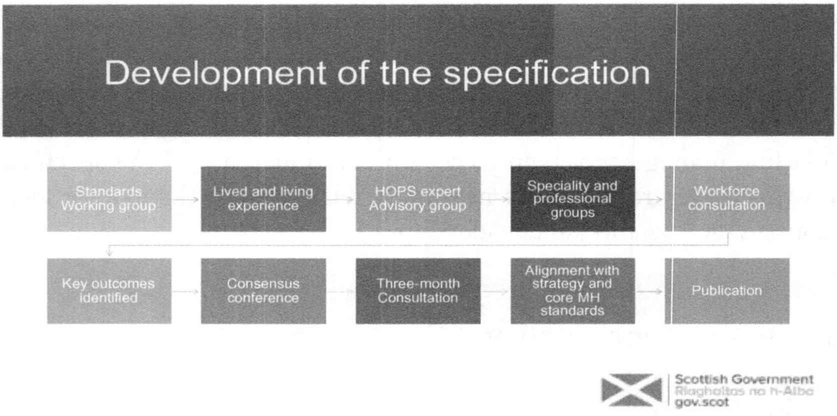

Figure 7.1 Engagement process for development of the specification.

enhance deliverable outcomes for the people it aims to help. Dr Caroline Cochrane, a **Chair of Heads of Psychology Services Scotland (HOPS),** shares how engagement with HOPS supported the development of the specification:

> *We have valued working closely with the Principal Psychology Officer and policy colleagues in the Mental Health Directorate as well as people with lived experience in contributing to the development of the specification. We are closely connected with all speciality groups and applied psychologists working in health and social care in Scotland, who also value the strategic intent and clarity this document brings. Psychological therapy plays an increasingly significant part in mental health treatment as well as being valued and evidence based in wider settings including for those who have long term conditions. This specification will ensure delivery of evidence based psychological treatments are safe, well governed, and accessible.*

Vision to Action – Milestones, Data, and Project Plans

Any big strategic idea needs to be evidenced, and the end product is not the end of the task. Implementation is as much a part of a vision as the product itself. The process of defining realistic timelines for milestones allows for flexibility but ensures that progress is made. The cornerstone of any work should be embedded in an assurance process where strategic objectives and risks are monitored. As any strategy or policy product moves forward, it is important to adjust and iterate based on feedback, changes, and new insights so it aligns with clear outcomes. This supports improved curious decision-making, risk management, and successful implementation.

Project management is a tool leaders can use to help execute, manage, track, and measure against an overall change aim. In Government, there are often various strategic objectives for different purposes, and alignment of shared goals helps mitigate risks, supports delivery, and supports clear accountable leadership. As stated in the Programme and Project Mandate Principles (2022) *a*lignment is crucial in making strategy happen – recognising that projects and programmes are tightly aligned to strategic objectives in order to ensure the delivery of strategy from every level. This Scottish Government guidance document sets out the key principles that are key to success with project delivery in policy (see Figure 7.2).

These principles set out how strategy (e.g. justification, alignment), process (e.g. benefits, risks), and people (e.g. roles, responsibilities) help to guide deliverable programmes of work. The aims of a proportionate approach are described within what is called a maturity matrix. The

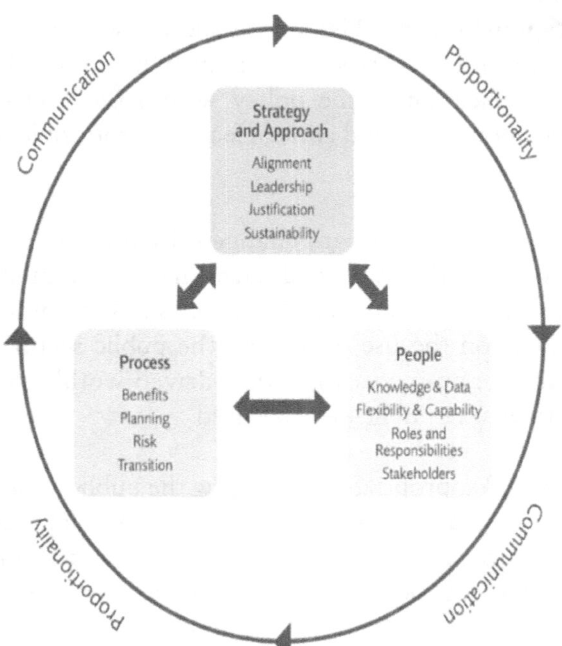

Figure 7.2 Strategy, people, and process factors that support programme management.

development and delivery of the specification were considered within this framework by taking an agile and adaptable approach.

Any vision, even with the best-laid project plan, can face unexpected challenges. Leading a national strategic vision requires skills of curious refinement, determination, strategic planning, and negotiation. It also requires leaders to take stakeholders with them on the change journey. Strategic leadership and agility were therefore crucial to reaching publication and implementation by considering the following programme principles:

- **Testing and adaptation:** An iterative approach to development, engagement, testing, and refining was used. The flexible adaptations combined the knowledge and capability to meet future and current challenges. This required clear communication, effective decision-making, negotiation, evidence, and problem-solving.
- **Keep the vision as the focus:** A balance was required between challenging the status quo, encouraging creative thinking, and pivoting where needed based on evidence. This required an approach of determination to focus on the core business case, and holding the strategic vision in mind.
- **Clear roles and responsibilities:** The key to success was to have the right people in the right roles with responsibilities for delivery – both for the publication of the policy within the Scottish Government and the operational and clinical leaders responsible for local implementation.

Another way to measure and drive forward change is by using reliable data. Data needs to be of good quality, avoid harm, have accountability, clarity of purpose, and public benefits. The Scottish Government published guidance in 2024 on the use of data by the public sector in Scotland, which states that in an increasingly data-driven world, good governance is required to ensure public data are used

> effectively, ethically and appropriately. Engaging the public – those whose data is used in research, planning and service development and delivery – helps to develop trustworthy and robust frameworks for how government and other agencies collect, analyse and use data.

Data is essential to governance and delivery within the public sector. Data can drive continuous improvement, support project plans, and enhance performance to support better outcomes. As with all elements of strategic change, data alone does not dictate improvement decisions, but once interpreted and analysed, it should inform actions. Data-driven approaches also support effective frameworks for action planning, setting progress, feedback, and review mechanisms. Using data to inform strategic aims drives forward innovation and strategic planning. Sarah Martin (**Unit Head for Data in the Mental Health Directorate in the Scottish Government**) shares why she feels the use of data is important:

> *Continuous monitoring and measurement is fundamental to achieving the best impact from public policy and to ensuring public spending delivers the intended outcomes. The fact is that we value what we measure, so we must measure what we value most and search beyond data that happens to be readily available. Converting information into data is not always easy or cost-neutral in practice. It requires resources and effort to robustly capture and use key knowledge around delivery and to look beyond appointment information to routinely collate what matters most in services: patient outcomes, staff wellbeing, views of patients with particular vulnerability, to name a few. And yet it is worth doing, as it is collecting this evidence that in turn creates a focus and drives improvement and sustainability.*

Hearing the Views of Those That Matter Most

There is little point in having a strategic vision that is not meaningful for those it is intended to help. Involving those with lived and living experience is therefore continuously required. Any leadership within health and social care should always review and consider if the vision and product produced will meet the needs of the people we are here to serve and help. Listening to the voices of those with lived and living experience, and their carers, is crucial. Any strategic vision should therefore be fit for purpose; otherwise, what is the point?

This can require an approach of constant evaluation and improvement. The term improvement is used in health and social care to refer broadly to any change which leads to an improvement in outcomes relative to historical norms. Quality Improvement (QI) is a tool defined in 2021 by the Health Foundation as giving the people closest to issues affecting care quality the time, permission, skills, and resources they need to solve them. To achieve meaningful change, it is critical to cascade best practice and making shared goals linked to the strategic plan and overall objectives. Staff working at all levels within the organisation can have really valuable insights and views. QI is therefore an approach that can help leaders manage to implement strategic change by listening to both experts by experience and experts by profession.

Strategic leaders should be inspired, motivated, and challenged by others' views and insights. Good leadership takes account of human factors in change processes, evidence, data, curiosity, refinement, and bold innovation. To turn any strategic vision into reality, therefore, requires strategic leadership skills of self-awareness, good communication, the capacity to see the bigger picture, regular engagement, adaptability, courageous decision-making, and situational awareness. Strategic leadership is often most successful when there is a humble, kind, and compassionate approach taken both with those who access services and those who work within them.

Conclusion

This chapter has described the strategic approaches used when working with Scottish Government, key clinical stakeholders, and those with lived and living experience, to turn a vision for a national specification for psychological delivery into reality. This vision was turned into reality through strategic drivers and was kept constantly informed and reviewed by key stakeholders – both by profession and experience. Strategic leadership requires skills to develop a clear vision for the future by building a shared culture that supports growth. Any change required should be collectively seen as a helpful endeavour and linked to clear objectives that will help influence positive deliverable change. These skills are inherent in training to become applied psychologists and can be harnessed to support change in organisational systems with the aim of helping the public achieve the outcomes they need and deserve.

Ideas in Brief

- **Bridge policy and practice**: Translate strategic vision into deliverable outcomes through stakeholder collaboration, quality improvement, and meaningful data use.
- **Lead with influence and purpose**: Use strategic leadership skills, including project planning, engagement, and evidence-based action – to drive organisational change.

- **Harness psychologists' expertise**: Applied psychologists bring unique strengths to strategic roles, offering system-level insight, relational leadership, and clarity of vision.
- **Centre lived experience**: Embed stakeholder and service-user voices to co-create policies that are informed, inclusive, and effective in real-world contexts.

References

Allen, S. (2020). *Creating space for compassion, empathy and learning.* King's Fund.

Bailey, B., & West, M. (2022). *Tired of being exhausted: Seven key actions for leaders In the NHS workforce crisis.* Kings Fund.

British Psychological Society. (2025, March 5). *Psychology matters. Influencing at the heart of government.* BPS.

Cairney, P. (2020). The 'Scottish approach' to policymaking. In M. Keating (Ed.), *Oxford handbook of Scottish politics* (pp. 369–386). Oxford University Press

Chartered Management Institute. (2011). *Setting smart goals checklist.* Chartered Management Institute.

Haslam, A., Reicher, S., & Platow, M. (2020). *The new psychology of leadership: Identify, influence and power.* Routledge

Hulk, S. (2020). *Heroic leadership: The order of the day?* The King's Fund.

Sharot, T. (2017). The influential mind: What the brain reveals about our power to change others. Henry Holt and Company.

IMD Business School. (2025, May). *Essential skills and approaches for strategic leadership.* Strategic Leadership: Essential Skills for Driving Long-Term Success.

Kotter, J. P. (1996). *Leading change.* Harvard Business School Press.

Lavender, T., & Hope, R. (2007). *New ways of working for applied psychologists in health and social care. Working Psychologically in Teams.* British Psychological Society.

Murray-Webster, R. (2020). *APM body of knowledge.* Association for Project Management.

Newitt, S. (2022, October). *How can managers and leaders support staff wellbeing In the NHS?* The King's Fund.

NHS Education for Scotland. (2023). *The Matrix: The guide to deliver evidence based psychological therapies and interventions in Scotland.* NHS Education for Scotland.

Public Health Scotland. (2023). *Psychological therapies and interventions waiting times standard definitions.* Public Health Scotland.

Scottish Government. (2022). *Programme and project mandate principles.* Programme and project management principles – gov.scot

Scottish Government. (2023). *Mental health and wellbeing strategy.* gov.scot

Scottish Government. (2023). *Psychological therapies and interventions specification.* gov.scot

Scottish Government. (2024). *Open data in Scotland: A blueprint for unlocking innovation, collaboration and impact.* gov.scot

Taylor, L. (2023). *No need for heroes. How can psychologists lead well.* British Psychological Society.

The Heath Foundation. (2021). *Quality improvement made simple.* The Health Foundation. www.health.org.uk/publications/quality-improvement-made-simple

West, M. A., Tjosvold, D., & Smith, K. G. (Eds.). (2003). *International handbook of organisational teamwork and co-operative working.* John Wiley & Sons, Ltd

Clinical Leadership within Systems **8**

Integrating Theory into Practice and Building Relationships to Enable Change

Dr Rachel Bradley and Dr Andrew Roberts

Psychologists as Leaders

The NHS Confederation (2023) describes clinical and care professional leadership as

> *'shaping health and care systems to ensure high-quality care for all'* and *'highlights the importance of the clinical voice at all levels of decision-making and the valuable contributions they make to improving our services'.*

Meanwhile, the Healthcare Leadership Model (NHS Leadership Academy, 2013) focuses on the leadership behaviours required for *'satisfied, loyal, productive and engaged employees'* resulting in *'high-quality, compassionate care, patient satisfaction and a successful and highly regarded service/organisation'.*

Clinical leadership can be exercised at a variety of levels, from the care of individual patients through working with teams, along clinical pathways, across organisations, and throughout regional systems, up to developing policy and strategy at a national level. However, it is crucial to identify the individuals/groups who are key to making the development successful – the 'stakeholders' (e.g. patients and carers/family, clinical, admin, and management staff within the team/organisation, and partners in the wider system) and to build effective working

DOI: 10.4324/9781003492399-11

relationships with them. The 'clinical' aspect of this type of leadership is rooted in the leader's own clinical practice experiences, combined with synthesising the best evidence with other qualitative factors, allowing psychologists to drive developments that can be demonstrably 'in the service of the patient'.

Psychologists are well placed to provide clinical leadership as their *'core psychological competencies and relationship expertise in engagement and collaboration can serve as valuable tools for effective leadership'* (Clinical Psychology Leadership Development Framework, British Psychological Society (BPS), 2010). However, the BPS (2021) also highlights that:

> *Particular challenges for psychologists in leadership roles are to embrace new work paradigms and roles, forge partnerships with stakeholders including experts by experience, address diversity gaps in the profession, take up non-traditional roles to influence, seek representation, build up cases for a sustainable workforce, assert professional autonomy, move beyond survival to thriving and adapt to an increasingly complex working environment.*

In practice, whilst some core clinical leadership skills may be part of psychologists' training, moving from a clinical focus to a clinical leadership focus is challenging and requires attention to the process of developing additional skills and experience.

Rao and Mason (2023) pose some helpful reflective questions:

- Reflecting upon your experience of leading and being led, what is leadership for you? What might hinder or foster leadership?
- What are your observations on being led by leaders?
- Do you consider leadership a solo task or one taken up in partnership with others?
- How is leadership influenced by the values we bring to work?
- What is your understanding of different types of leadership (e.g., strategic, professional, managerial, and clinical) and varied levels of authority in leadership roles?
- What are your thoughts on how power and authority are managed in leadership and followership roles?
- What key skills are required to adapt to the current leadership challenges?

More practically, NHS Improvement (2019) identify some 'key questions for leaders' and examples of tasks and support that may be helpful in this journey. The themes include how to help clinicians:

- build confidence in their ability to manage and lead
- gain leadership and management skills
- gain 'low-risk' leadership experience
- prepare as they take on new roles
- develop as leaders 'on the job'

Additionally, the BPS (2010) identifies how clinical, professional and strategic skills may be developed, held and utilised by trainee Clinical Psychologists through to Clinical Directors. From this, and our experience, examples of clinical leadership include:

- bringing a psychological perspective, advocating for patients, and being clear about the service offer in multi-agency meetings
- developing pathways to improve patient journeys
- leading audits and service improvement
- promoting co-production
- managing waiting lists and processes
- providing supervision and ensuring clinical governance
- supporting the development of clinical and reflective skills
- promoting evidence-based practice
- implementing broad approaches such as trauma-informed care
- addressing inequities in service provision
- developing best practice guidelines
- contributing to national policy and developments

The following sections explore how clinical leadership can improve patient care and services, engage and influence teams and systems, and translate policy and strategy into psychologically informed services. The intention is to bring together how psychologists might engage in clinical leadership with the kinds of tasks and challenges that may arise, illustrated through real-life examples.

Leadership in Direct Patient Care

Ensuring appropriate and high-quality care at an individual patient level is often the starting point for psychologists developing clinical leadership skills. Beyond this, balancing the needs of one patient with the wider patient population becomes increasingly important and requires the ability to set and flexibly adapt service boundaries. This involves a multitude of skills, and support from more experienced colleagues will be helpful.

Integrating perspectives

Development of an equitable diagnostic pathway, involving several community services, required a standardised approach. A senior Psychologist chaired the project (holding their own clear idea of 'best practice'). However, after several project meetings, the work became 'stuck', with no clear consensus or plan. Supervision and mentoring enabled the Psychologist to reflect on 'imposing' their views upon the process and disregarding the value of dissenting voices. Adopting a stance 'as though indifferent to the outcome' felt useful and enabled greater understanding of why standardising the process had been so difficult. The project progressed, developing shared perspectives and deliverable recommendations.

Reflections

- Leadership is not about imposing your own will or ideas.
- Reflective conversations with supervisors and mentors are invaluable.
- Including all colleagues in the process enabled progress.
- Adopting a 'stance' is an important skill.

To support teams in thinking about putting patients at the heart of service provision, Moullin (2002) developed '12 steps to a service culture'. These include deciding on your mission, values and vision, knowing your stakeholders, understanding the encounters that impact most on patients' perceptions of the service, learning from complaints, treating other staff well and recognising/rewarding service excellence, developing an improvement plan with performance standards and measures, and reflecting on progress and identifying next steps. Utilising this as a team can help to develop a shared purpose and support service development.

Developing the Offer

New team members had joined a psychological therapies team, bringing different therapeutic orientations, ways of working, and organisational experiences. The lead Psychologist wanted to develop the team identity, purpose, and ways of working to deliver improved patient experience.

For an extended meeting, the Psychologist developed questions from Moullin's 12 steps into write-on posters. Participants had 1 minute per poster to write ideas/suggestions before moving on. This was an efficient way of capturing different perspectives. Focused discussion of these ideas enabled the development of an improvement plan – team members also reported improved team cohesion.

Reflections

- The timing worked – with team members sufficiently integrated to understand current service provision but with enough 'newness' to challenge it.
- This approach provided more energy and interest than group discussion, aiding action planning.

Leading and Influencing to Transform and Develop Teams

Improving services for patients also requires work to improve team functioning. Drawing on formulation and therapy skills, psychologists are well placed to support teams in developing positive working relationships and becoming more integrated. This includes addressing conflict or 'splitting' – when two or more parts of the team have opposing views and struggle to come together and co-operate. Conflict can occur in relation to tasks, processes or relationships (NHS England and NHS Improvement, 2019) but often these are interconnected. Attending to the people involved and building relationships is more effective than focusing on the situation in isolation – 'coming alongside' can work better than trying to implement top-down ideas

Developing formulations and improving the patient journey

An assessment team (staffed and led by nurses, social workers, etc.) operated alongside a psychological therapies (PT) team (staffed and led by Psychological Professionals (PPs)). Waits for therapy were around 12 months, negatively affecting both patients, and the assessment team's workload/throughput. Staff morale deteriorated, and a split occurred between teams.

The PT lead Psychologist suggested that PT staff involvement in the assessment care plan could improve the patient journey and offered time to develop shared formulations. The assessment team initially rejected this, commenting, 'the best thing you can do is work through your waiting list more quickly'. However, PT staff often found that patients were not ready to start therapy, or the formulation was insufficient to identify the most appropriate therapy.

Two new Psychologists joined the team, and the PT lead suggested they focus on building relationships with the assessment team. Joint working increased across the teams, and patient care improved. Subsequently, the assessment team lead offered to part-fund an additional psychologist post *across* the two teams, enabling further development of this model.

Reflections

- Timing is important – if the time isn't right, patience and resilience are needed.
- Facilitating change successfully may mean others 'take credit' for the improvement, which can feel difficult.
- Focusing on relationships between staff enabled shared understanding and increased trust.

West and Lyubovnikova (2012) propose a helpful framework for thinking about team functioning by differentiating between pseudo and real teams. A pseudo team is a *'group of people working in an organization who call themselves or are called by others a team; who have differing accounts of team objectives; whose typical tasks require team members to work alone or in separate dyads towards disparate goals; whose team boundaries are highly permeable with individuals being uncertain over who is a team member, and who is not.'* In contrast, 'real team' members are clear about who is (and is not) a member of the team, work in a closely coordinated and timely manner towards common goals/objectives, have one or more clear shared team objectives, and systematically review performance and adapt future objectives and processes accordingly.

Conflict in the leadership team

The leadership team for a clinical service comprised a manager and several team leaders. A lead Psychologist joining them noticed regular conflict between team leaders, each feeling the actions and attitudes of other teams/team leaders threatened their team. Conflict arose from having limited resources, resulting in enforced boundaries to manage demand, sometimes to the detriment of patients.

The Psychologist modelled a 'yes, and' rather than a 'no, but' approach and offered reflective comments about the challenges in making decisions at individual patient/service levels with insufficient resources. As conflict reduced, the Psychologist facilitated conversations about shared objectives (for the leadership team) as opposed to individual objectives (for the team leaders/their teams). The concepts of 'pseudo' and 'real' teams were discussed once it seemed helpful to do so, and the leadership team recognised their journey from 'pseudo team' towards a 'real team'.

Over time, the leadership team became more empathic, conflict reduced, and issues were discussed collaboratively, enabling them to develop a service better able to meet patient needs within available resources.

Reflections

- It is important to model accepting different opinions and still working together.
- Conflict resolution requires time.
- To defuse conflict and increase empathy, systemic skills are key – highlighting areas of agreement and difference and the 'feelings behind' people's positions.
- Carefully consider the timing and method of introducing a framework.

A team's culture and dominant way of working often impacts its functioning. West (2012) differentiates between four types of teams: Type A – Resilient, with good levels of wellbeing and effective task completion; Type B – Complacent, warm and cohesive but struggling to be effective; Type C – Dysfunctional, with poor relationships and performance; Type D – Driven, focused on meeting objectives but with poor social functioning. Carter and West's Team Reflexivity Scale (1998) offers a tool to support thinking with a team about its emotional climate and approach to achieving goals. It has 16 questions, relating to either Task Reflexivity or Social Reflexivity.

Understanding the issues and developing a plan

A Consultant Psychologist joined a new service with about 60 staff and noticed conflicting views on aspects of service provision that staff found hard to share. The Psychologist asked staff to complete the Team Reflexivity Scale anonymously via an online form and received over 50 responses.

The average scores for 'Social' questions were higher than those for 'Task' questions – the team was categorised as 'Complacent'. On an away day, the Psychologist shared the results and organised staff into groups mixed across the service. The groups considered questions relating to making improvements based on the lowest scoring Reflexivity questions, writing their ideas down. The Psychologist identified themes and formed small working groups to further develop associated actions and improvements.

Reflections

- Team members valued providing feedback anonymously, which created more safety.
- Completing the questionnaire before the away day allowed a focus on improvements.
- Mixing staff enabled different conversations and new ideas.
- Having data about team functioning allows for comparison before and after improvements.

Leadership within Systems

When leading at a systems level, the identification of key stakeholders, the development of relationships, and understanding system culture are crucially important. Furthermore, the sense of being within a 'team' feels qualitatively different and is impacted by the maturity of the system or the strategic leadership goal.

Many healthcare services face challenges with demand exceeding capacity. Collaborative and creative working with partners is essential to understand the need and find new ways to meet it.

Managing the waiting list

An English Local Authority (LA) commissioned an NHS therapeutic service for Children in Care. Waiting times and the numbers waiting were increasing, causing frustration amongst Social Workers. The LA funded private assessments and therapy for some young people but found prioritising difficult. However, due to Social Workers making 'inappropriate' referrals, or the circumstances of those who were waiting significantly changing, the therapeutic staff felt some young people (and their carers) were unable to make the best use of the service.

A senior Psychologist quantified the team's capacity and demand. Without closing to new referrals, reducing the waiting list was impossible, and it would grow. The Psychologist proposed that the therapeutic service and social care collaborate at a monthly panel meeting, deciding who would be offered an assessment and/or therapy. This was agreed with senior social care managers and the commissioner, although good practice would have been to involve the young people and their carers, and may have led to additional ideas.

Prior to the panel starting, the waiting list was reviewed by the Psychologist and consultations were held with social workers to determine levels of need and a plan:

- brief indirect work could be sufficient
- other appropriate services were available
- referral to the Therapeutic Service was still needed – these cases were discussed at the first panel meeting.

Each month, the Therapeutic Service specified capacity for new assessments and therapy, and the Social Work teams submitted referrals. The panel reviewed them, deciding who was most in need and would most from support. This reduced conflict between the Therapeutic Service and Social Care. Clinical work started soon afterwards; there were no long waits, and timely intervention was offered.

Reflections

- Pre-existing relationships helped these discussions, i.e. knowing each other's strengths, limits, and pressures.
- Stakeholders required time to understand the disadvantages and advantages of the proposal.
- Joint leadership across systems enabled collaboration to address a shared problem.

Spending time identifying and engaging stakeholders is important, as understanding their different priorities or ideas creates opportunities for collaboration and avoids misalignment. NHS England and NHS Improvement (2019) suggest some helpful prompts, including considering stakeholders' financial or emotional interests, what motivates them, what communication they want, their current opinion of the work, who influences it, and how to manage opposition.

Engaging stakeholders around a national policy driver

Across an English ICS (Integrated Care System), a project was planned to scope the current provision of Psychological Therapies specified in the NHS Long-Term Plan (LTP)(2019) and consider whether any ICS-wide developments were needed, e.g., a 'supervision hub', sharing costs and responsibilities across the constituent Trusts.

A survey was designed with the most senior PPs across the ICS; however, the response rate was low. A Consultant Psychologist in an ICS-wide role took on the project and, using existing relationships and professional networks, contacted PP colleagues across the ICS in a targeted way. The number of survey questions was significantly reduced to decrease the burden on staff, and the approach changed to emails or brief conversations. This generated a more accurate and comprehensive data set. Additional feedback was that the narrow list of therapy models in the LTP seemed invalidating, with highly skilled and trained PPs already offering a comprehensive range of approaches.

In parallel, the psychologist liaised with colleagues in other ICS areas about their experiences of developing supervision hubs. An options appraisal paper was developed for delivering therapies sustainably within existing resources. This was successfully disseminated to an ICS-wide forum for senior PPs.

Reflections

- Using psychological formulation skills to refocus and reformulate the survey was crucial in responding quickly and effectively to stakeholders. Understanding *'who is this a problem for?'* and *'why now?'* was key to framing survey questions and articulating perspectives within the options appraisal.
- Being open, reflective, and non-defensive allowed space to express frustrations with aspects of the policy.
- Working from a position of realism rather than idealism allows for a more balanced perspective of the pros and cons of supervision hubs.
- Coming from a shared PP background and having delivered psychological interventions on the same pathways enabled understanding of the challenges of implementing this strategy.
- However, working in a role across the ICS meant coming from a position 'outside' of an organisation or team. This allowed engagement with no sense of having a 'vested interest' or agenda.

Systems Leadership thinking in health and social care (Edmonstone, 2019) emphasises that many challenges facing the NHS are complex and unlikely to be resolved through the efforts of single individuals or professional groups. These 'wicked' problems (Grint, 2008) are more prevalent in larger interdependent systems and require connectedness among leaders with the necessary understanding, skills, and influence, as well as considerable individual efforts. Important areas to address are:

- Clarifying the priorities at a system level
- Organising priorities into identifiable workstreams/projects
- Identifying stakeholders across the system
- Understanding stakeholders' needs and pressures
- Positioning yourself within this complex relationship structure
- Identifying 'common interests' across the System and connecting people
- Finding the 'open doors', going where there is 'good energy', and aligning with existing strategic priorities

Rather than being straightforward and linear, much of this work happens in parallel or involves circling back to earlier stages.

Developing interest in addressing system inequalities

Within an ICS, equitable access to psychological input within acute physical healthcare settings was a priority. Three of the constituent Places had District General Hospitals (DGHs) with little or no PP input to support patients, whereas the largest Place had two hospitals providing district, regional and national services, both with Clinical Health Psychology (CHP) departments.

The first task for the Consultant Psychologist leading this workstream was understanding the factors that enabled the successful development of CHP departments. Historic financial benefits associated with being within a large Teaching Hospital were important setting conditions, but the benefit of a CHP department model supported sustainable PP workforce development. However, the lead PPs in these Trusts were concerned about how the ICB (Integrated Care Board) might use detailed analysis of the variance in resources, so developing trust and relationships was an important component of the work.

Identifying key individuals interested in developing PP provision within the three DGHs occurred in parallel. Initially, their focus was on developing the existing limited (and often vacant) PP posts connected with specific clinical pathways. The challenges and frustrations within these acute care settings, including piecemeal funding allocations to services, became evident. The Psychologist was able to understand and articulate the recruitment and retention challenges, developing the shared view that a more radical model of recruitment and clinical governance was required.

The Psychologist connected CHP colleagues with their counterparts in other ICS areas, allowing constructively challenging conversations about how to adapt service development to the ICB commissioning landscape.

This culminated in a formal proposal document, which, alongside the relational work, resulted in connecting to ICB's 'sponsors' who had the will and influence to take the project forward.

Reflections

- Relationship building is fundamental to systems working, including being warm, enthusiastic, humorous (when appropriate), energetic, and grateful for colleagues' time.
- Preparation before meetings helps assure stakeholders that the meeting will be worthwhile.
- Actively listening to and responding to stakeholders' concerns builds trust and psychological safety.
- Defining the rationale for the project across different audiences is important.
- Identifying and influencing partners in the system who hold the power to move the project forward is crucial.

Summary and Final Reflections

Psychologists are well placed to lead at local, regional, and national levels and to translate policy into psychologically informed services, with patients at the centre. Changes may be supported by high-quality research evidence, but 'it's not enough to be right, you also have to be effective' (deGrasse Tyson, 2024), requiring attention to relationships, a clear understanding of the Psychological Professions, along with other leadership and service development skills.

This chapter includes the breadth of scenarios that psychologists may encounter across their careers. Where possible, we have removed identifying aspects to enable a greater focus on the more generalisable leadership skills. You may have noticed that the structure reflects the trajectory of personal and professional development in many psychologists' careers. We have included some personal reflections and hope these will be as helpful as the examples themselves.

Good luck with your leadership journey!

Ideas in Brief

- Clinical leadership is relevant to all psychologists regardless of level of experience or seniority within the organisation, but the nature of the activities will vary.
- A key part of effective clinical leadership is working collaboratively, understanding stakeholders, and building relationships.
- How ideas are gathered from others can make a difference to success, and often creative approaches are needed.
- It is important to consider your attributes and the 'stances' you can adopt when embarking on any development work.
- Opportunities to reflect on the work and gain a different perspective from peers, supervisors, or mentors, can make a difference when feeling stuck.

References

British Psychological Society. (2010). *Clinical psychology leadership development framework*. British Psychological Society.

British Psychological Society. (2021). *Leadership development and support for clinical psychologists working in health and social care*. British Psychological Society.

Carter, S. M., & West, M. A. (1998). Reflexivity, effectiveness, and mental health in BBC-TV production teams. *Small Group Research, 29*, 583–601.

deGrasse Tyson, N. (2024). *Communication: It's not enough to be right*. Retrieved April 19, 2025, from https://www.masterclass.com/classes/neil-degrasse-tyson-teaches-scientific-thinking-and-communication/chapters/communication-it-s-not-enough-to-be-right

Edmonstone, J. (2019). *Systems leadership in health and social care*. Routledge.

Grint, K. (2008). Wicked problems & clumsy solutions: The role of leadership. *Clinical Leader, 1*(2), 54–68.

Moullin, M. (2002). *Delivering excellence in health and social care*. Open University Press.

NHS Confederation. (2023, April). *What is clinical and care professional leadership?* https://www.nhsconfed.org/articles/what-clinical-and-care-professional-leadership

NHS England. (2023). *NHS long term workforce plan*. NHS England.

NHS England and NHS Improvement. (2019). *The handbook of quality, service improvement and redesign tools*. NHS England and NHS Improvement.

NHS Improvement. (2019). *Clinical leadership – A framework for action. A guide for senior leaders on developing professional diversity at board level*. NHS Improvement.

NHS Leadership Academy. (2011). *Leadership framework*. NHS Leadership Academy.

NHS Leadership Academy. (2013). *Healthcare leadership model: The nine dimensions of leadership behaviour*. NHS Leadership Academy.

NHS Staff Council Job Evaluation Group. (2023). *National profiles for clinical psychologists, counsellors & psychotherapists*. NHS Staff Council Job Evaluation Group.

Psychological Professions Network. (2020). *Leadership and* management *in the* psychological professions*: Discussion paper*. Psychological Professions Network.

Rao, A. S., & Mason, B. (2023). Examining leadership competencies. Are our leadership skills future ready? *Clinical Psychology Forum, 363*, 63–73.

West, M. A. (2012). *Effective teamwork: Practical* lessons from organizational research (3rd ed.). John Wiley & Sons.

West, M. A., & Lyubovnikova, J. (2012). Real teams or pseudo teams? The changing landscape needs a better map. Industrial and Organizational Psychology, 5(1), 25–55.

9 Fostering Transactional Business Skills, Creativity and Psychological Principles to Lead Well

Professor Aimée Aubeeluck

Transactional Business Skills in Leadership Roles

If we consider the activities we engage in to navigate the world and handle day-to-day human exchanges, many of these actions can become automated and driven by habits that allow us to interact with others with minimal cognitive effort. However, honing these skills can maximise our success in having and maintaining smooth, efficient, authentic, and mutually profitable transactions important in our personal and work lives. Taking up leadership roles can be enhanced by employing transactional business skills in today's organisations where efficiency, structure, and outcomes, and effective operational structures are emphasised. Psychologists bring a variety of skills to leadership roles from a broad knowledge base and a commitment to ongoing learning, including embracing the space where psychology meets business models. Examples of relevant transactional business skills are provided with a focus on Health Psychology, although these are likely to apply to many branches of applied psychology.

Operations Management

Operations management can broadly be defined as the oversight and control of the processes that convert inputs, such as human resources,

DOI: 10.4324/9781003492399-12

to outputs such as products or services. Within this remit lies, for example, how we design and optimise our processes, how we manage supply chains, build capacity, allocate our resources, and deliver to a high quality, seeking opportunities for continuous improvement. As such, effective operations management should be efficient, reduce costs, and improve quality and consumer satisfaction.

There are many methodologies and underlying principles that seek to minimise surplus whilst maximising quality and productivity. The methodology of Lean management (Liker, 2018; Holt, 2019) is considered a systematic approach to identifying and eliminating waste or non-value-added activities within organisations with the goal of creating more value for customers with fewer resources.

The principles of Lean Management lend themselves to a cyclical process that allows for continuous improvement and considers overarching value, value streams, flow, pull, and perfection in the pursuit of adding improvement with limited 'waste' (see Table 9.1).

So, what does waste mean within this context? There are seven key types of waste that can be identified within Lean management as follows:

1. Overproduction: Producing more than is needed
2. Waiting: Idle time between process steps
3. Transportation: Unnecessary movement of materials or information
4. Inventory: Excess raw materials, work-in-progress, or finished goods
5. Motion: Unnecessary human movements or ergonomic inefficiencies
6. Over-processing: Doing more work than the customer requires
7. Defects: Rework, scrap, or correction of errors

One of the most utilised tools for lean management is Six Sigma (George, 2004), a data-driven approach to eliminating defects and reducing waste variability in processes. The Six Sigma methodology was originally developed by Motorola in the 1980s and has since been widely adopted

Table 9.1 Key principles of lean management

Value	Clear definition of value from a customer's perspective
Value Stream	Identification and mapping of end process to deliver that value
Flow	Ensuring a smooth continuous flow of work through the value stream
Pull	Align product with customer demand
Perfection	Seek continuous and incremental improvements

by organisations across various industries, including Higher Education Institutions (Balzer & Sinha, 2023).

At the core of Six Sigma is the Define, Measure, Analyse, Improve, Control (DMAIC) methodology (see Table 9.2).

Six Sigma places focus on customer needs, uses data to drive decision-making, prioritising standardisation and improvement. Six Sigma is an investment in time at the forefront of a process to allow for improved quality, replicability, customer satisfaction, a reduction in costs by eliminating waste and defects, an increase in productivity and efficiency, and more broadly, the development of a culture of continuous improvement. As psychologists, our education and training lend themselves to transparent, rigorous, and data-driven processes that can facilitate this way of working, with our customer being the patient, client, or maybe the learner we are there to support.

Negotiation

The art of negotiation is a critical skill in transactional business communications, requiring a number of skills to be executed efficiently;

- Preparation: Diligence in terms of understanding your and others' positions
- Active listening: Meaningful understanding of others' needs and concerns
- Problem-solving: Establishing creative solutions for stakeholders' benefit

Table 9.2 Outline of define, measure, analyse, improve, control DMAIC methodology

Define	Define the problem/opportunity for improvement, project goals, and any critical-to-quality (CTQ) characteristics.
Measure	Collect and analyse data to understand current process performance and identify root causes of defects.
Analyse	Analyse data to determine the key factors influencing the process.
Improve	Establish and implement solutions to address the root causes and improve the process.
Control	Establish controls that allow for maintenance and improvement of newly established process.

- Emotional intelligence: Understanding others and the importance of developing meaningful relationships
- Patience and persistence: Being willing and able to work through disagreements
- Strategic concessions: Understanding when and how to make strategic trade-offs
- Building relationships: Fostering long-term trust through fair negotiations

These skills are rarely intrinsic to us as individuals and are likely to be developed and honed over time. Health Psychologists have extensive knowledge and experience in behaviour change activities that can be used to understand how we can change our behaviours to develop these skills, forming habits with our negotiations that lead to success through practice and consistency. One example of using negotiation skills optimally comes from the Best Alternative to a Negotiation Agreement (BATNA) model (Nolan-Hayley, 2013) which accentuates the importance of understanding fallback positions to strengthen the power of negotiation. Using this model allows for flexible thinking by having a considered and favourable alternative when an agreement between parties is unable to be reached. In knowing your own BATNA, you arm yourself with power and insight into the minimum requirements that are acceptable to you within any given negotiation (see Table 9.3).

To develop a strong BATNA, there is a need to thoroughly research all options and alternatives; an objective assessment of the quality and value of these, ongoing refinement throughout negotiations, and to be ok with walking away if an agreement does not meet the minimum requirements. Some common examples might include being able to procure from another supplier or being able to solve a problem internally

Table 9.3 Knowing your BATNA

Action	Outcome
Assess the value of a potential agreement (financial or otherwise)	Ability to compare a proposed agreement determining if it meets requirements
Set up reservation points	A clear understanding of minimum bar
Gain negotiation leverage	Strengthens position and allows assertion when required
Guard against making poor agreements	Know when to walk away

rather than outsourcing. Having alternatives in the back pocket allows us to have all the required information and leverage to hand to secure the best possible outcome.

Using Data to Inform Decision-Making

Using data to inform decisions or data-driven decision-making requires a number of steps that allow for the making of the best decisions with the information in front of us (see Table 9.4).

Many branches of applied psychology equip psychologists with these areas of competence. For instance, health psychologists often utilise 'big data' to understand patterns, trends, and associations to comprehend health outcomes on a population level and work towards models of preventative health care. Big data are large and complex data sets and can be characterised by the "3 Vs" (Laney, 2001):

- Volume – sheer volume data being generated and collected
- Variety – different types of data, e.g., structured, unstructured, and semi-structured
- Velocity – speed at which data is being created, collected, and processed

In applied psychology, such data allows for predictive illness/risk modelling, client outcomes analysis, and treatment developments, but it also creates several challenges in use and manipulation. For example, how to store, process, analyse, and extract meaningful findings promptly. Moreover, it is important to consider how new knowledge can be

Table 9.4 Data-driven decision-making process

Collection	Gathering relevant information from various sources
Analysis	Using statistical and analytical tools to interpret data
Identifying trends and patterns	Recognising important insights in the data
Predictive analysis	Utilising data to forecast future trends
Risk assessment	Evaluating potential outcomes
Performance measurement	Utilising metrics to track and improve performance
Visualisation	Presenting and feeding back data clearly

integrated and linked to existing data sources to fully understand, contextualise, and benefit from its availability. To address such challenges, organisations can employ a variety of tools and technologies such as distributed computing frameworks, in-memory data processing, machine learning, predictive analytics, data visualisation, and dashboards. The use of big data can, therefore, provide a number of benefits that include:

- Improved decision-making via data-driven insights
- Enhanced operational efficiency and financial savings
- Tailored client experiences
- Identification of new opportunities or ways of working
- Predictive and prescriptive analytics for proactive problem solving

The volume and complexity of the data available are only set to grow, and as such, the effective management and analysis of Big Data are essential to ensuring that organisations and individuals can drive innovation in the future.

Communication

When we consider effective communication in work/business transactions, we need to reconsider sequencing our information in the form of an introduction, main details, conclusion, and finding ways to get to the point at pace. The key elements of effective communication require us to hone both our verbal, written, and non-verbal communication skills and focus on the following:

- Clear and concise messaging – How can I convey information accurately and efficiently?
- Active listening – Am I focused on understanding, and responding to the speaker?
- Non-verbal communication – Do I understand and use body language effectively?
- Written communication – Have I honed the craft of producing clear emails and other documents?
- Presentation skills – Can I orate and effectively convey information to others?
- Interpersonal skills – How can I build rapport and relationships?
- Cross-cultural communication – How can I adapt my style for diverse audiences?

- Feedback – Can I 'disagree well', giving and receiving constructive feedback?

Psychologists can employ the use of storytelling in work interactions (Kemp et al., 2023), drawing on narrative techniques to make data and ideas more engaging. Indeed, storytelling can be a powerful tool to engage audiences, convey information, and influence decision-making. This style of communication moves beyond presenting facts and data and uses stories to make ideas more compelling, memorable, and impactful (see Table 9.5).

Psychologists can utilise storytelling to create emotional connections, motivate and guide others in training and development, enhance social responsibility, and foster a sense of community, culture, and shared purpose.

So what are the key elements of effective storytelling in leadership? Being relatable, compelling and providing emotional appeal that helps to drive a message home are excellent starting points. However, the story also needs to be authentic, credible and have relevance to the listener. In mastering the art of storytelling, organisations can significantly enhance their ability to communicate, persuade and connect with their stakeholders to drive better business outcomes. Being an effective storyteller requires emotional intelligence (EQ) (Goleman, 2005), i.e. that we understand and are able to manage emotions in ourselves and in others. EQ is an essential part of effective communication that requires several cognitive and psychological components as outlined in Table 9.6.

Honing EQ skills in leadership roles improves rapport and connections, allowing us to navigate difficult conversations, persuade and influence. By adjusting style as necessary, the likelihood of miscommunication, misunderstandings, and breakdowns in communication is

Table 9.5 Benefits of storytelling in business

Increased engagement	Capture attention, making the audience more receptive to the message
Improved communication	Translating complex information into a simpler format
Enhanced persuasion	Compelling stories tap into emotions and build trust
Improved retention	Less abstract and easier to remember
Differentiation	Helps the information to 'stand out in the crowd'

Table 9.6 The key components of EQ

Self-awareness	How our own emotions impact our behaviour and communications
Empathy	Recognising and understanding the emotions of others
Emotional regulation	The ability to manage and express emotions appropriately
Social Skills	The ability to communicate effectively and build strong relationships

reduced, enhancing impact, improving outcomes, and building stronger relationships for greater success.

Creativity

Creativity in business and leadership transactions refers to the ability to think outside the box, identify innovative solutions, and approach problem-solving in unique ways. Incorporating creativity into work transactions can provide many important benefits and innovative solutions. The following section addresses three ways of harnessing creativity through service innovation, problem-solving, and process improvement.

Service Innovation

Within the context of psychology, there are a number of effective strategies that we can utilise to foster creativity and innovation as outlined in Table 9.7.

These strategies can foster a culture of creativity to empower those we work alongside to take risks and recognise innovative contributions. By balancing structure and discipline with a creative and exploratory mindset, we engender a culture that spurs innovation for the benefit of stakeholders within the wider healthcare context.

Problem Solving

Creativity is also highly beneficial in solving some of the 'wicked problems' that we encounter as Applied Psychologists. There are a variety

Table 9.7 Fostering creativity and innovation

Encourage Diverse Perspectives	Assemble cross-functional teams with people from different backgrounds, experiences, and areas of expertise to spark new ideas and challenge assumptions
Design Thinking Workshops	Employ empathy mapping, journey mapping, and ideation sessions (Çeviker-Ç ınar et al., 2017) to deeply understand needs and generate creative solutions
Experimental Mindset	Create psychologically safe spaces to take calculated risks and experiment with new ideas
Creative Problem-Solving Tools	Utilise mind mapping and lateral thinking techniques (e.g. Clark, 1998) to increase innovative thinking
Understand the Customer Experience	Shadow activities and experience services first hand to uncover insights and inspiration
Encourage Unstructured Ideation	Engage in open-ended ideation sessions without predefined constraints to allow ideas to flow freely before evaluating and refining
Collaborate with External Partners	Invite stakeholders and competitors to co-create new service concepts
Analyse Analogous Experiences	Study how others have approached similar challenges. Look for creative context specific solutions
Leverage Emerging Technologies	Consider how the latest technological advancements can be incorporated into new services

of strategies that we can utilise from both the worlds of business and psychology, as follows:

Reframing (Clark, 1998): A key element of creative problem solving is the ability to reframe the problem, taking a step back and exploring different and alternative ways of framing the challenge. This opens up new perspectives and solution paths.

Divergent thinking (Clark, 1998): This can help to generate a wide range of ideas to explore conventional solutions. Whilst we can problem-solve on our own, it can also be highly beneficial to bring together diverse team members to cross-pollinate ideas. Such collaborative ideation across different backgrounds, experiences, and areas of expertise can lead to highly creative solutions and buy-in from the wider team. Drawing on inspiration from other industries and challenging assumptions also helps to spark novel connections and uncover new possibilities.

Tolerating ambiguity (Hoffmann et al., 2022): Whilst we endeavour to solve problems creatively, it is important to have a mindset that allows us to be comfortable with a degree of ambiguity as we move through the process, resisting the urge to jump to conclusions too quickly and allowing space for the unexpected. It can help to incorporate elements of fun and playfulness to reduce mental blocks and stimulate innovative thinking.

Failure as a learning opportunity (Mitchell et al., 2008): Of utmost importance is the ability to accept failure as a learning opportunity, analysing unsuccessful ideas to understand what didn't work and why. Failures as an opportunity open learning, refinement and generative ideas to unlock innovative solutions to even the most complex individual and organisational challenges.

Process Improvement

Some of the key strategies considered earlier also fit nicely into the utilisation of creativity in process improvement. By combining creative thinking and analytical rigour, we can establish many opportunities to streamline operations, enhance quality, and drive continuous process improvement. The psychology of change management (Kotter & Schlesinger, 1979) is integral to our understanding of process improvement and draws on both human and technical elements to facilitate a culture of improvement. To foster creativity, there are a variety of ways we can enhance the likelihood of success. Table 9.8 below, outlines a number of the key tools that are utilised regularly in facilitating change (see also Noble & Tarrant, 2022; Dawson et al., 2024).

Fostering creativity in our communications and transactions requires us to champion a culture of innovation and experimentation. We need to be willing to invest in training and tools to develop creative problem-solving skills, gather diverse perspectives, and challenge assumptions, analyse our successes and failures, and seek continuous improvement. Moreover, it requires monitoring trends and feedback to identify unmet needs and empower others to take calculated risks and try new approaches.

Table 9.8 Tools to support the management of change (Balzer & Sinha, 2023)

Process mapping	Tools like process flow diagrams and value stream maps provide a clear, visual understanding of existing process
Observation	Observe process first hand. Talk to the people that do the work to bring it to life
Challenge current assumptions	Identify and question the underlying assumptions that may be limiting the current process design
Look outwards	Creative solutions can be found by considering how other industries function
Be experimental	Take calculated risks and test out creative process improvement ideas
Analyse process data creatively	Use data visualisation, trend analysis, and predictive modelling to discover patterns and insights to inspire innovation

Applied Psychologists may draw on models of creativity in work transactions to improve the patient or client experience by identifying novel ways to tailor health care to the individual and address their specific needs; to implement process improvements or technological solutions to streamline transactions and communications and provide consultancy solutions to broader systems and organisations. If we embrace creativity, we can unlock new avenues for growth, enhance our competitive positioning, and deliver greater value to clients through more innovative and effective work transactions.

Conclusion

By integrating psychological concepts, best practices, and learning from other relevant fields such as business management, leaders can develop a more nuanced understanding of human behaviour and support others in reaching their full potential. Table 9.9 outlines several key leadership qualities that may enhance our transactional business skills, creativity and psychological skills in our endeavours to lead well (see e.g., Brown, 2018; Noble & Tarrant, 2022.

Table 9.9 Qualities that enhance our ability to lead well – Is there a reference?

Self-awareness	understanding own personality, strengths, weaknesses, biases, and emotional intelligence
Emotional intelligence	ability to recognize, understand, and manage emotions in oneself and others
Motivation and engagement	designing work environments and incentive structures that intrinsically motivate others
Team dynamics	knowledge of group dynamics, conflict resolution, and team-building fosters cohesive and high-performing teams
Change management	understanding the psychological factors that drive human resistance to change
Decision making	awareness of unconscious influences on decision-making.
Coaching and feedback	providing feedback, coaching, and mentoring to others
Cultivating a positive culture	creating an environment that fosters well-being, resilience, and allows others to flourish

Self-awareness allows leaders to play to their strengths, manage their weaknesses, and model the behaviours they want to see in others. Emotional intelligence engenders psychologically safe spaces that allow for empathetic communication, trust, and collaboration. Work environments that intrinsically motivate and foster a team-building culture can boost engagement and productivity. Understanding why individuals can be resistant to change helps leaders navigate organisational transformation more effectively and can mitigate some of the cognitive biases that influence decision-making to make better choices.

Leadership underpinned by psychology is also situated in a growth mindset and considers how to provide feedback, coaching, and mentoring to foster greater personal and professional growth, allowing others to flourish. Psychology-informed leadership can therefore lead to increased engagement, innovation, and organisational performance, having a profound impact on organisational success.

Ideas in Brief

- Psychological theory in combination with business management models can provide a powerful vehicle for leading well
- Integrating 'lean practice' into your day-to-day life helps to eliminate unnecessary processes and frees up time for creativity and innovation
- The importance of excellent communication cannot be underestimated – successful leaders invest time in honing their ability to listen, build relationships, and adapt their style to their audience.
- Psychology-informed leadership that considers how to negotiate, provide feedback, and mentor others can lead to increased engagement, innovation, and organisational success.

References

Balzer, W. K., & Sinha, T. (2023). *Hoshin Kanri in higher education: A guide to strategy development, deployment, and management*. Routledge.

Brown, B. (2018). *Dare to lead: Brave work, tough conversations, whole hearts*. Vermilion.

Çeviker-Çınar, G., Mura, G., & Demirbağ-Kaplan, M. (2017). Design thinking: A new road map in business education. *The Design Journal, 20*(sup1), S977–S987.

Clark, A. J. (1998). Reframing: A therapeutic technique in group counseling. *The Journal for Specialists in Group Work, 23*(1), 66–73. https://doi.org/10.1080/01933929808411382

Dawson, P., Andriopoulos, C., & Pattinson, S. (2024). *Managing change, creativity and innovation*. Sage Publications.

George, M. L. (2004). *The lean Six Sigma pocket toolbook: A quick reference guide to 100 tools for improving quality and speed* (1st ed.). McGraw-Hill Education.

Goleman, D. (2005). *Emotional intelligence: Why it can matter more than IQ*. Bantam Books.

Hoffmann, J. D., McGarry, J., & Seibyl, J. (2022). Beyond tolerating ambiguity: How emotionally intelligent people can channel uncertainty into creativity. In R. A. Beghetto & G. J. Jaeger (Eds.), *Uncertainty: A catalyst for creativity, learning and development* (Vol. 6). Springer. https://doi.org/10.1007/978-3-030-97134-7_4

Holt, P. (2019). *The simplicity of Lean: Defeating complexity, delivering excellence.* Management Impact Publishing.

Kemp, A., Gravois, R., Syrdal, H., & McDougal, E. (2023). Storytelling is not just for marketing: Cultivating a storytelling culture throughout the organization. *Business Horizons, 66*(3), 313–324. https://doi.org/10.1016/j.bushor.2023.01.003

Kotter, J. P., & Schlesinger, L. A. (1979). Choosing strategies for change. *Harvard Business Review.* https://hbr.org/1979/07/choosing-strategies-for-change

Laney, D. (2001, February 6). *3D data management: Controlling data volume, velocity, and variety.* META Group.

Liker, J. K. (2018). *The Toyota way (2nd ed.): 14 management principles from the world's greatest manufacturer.* McGraw Hill.

Mitchell, R. K., Mitchell, J. R., & Smith, J. B. (2008). Inside opportunity formation: Enterprise failure, cognition and the creation of opportunities. *Strategic Enterprise Journal, 2*, 225–242.

Noble, S., & Tarrant, A. (2022). *Coaching people through organizational change: Practical tools to support employees through business transformation.* Kogan Page.

Nolan-Haley, J. (2013). *Alternative dispute resolution in a nutshell* (4th ed.). West Academic Publishing.

How Business Skills Can Strengthen Effective and Impactful Leadership 10

Dr Rosie Gilderthorp and Dr Amra Saleem Rao

Bridging Psychology and Business Skills for Impactful Leadership

The integration of psychological expertise with business acumen can elevate leadership effectiveness. Psychologists, equipped with scientific training and specialist skills, play a crucial role in shaping values-driven organisations that foster diversity and transform lives.

While psychology naturally enhances leadership skills, such as strategic thinking, governance, and operational management, these can be further strengthened by incorporating principles from economics and business management. This chapter takes a broader perspective, examining how these business disciplines and psychological knowledge can support practitioner psychologists in healthcare leadership.

Sustainability through Open Strategy

COVID-19 shattered long-held assumptions in public service planning, exposing vulnerabilities and intensifying mental health challenges. Yet, the crisis also drove unprecedented innovation and technological advancement in businesses, demonstrating the power of creative reinvention when assumptions are abandoned to re-focus on a purpose.

Strategy aligns an organisation's activities with its purpose. A strong strategy provides a roadmap for achieving organisational aims, outlining

DOI: 10.4324/9781003492399-13

the competencies required, key personnel, measurable outcomes, and necessary cultural shifts. However, public sector leaders face a unique challenge as there is pressure to be "ambidextrous" and continue delivering the services people expect while simultaneously responding to new and emerging needs (Heracleous & Werres, 2016).

Such a balance can prove daunting even for corporate giants with substantial budgets (Heracleous et al., 2017).

Utilising strategic tools commonly taught in business schools, combined with psychological understanding, can help to manage these tensions and forge a purpose-driven path for the future. One approach that aligns particularly well with psychological thinking is Open Strategy (Stadler et al., 2021). Open Strategy is a framework for the development of strategy that emphasises transparency, inclusivity, and participation, along with a commitment to engaging stakeholders at all levels as its guiding principles. Open Strategy begins by seeking diverse knowledge to anticipate shifts and identify trends before running challenges and exercises with groups of divergent thinkers to solve problems and unlock new opportunities (Hautz et al., 2017).

Reflecting on past decisions illustrates how a more inclusive and forward-thinking approach might have reshaped mental health services:

- Could the NHS have embraced online therapy earlier if technology experts had been part of strategic discussions in 2015?
- Might child and adolescent mental health services (CAMHS) have mitigated social media's impact by consulting app developers in 2012?
- Could triage systems operate more effectively by learning from industries like logistics?

While Open Strategy fosters innovation and engagement, implementation is not without challenges. Meaningful participation demands time and resources—to involve staff, remunerate external experts, and ensure diverse user representation. Aligning strategy with broader organisational and governmental priorities can be difficult. The pressure of managing long waiting lists and strained resources often forces leaders into short-term firefighting rather than long-term visioning (Heracleous et al., 2017).

However, history reminds us that bold change is possible. Just 75 years ago, the NHS itself was a radical concept that defied entrenched norms. Radical transformation—such as service redesign—requires not just strategic frameworks but also strong political will and bold leadership

(Heracleous & Werres, 2016). When political resolve meets the necessity for transformation, frameworks like Open Strategy ensure that innovation is not just an aspiration but a reality—one that places communities at the heart of progress.

Useful Resources

Stadler (2021) *Open Strategy*

HBR podcast - https://hbr.org/podcasts/on-strategy

The Business of Psychology Podcast – https://psychologybusinessschool.com/the-business-of-psychology/

The Overlooked Role of Economics in Leadership

Effective leadership requires a deep understanding of the forces shaping an organisation. While psychology equips us with behavioural insights, economics provides a framework for decision-making in resource-constrained environments. Many leaders instinctively engage with social and political factors but often overlook the economic forces shaping their organisations. However, as we progress in our careers, it becomes clear that psychology and economics are deeply intertwined—both disciplines seek to explain human behaviour through empirical study, and neither offers a complete picture on its own.

Leaders who grasp the economic dynamics within their organisations are far more successful in advocating for priorities and ensuring long-term sustainability. By aligning financial realities with service needs, they can drive meaningful change rather than reacting to funding pressures.

Supply and Demand in Healthcare

Austerity-driven "efficiency savings" often feel counterintuitive, leaving frontline staff demoralised while executives struggle with financial constraints. One[1] of us recalls working as a newly qualified Clinical Psychologist in a Learning Disability service where, despite relentless dedication, the team felt powerless in the face of social care cuts. Over years of austerity, a disconnect emerged between executives making financial decisions and clinicians overwhelmed by unmanageable workloads and burnout.

Understanding healthcare economics can help to make sense of the thought processes behind executive decisions in such contexts. Leaders require awareness of emerging economic challenges as well as connection with their teams. This can facilitate team alignment with policy changes but also allows leaders to advocate for change more effectively when professional priorities conflict with financial policies. For instance, the ageing population and rising chronic health conditions—mental health included—have dramatically increased healthcare costs (Phillips, 2024). However, funding constraints, workforce shortages, and systemic inefficiencies have left the public sector struggling to meet demand. This imbalance has fuelled a shift towards private healthcare, with NHS services increasingly outsourced (IBISWorld, 2023). Some economists argue that competition in healthcare should drive better services, as monopolies often fail to prioritise customer value (The Health Foundation, 2011). However, healthcare is not a truly free market. High costs, regulatory barriers, and the exclusion of high-need, low-income patients limit the effectiveness of competition. Furthermore, the private healthcare sector remains concentrated among a few dominant providers, reducing the theoretical benefits of competition.

The consequences of this supply-demand gap are visible in long waiting times, rising health inequalities, and staff burnout (The King's Fund & Nuffield Trust, 2023; NHS England, 2023). Lord Darzi's 2024 report highlights how chronic underfunding, poor management, and disengagement from frontline staff have eroded care quality, patient satisfaction, and workforce well-being. In response, NHS England is undergoing structural changes, including its disbandment, to streamline decision-making and reduce inefficiencies.

Such a context highlights the complexity of balancing supply and demand. Psychologists bring critical skills to healthcare leadership—formulation, data analysis, service planning, and behaviour change strategies. By reviewing economic trends, psychology leaders are well equipped to manage the complexity and develop services minimising waste and allocating resources efficiently. A deeper understanding of market structures and political forces also enables psychologists to anticipate and communicate the risks and benefits of decisions like privatisation, playing a more credible role in shaping service strategy.

Rethinking Cost Structures for Long-Term Sustainability

Given the increasing demand for services and limited financial resources, psychology leaders are often required to navigate the tension between cost efficiency and service quality. A key aspect of this is understanding cost structures—the balance between fixed costs (e.g., staff salaries, facilities) and variable costs (e.g., therapeutic materials, consumables).

Many psychology-led services are heavy on fixed costs, with most of the expenditure centred on staff costs and premises. This explains why historically, there has been significant pressure to find savings through a reduction in staff costs and office space. Due to the workforce pressures, this is unlikely to be an effective strategy going forward. Looking for areas where expensive resources may be under-utilised or where contracts could be renegotiated should always be the first step when seeking efficiency savings. As we have had many years in this cost-conscious environment, many leaders feel there are no more leaks to plug in the financial bucket. However, given enough political motivation, investment in innovation, service re-design with meaningful staff engagement, the use of AI, radical change, and improved efficiency are possible.

Psychology itself can also provide creative routes to improved efficiency. For instance, applying behavioural economics to resource allocation alongside formulation and data analysis skills can improve engagement and reduce inefficiencies. Studies show that patient no-show rates decrease significantly when behavioural nudges—such as personalised appointment reminders—are used. These cost-effective strategies, informed by psychology, can enhance service delivery without requiring additional funding, targeting resources to the groups that need them most.

The Economics of Healthcare

As leaders, advocating for the value of our services and ensuring the protection of quality care can be challenging—especially when mental health services are perceived as costly and unappealing to politicians and the media. However, a strong understanding of the economics within our area of expertise can help make a compelling case. The 2023 NHS Confederation report, *The Economic and Social Costs of Mental Ill Health*, provides clear examples of how investing in services that may seem like financial "pits" on paper can ultimately improve overall societal wealth and health.

For example, mental health problems cost the UK economy at least £117.9 billion annually. The majority of those costs are caused by reductions in productivity and decreases in well-being rather than healthcare costs (NHS Confederation: Mental Health Network, 2023). Epidemiological and economic estimates indicate that the global burden of mental disorders is considerable, both in its impacts on human health and losses to societal welfare. The economic case for investment in mental health is strong: for every $1 invested in scaled-up treatment for depression and anxiety, there is a $4 return in better health and productivity (World Health Organization 2016). mental health problems cost the UK economy at least £117.9 billion annually, equivalent to around 5% of the UK's GDP. Figures like these can help leaders in budget discussions and business bids to make an economic case for investment in mental health (Mental Health Foundation & London School of Economics and Political Science, 2022).

Behavioural Economics in Service Design

Behavioural economics blends psychological and economic principles to understand how people make decisions on issues like spending, education, and health—decisions that ultimately impact the broader economy. Grasping its key concepts is crucial for effective service design and evaluation. For instance, if a service struggles with high staff costs, long waiting lists, and non-attendance, behavioural economics can offer strategies to improve productivity, outcomes, and user experience. Psychologists, with their expertise in cognitive biases, bounded rationality, discrimination, and group behaviour, are well positioned to identify and address these issues. By framing problems through a behavioural lens, psychologists can develop impactful solutions that can be tested and refined through a Quality Improvement process.

Moreover, behavioural economics can inform leadership communication strategies, particularly in how information about risk and uncertainty is presented. Understanding how people process such information—and how to help them contextualise it—can lead to improved patient health, employee safety, and overall organisational culture.

Beyond Cost-Cutting—Strategic Leadership for the Future

The future of healthcare leadership demands more than cost-cutting; it requires data-driven, psychology-informed, and economically sound decision-making. By integrating behavioural insights with economic realities, leaders can drive sustainable service redesign that aligns financial constraints with patient needs.

Psychologists, with their expertise in behavioural analysis and change management, are well positioned to shape the next generation of healthcare leadership. However, to do so effectively, they need to anticipate and engage proactively with change, economic and strategic decision-making, ensuring that services remain both financially viable and patient-centred.

This brief skim of economics is intended to help balance financial prudence with a deep understanding of human behavioural psychology to transform economic constraints from a limiting factor into an opportunity for innovation and impact. As it does not delve deeply into the latest economic trends or innovations in behavioural economics, the resources provided below are added for further exploration.

- Inside Behavioural Economics database (Inside BE, 2024)—https://insidebe.com/database?s=appointment+attendance
- NHS Confederation: The economic and social costs of mental ill health (NHS Confederation: Mental Health Network, 2023)
- The Rest is Money podcast—https://podcasts.apple.com/lu/podcast/the-rest-is-money/id1703785141
- The King's Fund
- The Nuffield Trust
- Nudge Podcast—https://www.nudgepodcast.com/
- ELFT Quality Improvement resources (East London NHS Foundation Trust, 2024)
- Mental health matters

Project Management and Budgeting Knowledge

Project management and budgeting are key leadership skills, enabling leaders to achieve objectives on time and within budget. Essential skills like communication, resource allocation, and stakeholder engagement are critical for success (Project Management Institute, 2017). Incorporating the models below, alongside budgeting, can help psychologists enhance their strategic impact and efficiency.

The Lean Business Model focuses on eliminating inefficiencies and managing costs (Womack & Jones, 2003). It helps psychologists track costs, ensuring funds are spent on high-impact activities while avoiding unnecessary overheads.

The Business Canvas Model outlines key components of a project, such as resources, value propositions, customer segments, and revenue streams (Osterwalder & Pigneur, 2010). Psychologists can use it to ensure strategic, financial, and operational goals are aligned by forecasting how funds are allocated.

The Agile Model emphasises flexibility, iteration, and continuous improvement, allowing for adjustments based on emerging challenges (Highsmith, 2002), while dynamic budgeting accommodates evolving priorities.

SWOT (Strengths, Weaknesses, Opportunities, Threats) Analysis helps psychologists assess internal and external factors to inform decision-making (Humphrey, 2005). It aids in strategic development, evaluating solutions, and preparing investment bids. SWOT analysis helps psychologists assess internal and external factors to inform decision-making (Humphrey, 2005). It aids in strategic development, evaluating solutions, and preparing investment bids.

Effective budgeting ensures resource allocation aligns with strategic goals, keeping stakeholders confident in a project's viability (Kerzner, 2017). Integrating business models with budgeting practices like cost estimation, expense tracking, and budget adjustments equips leaders to deliver sustainable outcomes, remain aligned with goals, and maximise impact (Gray & Larson, 2020). These skills are essential for good governance, and psychologists should develop them through training and development as they take on leadership roles.

Marketing and Communication Skills

In our work as business mentors, coaches, and consultants, we often observe that many psychologists feel uncomfortable with the concept of "marketing." This response is understandable, given the aggressive and unethical marketing tactics we encounter daily, which can distort the true purpose of marketing.

At its core, marketing is about understanding the people we serve and ensuring our services meet their needs effectively. This applies whether we are working within the NHS, offering private psychology-informed antenatal classes, or engaging in organisational development work. When marketing is approached with a focus on societal or beneficiary outcomes, it becomes what is known as "social marketing" (Lee & Kotler, 2019). Psychologists are well-equipped with many of the essential "soft" marketing skills, such as creativity, communication, empathy, and problem-solving. Additionally, the "hard" marketing skills—such as data analysis, content creation, social media, and consultative selling—are increasingly part of the applied psychologist's toolkit. Marketing can be a powerful tool for psychologists in leadership roles, particularly in three key areas: segmenting client groups, outreach, and engagement.

Segmenting Client Groups

In our work with mental health teams, we've observed assumptions that certain client groups, such as those from the Afghan or Chinese diaspora, would never seek services. These groups weren't accessing primary care either. This reflects a common problem in service engagement. By breaking down the task of engagement into actionable, evidence-based steps, we can begin to address these challenges.

Every service, even those that seem homogeneous, should segment its client base to gain a deeper understanding of the people it serves. Segmentation can be based on demographics or the types of problems clients face. Larger organisations, such as secondary mental health services or professional bodies, require multiple segments to reflect the diverse challenges and perspectives of their target populations.

Once segments are identified, creating "customer personas" or profiles helps represent each group. These personas detail how a segment perceives its problems, what motivates them to seek change, the solutions they have already attempted, and whom they trust for advice (Jobber & Ellis-Chadwick, 2024).

Psychologists are well suited to lead this process due to their expertise in scientific research methods. One particularly effective approach is ethnography—the systematic study of people and cultures—which helps uncover cultural phenomena that influence service engagement, such as why certain groups may not access healthcare (Jobber & Ellis-Chadwick, 2024). Common ethnographic methods, including observations, interviews, focus groups, archival research, and life history interviews, offer valuable insights. Unlike traditional service user consultation groups, which often fail to capture those who do not engage with services, ethnographic research enables leaders to identify and address the barriers preventing full participation.

Outreach: Meeting Clients Where They Are

Customer personas can guide our outreach efforts by identifying where clients who aren't currently accessing services are most likely to go. For example, if a persona indicates that a segment is seeking help from their GP but isn't being referred, efforts can be focused on educating GPs and improving the referral process. Alternatively, for groups unlikely to visit a GP, outreach can involve building relationships with influential community members, schools, or social media platforms to spread awareness. Throughout the outreach process, success should be tracked using metrics and frameworks such as those offered by the East London Foundation Trust (2024).

Engagement: Removing Barriers and Enhancing Experience

Engagement goes beyond simply raising awareness; it involves removing barriers that prevent clients from accessing services. Marketing research indicates that even small "frictions" can become significant obstacles. For instance, a late appointment letter or limited public transport could be enough to prevent a client from attending. To improve engagement, customer personas can help identify and address these barriers, focusing on the most achievable first, before tackling more complex issues (Halpern, 2016).

Appreciating Client Experiences

A positive client experience is key to effective marketing, yet 71% of NHS mental health service users report dissatisfaction (Gilburt & Saoirsie, 2024), leading to disengagement and reputational harm. Creating detailed customer profiles helps align services with client needs, making marketing a tool for service improvement. Open Strategy frameworks facilitate co-creation with communities, using focus groups and a Quality Improvement (QI) approach to enhance engagement.

Despite resource limitations, even small improvements can have a significant impact. For example, one of the authors spoke with a mother who had a distressing experience with community paediatrics. Her challenges included long waiting times, short-notice appointments, inconvenient locations, unresponsive admin staff, and waiting areas that didn't accommodate her neurodivergent son. Had she faced just one additional barrier, such as financial constraints, she would have likely become a "Did Not Attend" statistic. As leaders, it is our ethical duty to address health inequalities by removing access barriers, ensuring services are inclusive, effective, and responsive to client needs.

Useful Marketing Resources

- Nudge podcast—https://www.nudgepodcast.com/
- The marketing meetup podcast—https://themarketingmeetup.com/podcast/
- The Business of Psychology podcast—https://psychologybusinessschool.com/the-business-of-psychology/

Thought Leadership

In the past, antibiotics might have been seen as a "nice to have," but a group of medical experts recognised their critical importance and advocated for their widespread use. Similarly, entrepreneurs often convince investors of the potential of untested ideas, using their vision to secure funding. These examples illustrate the power of "thought leadership" (Bendell & Kipping, 2018), which is the capacity to shape discourse by bringing alternative views, influencing and empowering others while enhancing the profession's visibility. Many of the skills required for thought leadership align closely with the core competencies of applied psychologists. So why, then, do we struggle to confidently claim authority in policy discussions or public discourse? It is beyond the scope of this chapter to fully investigate our professional psychology, but we must consider both confidence and platforms to influence. The medical profession's thought leadership is often the result of well-organised efforts by their professional bodies, with many medical professionals occupying influential positions in government. Our platform, and our willingness to step onto it, appear less secure and inconsistent.

Historically, thought leadership in psychology has been associated with figures like Freud, Skinner, Bandura, Rogers, and Seligman. Effective leadership in today's world requires a more diverse and contemporary range of voices that reflect evolving challenges and applications of psychology in a complex context. If every leader in psychology embraced the principles of thought leadership and cultivated these abilities in others, we could collectively elevate the profession and drive more radical change.

Many psychologists are already driving change, conducting innovative research, and implementing transformative practices. However, we have observed a widespread lack of confidence and fear of judgement that stifles their willingness to publish and engage publicly. This anxiety is understandable but limiting. If you are reading this book, you may have witnessed scenarios that illustrate this hesitation.

Unfortunately, this fear often leads psychologists to hold back from sharing their insights on public platforms. It is therefore essential for those in leadership positions to foster an environment where thought leadership can thrive—one that is safe, supportive, and compassionate. Mistakes should be expected and tolerated, and ideas should be celebrated. Creating structured platforms for expression and investing in training and mentoring can help build confidence, enhance visibility, and strengthen professional networks.

However, without strategic positioning, individual contributions risk remaining fragmented and underutilised. If more psychology leaders actively embraced thought leadership—by empowering others, engaging in public discourse, and confidently positioning their expertise—psychology could play a far greater role in shaping policy, practice, and the future of leadership itself.

Conclusion

Applied psychologists possess a wealth of skills that are essential for developing impactful strategies, influencing policy, and engaging with communities. We hope that this exploration of strategy development, economics, project management, and marketing has sparked new insights and inspiration for psychologists to leverage business skills in their leadership roles.

By integrating business principles—including strategic communication, financial and economic acumen, advocacy, and professional influence—psychologists can expand their leadership impact far beyond their immediate roles. Thought leadership is not about personal recognition alone; it is about ensuring psychology remains a driving force in shaping healthcare, policy, and organisational strategy.

Now is the time to harness these tools, not only to strengthen our practice but also to shape the future of the profession in an increasingly complex world.

Ideas in Brief

- Integrating psychological expertise with business acumen enhances leadership effectiveness, enabling the creation of values-driven, inclusive organisations that foster diversity and transform lives.
- Strategic thinking for sustainable services requires leaders to plan services ambidextrously—meeting current needs while proactively preparing for emerging future demands.
- Economic and business literacy equips leaders to advocate with decision-makers, engage communities, and design impactful services.
- Psychology has the potential for greater influence in shaping policy, practice, and leadership, ensuring the protection of value-driven, high-quality services.
- Psychologists have much to offer as thought leaders, ensuring psychology remains a powerful force in shaping healthcare, policy, and organisational strategy.

Note

1 Dr Rosie Gilderthorp.

References

Bendell, J., & Kipping, M. (2018). The power of thought leadership in business: From concept to reality. *Journal of Business Research, 70*, 80–92. Retrieved April 20, 2025, from https://doi.org/10.1016/j.jbusres.2016.10.002

East London NHS Foundation Trust. (2024). *QI at a glance*. Retrieved April 20, 2025, from https://qi.elft.nhs.uk/stories/

Gilburt, H., & Saoirsie, M. (2024). *Mental health 360: Quality and patient experience*. The King's Fund.

Gray, C. F., & Larson, E. W. (2020). *Project management: The managerial process* (8th ed.). McGraw-Hill Education.

Halpern, D. (2016). *Inside the nudge unit: How small changes can make a big difference*. Random House.

Hautz, J., Seidl, D., & Whittington, R. (2017). Open strategy: Dimensions, dilemmas, dynamics. *Long Range Planning, 50*(3), 298–309. https://doi.org/10.1016/j.lrp.2016.12.001

Heracleous, L., & Werres, K. (2016). On the road to disaster: Strategic misalignments and corporate failure. *Long Range Planning, 49*(4), 491–506. https://doi.org/10.1016/j.lrp.2015.08.006

Heracleous, L., Papachroni, A., Andriopoulos, C., & Gotsi, M. (2017). Structural ambidexterity and competency traps: Insights from Xerox PARC. *Technological Forecasting and Social Change, 117*, 327–338. https://doi.org/10.1016/j.techfore.2016.11.008

Highsmith, J. (2002). *Agile software development ecosystems*. Addison-Wesley Professional.

Humphrey, A. S. (2005). *SWOT analysis for management consulting*. SRI Alumni Association.

IBISWorld. (2023). *Hospitals in the UK*. Retrieved April 19, 2025, from https://0-my-ibisworld-com.pugwash.lib.warwick.ac.uk/uk/en/industry/q86.101/at-a-glance

Inside BE. (2024). *Inside behavioural economics: Database*. Retrieved April 19, 2025, from https://insidebe.com/database/

Jobber, D., & Ellis-Chadwick, F. (2024). *Principles and practice of marketing* (10th ed.). McGraw Hill.

Kerzner, H. (2017). *Project management: A systems approach to planning, scheduling, and controlling* (12th ed.). Wiley.

Lee, N. R., & Kotler, P. (2019). *Social marketing: Behavior change for social good*. Sage Publications.

Lord Darzi. (2024). *Independent investigation of the National Health Service in England*. GOV.UK. https://www.gov.uk/government/publications/independent-investigation-of-the-nhs-in-england

Mental Health Foundation & London School of Economics and Political Science. (2022). *The economic case for investing in the prevention of mental health conditions in the UK*. Mental Health Foundation. Retrieved from https://www.mentalhealth.org.uk/explore-mental-health/publications/economic-case-investing-prevention-mental-health-conditions-UK

NHS Confederation: Mental Health Network. (2023). *The economic and social costs of mental ill health*. Retrieved April 19, 2025, from https://www.centreformentalhealth.org.uk/wp-content/uploads/2024/03/CentreforMH_TheEconomicSocialCostsofMentalIllHealth.pdf

NHS England. (2023). *The NHS in England at 75: Report summary*. Retrieved April 19, 2025, from https://www.england.nhs.uk/long-read/the-nhs-in-england-at-75-report-summary/

Osterwalder, A., & Pigneur, Y. (2010). *Business model generation: A handbook for visionaries, game changers, and challengers*. Wiley.

Phillips, D. (2024). Health spending planned to fall in England and Scotland in 2024–25, suggesting a top-up likely. *The Institute for Fiscal Studies*. Retrieved March 4, 2024, from https://ifs.org.uk/articles/health-spending-planned-fall-england-and-scotland-2024-25-suggesting-top-likely

Project Management Institute. (2017). *A guide to the project management body of knowledge (PMBOK Guide)* (6th ed.). Project Management Institute.

Rosenhan, D. L. (1973). On being sane in insane places. *Science, 179*(4070), 250–258. https://doi.org/10.1126/science.179.4070.250

Stadler, C., Hautz, J., Matzler, K., & von den Eichen, S. F. (2021). *Open strategy: Mastering disruption from outside the C-suite*. MIT Press.

Statista. (2023). Private healthcare expenditure (including out-of-pocket and voluntary health insurance schemes) in the United Kingdom from 1997 to 2022 (in billion GBP). Retrieved March 2, 2024, from https://www.statista.com/statistics/317868/private-healthcare-expenditure-in-the-united-kingdom-by-sector/

The Health Foundation. (2011). Competition in healthcare. The Health Foundation.https://www.health.org.uk/sites/default/files/CompetitionInHealthcare.pdf

The Kings Fund, & Nuffield Trust. (2023). *Public satisfaction with the NHS and social care in 2022*. Retrieved April 19, 2025, from https://www.nuffieldtrust.org.uk/sites/default/files/2023-04/Public%20satisfaction%20with%20the%20NHS%20and%20social%20care%20in%202022_FINAL%20FOR%20WEB.pdf

Tufano, P. (2001). Financial innovation and first-mover advantage. *Journal of Financial Economics, 56*(2), 313–326. https://doi.org/10.1016/S0304-405X(00)00101-5

Womack, J. P., & Jones, D. T. (2003). *Lean thinking: Banish waste and create wealth in your corporation*. Free Press.

World Health Organization. (2016). *Investing in treatment for depression and anxiety leads to fourfold return*. Retrieved from https://www.who.int/news/item/13-04-2016-investing-in-treatment-for-depression-and-anxiety-leads-to-fourfold-return

Zhang, R., & Bohlen, J. (2023). Healthcare business budgeting. In *StatPearls* [Internet]. Treasure Island (FL): StatPearls Publishing. Retrieved January 7, 2025, from https://www.ncbi.nlm.nih.gov/books/NBK589707/

11

What Does Good Leadership Look Like?

Interview with a Leader

Professor Aimée Aubeeluck and Dr Elizabeth Jenkinson

Introduction

How can applying psychological principles and insights help us to grow as leaders? What impact can self-reflection, applied psychological expertise and transactional skills have on our development and trajectory? How are these journeys unique but often also have many common themes? Following on from Chapter 9, 'Fostering transactional business skills, creativity and psychological principles to lead well', the interview attempts to illustrate unique perspectives and experiences that we may have as leaders, as well as the use of transactional skills on the complex metrics of leadership in practice through a conversation with an experienced Health Psychologist and academic leader.

Dr Elizabeth[1] Jenkinson is a National Training Director for Health Psychology at NHS England and Associate Professor in Health Psychology at the University of the West of England. The conversation with Dr Jenkinson provides an authentic insight into what leading well looks like to her, how everyone has the potential to lead and the importance of believing in yourself and those around you. The importance of self-awareness, reflective practice and harnessing of strengths alongside seizing opportunities to grow are explored.

Dr Jenkinson draws on her education in Health Psychology, her exposure to other fields of psychology, her work within the NHS and Higher Education and her business acumen to lead well. She emphasizes the

DOI: 10.4324/9781003492399-14

importance of knowing oneself to coach, support and mentor others and draws upon her emotional intelligence to build trust and collaboration in the workplace. Her practitioner psychologist status provides her with an excellent understanding of human behaviour and the need to motivate others and build teams to increase productivity and organizational performance.

Aimee Aubeeluck: Thank You for Speaking with Me Today. Tell Us about Your Career Path and Leadership Journey.

Dr Elizabeth Jenkinson: Following my undergraduate Psychology degree, I wanted to work in the NHS or the charity sector with patients or their families. In the earlier stages of my career, I immersed myself in the NHS, in assistant psychologist posts in primary care and secondary NHS mental health services, applied research at Oxford University and worked in the charity sector, all while working in multidisciplinary teams. In these roles, I developed my leadership skills and was mentored by senior psychological practitioners and NHS leaders, many of whom still inspire my work today.

I moved into university-based research and lecturing in 2005 and completed my doctoral health psychology training in 2012. Since joining the University of the West of England, Bristol, I have held leadership roles in research, teaching and learning in health psychology, recently being promoted to Associate Professor. I am currently seconded to NHS England, leading the Health Psychology and Workforce Redesign Programme as the National Training Director for Health Psychology.

Aimee Aubeeluck: How Has This Breadth of Experience Contributed to Your Career Development?

There have been points in my career where I have felt more valued because of my broad understanding. However, sometimes it can also be hard to progress to the senior levels of leadership when you haven't got one obvious track. For me personally and professionally, I do feel my breadth of experience gives me a more credible and authentic kind of presence, bringing together a lot of different strands and skills that I've developed across a variety of different roles. The topics or the environment have been varied, but the skills I have all come together to inform my approach.

Aimee Aubeeluck: How Has Your Health Psychology-Specific Education and Training Underpinned Your Leadership Roles?

Dr Elizabeth Jenkinson: My health psychology training absolutely underpins my leadership approach and the roles that I have undertaken. You might not realize it at the time, but the competencies that you have to undertake for your training in health psychology provide the building blocks to have the confidence at a senior level and the skills that are required. I undertook a professional doctorate to become registered with the Health and Care Professionals Council (HCPC) as a Practitioner Psychologist and with the British Psychological Society (BPS) as a Chartered Psychologist.

The depth and breadth of learning from these qualifications are applied in every aspect of my work. For example, I utilize research skills and the evidence base to underpin my practice. Being competent in psychological intervention and behaviour change is a highly prized skill that organizations often seek to know to work more effectively.

I also use my consultancy skills in my current role, negotiating contracts and considering issues around data protection and ethics. I know that may not be a skill set covered in depth in all psychologists' training in applied psychology, but it is part of health psychologists' core training.

Aimee Aubeeluck: What Does 'Good Leadership' Look Like to You?

Dr Elizabeth Jenkinson: An important thing to me is to be authentic, credible and accountable for the work that I do.

As a leader, I think it's important to continuously develop your skills because we're not going to get things right all of the time. We will inevitably make mistakes, and I think we need to be accountable and think about how we could do things differently using reflective practice.

As a psychologist, compassion, empathy, respect and inclusivity are close to my professional heart. For me, it is important to lead with kindness and understanding to remember that we are role models for other people, even though it might not feel like it. I sometimes still feel like I am quite early on in my career, but many other people are looking up and across for mentorship or supervision. In that sense, you're showing people how to lead and how to supervise. In terms of the legacy of our profession and our teams, it's important to role model what you would like to see emulated. It's important to show balance as well. We've all worked hard to get where we are, but there is something powerful in role modelling work-life balance, showing that you know this is a job and that we all have responsibilities outside of work. That goes back to being authentic, to lead in a way that doesn't expect others to be putting in very long hours and compromising their own well-being.

There's a lot written about collaborative ways to lead, and that's important. You have an investment in the team's interests and the direction you are going. Having common goals and agreeing on what you're all working towards are essential. Sometimes that is built in. For example, in a research centre or an NHS team where you have key performance indicators you're all working towards. However, it might be less clear in some teams, so it becomes important to be working towards a goal that you all believe in and aspire to. There is also a place for individual contributions and individual goals. If we're only ever thinking about the 'we', we might miss the person who wants to progress and do something different. I think we need to communicate and discuss to make sure that team members feel they have the psychological safety to disagree or say, 'this isn't where I'm going'.

Aimee Aubeeluck: What Health Psychology-Specific and Other Related Models and Theories Do You Draw upon When You Are Leading Others?

Dr Elizabeth Jenkinson: Good communication skills and clinical skills like motivational interviewing, CBT or Socratic Questioning are all elements that I use. I use reflective practice as part of my involvement in qualitative psychological research. I think a lot about 'who I am', my positioning, what views and experiences I'm bringing to the table and how that might influence the way I respond to situations. I like reflective practice models that are very hands-on and used a lot in healthcare like Gibbs (1998), Rolf et al. (2001) and Schön (1991). These include many curious questions – what happened?

- How did you feel?
- What are you going to do differently in the future?
- What can I learn from this situation?
- How could I approach it differently next time?
- What are the thoughts and feelings that I'm having as a result?
- What is personal to me and what might be shared by others?

I also like the idea of self-efficacy and building it as a concept and as a leader. Particularly if I'm mentoring or supervising someone, I aim to make them feel that they have built confidence in their ability to engage in the actions required of their task.

Behaviour change models such as the COM-B (Michie et al., 2011) help us understand how people's capability, opportunity and motivation might drive their behaviour. If you're looking at behaviour change in organizations or with patients, learners or colleagues, you can explore it in a number of ways. Some of the questions to consider would include:

- Do they have the capability?
- Do they know how to do it?
- Do they have the motivation?
- Do they want to do it differently?
- Do they have the opportunity to change that?
- Do they have access to the tools they might need?
- Is this likely to happen, or is this less likely to happen?
- And if it's not likely to happen, how can we foster each of those elements to make behaviour change more likely?

The one thing I have used recently that isn't from health psychology but is more from the business world is Cope's (2012) Seven Cs of consultancy (Client, Clarify, Create, Change, Confirm, Continue, Close). It's a helpful model, especially if you're a new consultant, to help prompt certain conversations along the way. I've also used several change tools such as the Health Education England Star model (https://heestar.e-lfh.org.uk/) (HEE 2021) as part of my NHS workforce projects. It's interesting as some of the models and theories that you think of as psychology are models that other people think of as business models – there's a lot of overlap! Working in an NHS setting, you've got continuous improvement and lean/Six Sigma principles (Miller, 2005); such frameworks sit in that space where business meets psychology.

Aimee Aubeeluck: What Advice Would You Give to Others Interested in Leadership and Leading Well?

Dr Elizabeth Jenkinson: For someone just coming to leadership, I would say, you might never feel ready for it, but you have probably been leading already even if it's not in a formal role. We've usually led in our lives outside of work; maybe you run a home or lead a group. There are all kinds of things that you may have done; you've probably done more leadership than you think. It's about not being afraid and allowing yourself to grow into a role. You're not going to come fully formed as the leader you want to be. If you move into a leadership role, you can develop leadership skills, particularly if you reflect on where you may be least experienced and confident and seek out opportunities to develop.

Leadership training with peers is also important. I would recommend people consider going on some form of formal leadership training. I was able to do some leadership training with AdvanceHE (www.advance-he.ac.uk) which built my confidence and gave me some space for reflection with other people on their leadership journey. I found training specific to women in leadership particularly helpful – it's important to consider what might work best for you. It's also important to engage in reflective practice – I've mentioned this throughout. This comes very much from my psychology background. Engaging in reflective practice and continuing your professional development supports you to carry on learning about leadership and yourself as a leader.

Finally, take note of the practices of the leaders you aspire to be. Consider engaging in being mentored by those who have valuable experience and qualities you want to exude. Grow into a leader that you can be proud of.

Note

1 Dr Jenkinson is an experienced registered practitioner health psychologist (HCPC), chartered psychologist (BPS) and senior academic (SFHEA), skilled in clinical applications of health psychology, research, teaching, supervision and practice. Liz currently leads research, teaching and knowledge exchange at UWE, Bristol, as an associate professor, and leads innovation in Health Psychology at NHS England as the National Training Director for Health Psychology in Workforce Redesign.

References

AdvanceHE. (n.d.). *Advance HE.* Retrieved April 19, 2025, from https://www.advance-he.ac.uk

Cope, M. (2012). *The seven Cs of consulting* (3rd ed.). Prentice Hall.

Gibbs, G. (1988). *Learning by doing: A guide to teaching and learning methods.* Oxford Brookes University.

Health Education England (HEE). (2020). *The STAR model.* Retrieved April 19, 2025, from https://heestar.e-lfh.org.uk/

Michie, S., Van Stralen, M. M., & West, R. (2011). The behaviour change wheel: A new method for characterising and designing behaviour change interventions. *Implementation Science, 6*(1), 42. https://doi.org/10.1186/1748-5908-6-42

Miller, D. (2005). *Going lean in healthcare* (IHI white paper). Institute for Healthcare Improvement.

Rolfe, G., Freshwater, D., & Jasper, M. (2001). *Critical reflection for nursing and the helping professions: A user's guide.* Palgrave Macmillan.

Schön, D. A. (1991). *The reflective practitioner: How professionals think in action.* Ashgate Publishing.

PART THREE

PHOENIX LEADERSHIP

Navigating through Change, Renewal, and Transformation

12 A Model for Understanding Organisational Leadership and Change and Its Application in Health and Social Care

Professor Emeritus Tony Lavender

Introduction

The sheer amount of academic and professional literature on the topics of leadership and management can be rather overwhelming. Organisations are the places where most of us spend much of our working lives; they influence our sense of satisfaction with our lives and our purpose. They impact our wellbeing and sense of contribution to our communities and society. Given their importance, it is surprising that, as Mintzberg (1989) points out, we spend a lot of time planning to get out of them for holidays and eventually retirement. Organisations are essentially communities to which we should enjoy belonging, and which at their best, bring satisfaction and wellbeing to our lives (Rao et.al, 2021. If this is how you feel, then you don't have a problem; if it isn't, there is something to work on.

This chapter discusses a framework to understand organisational leadership and change. NHS England, in its current 2024/5 form, is put forward as an example, with a reference to the recent announcements by the Prime Minister in March 2025 to abolish the organisation. This model is, however, relevant to other settings outside NHS settings

DOI: 10.4324/9781003492399-16

(Burke & Litwin, 1992). In this chapter, I would also like to argue, in agreement with Mintzberg (2009), that we shouldn't underestimate the importance of management experience both in preparation for and in operating successfully in "organisational leadership" roles.

Organisational Boundaries

At its simplest, it is important to identify the organisational boundaries and what the internal and external environmental factors are that influence the functioning of the organisation. This can be rather more complicated than it might appear at first, although it remains important to understand. With the NHS, it is both an organisation subject to external forces that influence its functioning, including the state of the economy, globally and nationally (how much money the country has to potentially spend on healthcare), the political willingness of the party-controlled government to invest in that organisation (Darzi, 2024) and public opinions and perceptions of the service as a whole and particular aspects of the service (e.g. waiting times). These are but three factors that the NHS, as an organisation must seek to understand, respond to, and where possible, influence. If these are ignored or not worked with, the organisation would begin to operate like a "closed system", which quickly becomes maladaptive, unhealthy, and faces existential crises (Roberts, 2019). Whilst recognising that the organisational boundaries should not be impermeable, it is important to develop a working understanding of what is inside and outside the organisation (Roberts, 2019).

Organisational Model

Given the significance of organisations, and how there is usually a drive to try to change and improve them, it seems important to have a model of how they work. A model can help you to think about an organisation as a whole system and to locate your place in that system and where you can contribute. Psychologists operate with a variety of models about individuals and indeed families but less often about organisations. There are numerous models, but the model I have found most useful is that of Burke and Litwin (1992), which was developed to understand and help facilitate organisational change (Figure 12.1). They make an important distinction between the variables that influence "transformational

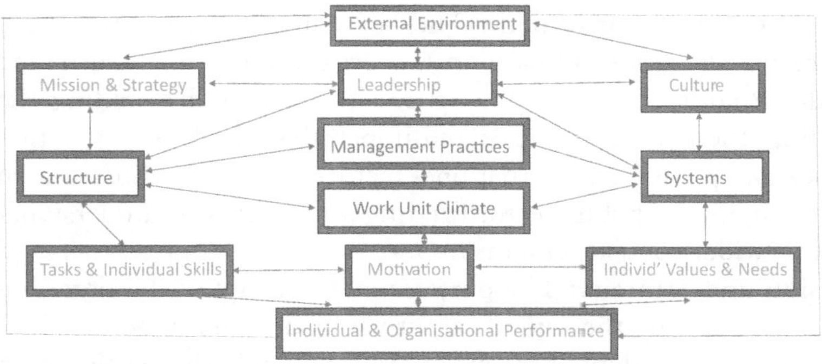

Figure 12.1 Burke and Litwin's causal model of organisational change.

change" and those that influence "transactional change", which in turn influence the "individual and personal" factors. Ultimately, these variables or factors impact on the performance of the organisation and its staff members. Burke and Litwin emphasise the significance of knowing which type of variables you are influencing and, therefore, what type of change processes you are likely to be engaged in.

The NHS is rife with talk about transformational change, but in Burke and Litwin's terms, much of it is transactional change. Transformational change occurs as a response to changes in the external environment that impact directly on the organisations' purpose, strategy, leadership, and culture.

The transactional factors of structure, management practices, systems, and climate are always impacted by transformational change but are extremely important in determining the motivation and wellbeing of staff and the effectiveness of organisations. *These internal organisational factors will not be transformative for the organisation.*

When trying to think organisationally, the first point to consider is what the organisation, or in systemic terms, what is the system? This is not as simple as may first appear, particularly in the NHS where Trusts/Health Boards are embedded in wider National NHS Organisations, but leaving this aside, for the purposes of this chapter I'm referring to a Trust/Health Board. So, what are these variables?

Transformation Variables

In Burke and Litwin's model, the transformational variables (Figure 12.1) include:

- **The External Environment:** The key external factors that have a direct and indirect impact on the organisation. For Trusts and Health Boards, it is the funding and the bodies distributing the funding, the national policies and imperatives, and the inspection bodies and processes. The national picture is clearly influenced, in the main, by the public sector funding settlements, so understanding this wider context remains important.
- **Mission and Strategy:** The purpose and strategy of the organisation, as agreed by the senior executives/board and understood by employees. The extent of employee engagement in the development of and knowledge about the purpose is significant in terms of meeting the purpose and delivering the strategy.
- **Leadership:** Organisational leadership refers to the direction provided by the executives and board to implement the strategy and display the values and behaviour that are espoused by the organisation. In understanding change processes in organisations, it is important to understand these leadership arrangements and how they work. It is worthy of note that effective leaders do not sit passively in relation to the external environment and do work to shape it by their influence on national policies and priorities.
- **Organisational Culture:** Put simply, this is "the way things are done around here". An organisational culture is the explicit as well as the implied rules, regulations, customs, principles, and values that influence organisational behaviour. Knowing an organisation's history is often a key to understanding how the culture has emerged and developed. Within NHS organisations, there is both a national and local perspective to consider.

The most important factor in terms of transformational change is the external environment. For the NHS, this has occasionally arisen when governments have considered if there are alternative ways to run things, such as transferring to an insurance-based funding model under PM Thatcher (Timmins, 1992), but the perceived popularity of the current funding model has always meant this was never implemented. Change in executive leadership can have transformative potential, especially if brought about by difficulties in the external environment (e.g. poor CQC ratings, financial failure). It is the "organisational leaders" appointed at the executive/board level whose job it is to work on these factors which, even if not resulting in transformational change, have a deeply significant impact on the transactional factors, the satisfaction of staff, and the effectiveness of the organisation.

It is for this reason that there has been increased recognition that without psychological professional appointments at an Executive/Board level (PPN, 2022) it is going to be difficult to influence and change the organisations to adopt and deliver more psychologically informed services that are called for by policy and by considering what should be happening if NICE Guidance were followed. Heads of Services do a remarkable job of trying to change things in this direction but are often limited (and I might add frustrated) by their organisational position. A symptom of this has been, and in some nations still is, the difficulties in establishing at a national level within the NHS Chief Psychological Officers. This is work in progress at a Trust/Health Board and national level but is important to continue so that services are better able to deliver the psychological interventions and psychologically informed culture that service users need and deserve.

These transformational variables are associated with "organisational leadership" and concern understanding the external environment and setting the vision, the values, and the strategy to deliver that vision. As stated in the PPN Discussion document (2021) management and leadership are terms that are often used interchangeably. Indeed, as Mintzberg (2007) points out, people in "organisational leadership" roles spend a good deal of their time managing. There are other individuals in positions where they manage people in the organisation, and indeed can act in ways that leaders should, for example acting in congruence with the espoused values, but this is not the same as holding formal organisational leadership roles. In the context of "organisational leadership", this attempt to emphasise the point that all staff are leaders can obscure the importance of the organisational hierarchy. Categorising all staff as leaders does not help improve our understanding of the processes of organisational change.

Transactional Variables

The heart of organisational management is what Burke and Litwin identify as the "transactional variables", and these are concerned with the delivery of the organisation's vision, values, and strategy. It is in this area of organisational management that most psychological professionals work, and it is vital both to the effectiveness of the organisation and to their development as potential organisational leaders. So, what are these variables:

- **Structure:** This refers to the arrangements of functions and people into particular areas with their associated levels of responsibility, authority, communication channels, and relationships to ensure the delivery of the strategy in a way that embraces the organisation's espoused values. How effective the management hierarchical structures are appropriate to deliver the organisational strategy is frequently brought into question and has been the subject of numerous NHS reorganisations since the first NHS reorganisation in 1974. Yes, the NHS went from 1948 to 1974 without a reorganisation but has been going through many structural reorganisations since.
- **Systems:** This refers to the policies and processes that enable the work and include the reward systems (remuneration and other types of reward), appraisal/job planning arrangements, management information systems, budget development arrangements and human resource allocation (including recruitment processes). The systems area covers many aspects, and care needs to be taken so that systems are reviewed, amended, and discarded when interfering with the effectiveness of the organisation.
- **Management Practices:** This is what managers do in the normal course of their work to enable the people and the use of physical resources to deliver the organisation's strategic goals. Whether managers are clear about what they are is often an interesting question. How managers go about supporting and encouraging staff in their work is key to the immediate "work climate" but also to the individual motivation of staff. We all probably have good and poor examples of this in practice.

There are opportunities for psychologists, and indeed many are, to get involved in each of these areas and help make the organisation a better place to work if done well. It seems important for psychologists to become involved in these areas (including managing staff and reviewing policies and processes) to both try to improve the effectiveness of the organisation and to further their understanding of how organisations work as preparation for taking up formal organisational leadership roles.

Individual Variables and Organisational Performance

Finally, the model involves individual/personal factors which include:

- **Climate:** This is a collective current, impression, feelings, and expectations of staff in a team/unit which affect their relationships with each other, with the team leader/manager, and with other teams. It is members' perceptions of how well the team/unit is managed and how effectively they work together on their collective task. Climate is more subject to change and variation than the culture, which is more enduring (Burke and Litwin, 1992). Psychologists can find themselves in roles as team managers or team members and can by their actions contribute to creating a positive and constructive climate. They can also get involved in helping to address climate issues as consultants/facilitators trying to improve teams' effectiveness in delivering the task and improving working relationships. Attempts to do this, if the psychologist is also a team member, are fraught with boundary difficulties, and it is almost certainly best with teams where the psychologist is not a member.
- **Tasks and Skills:** This involves the match between the job requirements and the ability/competence of the individual to meet those requirements, that is, how well jobs and employees have been matched. The processes of recruitment/selection are clearly important here, but so are the ongoing management and development processes. The psychologist, as a manager, needs to support staff post-recruitment to develop new competencies as the job evolves.
- **Motivation:** This is about the desire/drive of the individual to carry out the work and is impacted by all the factors in the model, but in the most immediate way by the individual needs and values. The manager has an important and direct impact on motivation, although outside work factors also come into play.
- **Individual Values and Needs:** This concerns the individual's values that make the job seem worthwhile (or not) and the psychological needs that influence their desire to do the job. It is a dimension that is concerned with the staff member's opinion about their work and the quality of the work context. The influence of an individual's background on their values and opinion of their work is important for the manager to be aware of to understand their motivation.

In the end, the **Individual and Organisational Performance** is what counts. All organisations have indicators of performance, at individual and organisational levels, in key areas like productivity, quality, efficiency, budget, and client and staff satisfaction. For individuals, it is often discussed and judged at appraisals/job planning processes. For NHS organisations, many performance indicators are externally set by the Government or the NHS Executive. There are external quality checks through the CQC and by commissioners in terms of fulfilling contracts. There are also internal organisational indicators agreed upon at the Board level. Psychologists need to understand these organisational performance indicators, whether or not they are interested in organisational leadership roles, in order to improve their understanding of the organisation and how they might individually contribute to that performance.

Model in Action: The NHS

NHS Boundaries, Organisational Leadership, Mission, and Culture

In the next section, an attempt is made to use the model to understand how the NHS in England works as an organisation.

The question is how to delineate the boundaries of the NHS and its associated organisations. It is helpful to start this process by understanding how the NHS works, including the key structures and organisations that make up the NHS. There are differences in arrangements between England and the other UK nations, and here, for illustration purposes, I will refer to those in England. Unlike most organisations, the Head is a political appointment in the form of the Secretary of State for Health and Social Care in England, operating through the Department of Health (DoH) and National Health Service England (NHSE). The boundaries of the NHS include these top structures and all the organisations that fall under these structures (see below).

When looking at Organisational Leadership, it is usual to identify the leader most often called a Chief Executive Officer (CEO), but the NHS arrangements are less straightforward. The Department of Health is led by a Permanent Secretary (a civil servant) who reports to the Secretary of State. NHSE is led by a CEO who is also considered to be a civil servant recruited because of their leadership and management expertise and knowledge of the Health Service. NHSE has a number of Directorates (Transformation, Education and Training, etc.) which are managed by the CEO.

This somewhat divided leadership is not what is seen in most organisations and the Head is a minister, an elected MP who is at the heart of Government in that they are a member of the ruling cabinet. They are thus operating across the NHS boundary with a dual role as both leader of NHS and Social Care and a member of a cabinet whose task is to run all aspects of the country, including the economy. The amount of funds made available to the NHS is a political decision made with the involvement of the minister but powerfully affected by the decisions of the Treasury, as Darzi (2024) has eloquently pointed out. It is vital that the Minister as the ultimate leader of the service manages this boundary effectively.

The mission/strategy for the NHS is ultimately the responsibility of the Secretary of State but is developed with advice from both DoH and NHSE. It is primarily NHSE's responsibility to deliver that mission/strategy. The mission of the NHS is defined in the NHS constitution. The mission is contained in the first line of the constitution: *"It is there to improve our health and wellbeing, supporting us to keep mentally and physically well, to get better when we are ill and, when we cannot fully recover, to stay as well as we can to the end of our lives"*. An ambitious goal for an organisation that sets the size of the task considerably larger than any other organisation in the UK.

In terms of the intended culture, it is also contained in the NHS constitution (DoH, 2012) embedded in the seven stated principles:

- comprehensive service for all,
- access based on clinical need, not ability of the individual to pay,
- aspires to high standards of excellence and professionalism,
- patients at the heart of everything done,
- works across organisational boundaries,
- providing best value to taxpayers,
- accountable to the public, communities, and patients it serves.

and six values:

- working together for patients,
- respect and dignity to all,
- commitment to quality care,
- compassion is central to care,
- improve health and wellbeing of all,
- everyone counts.

These principles and values sit alongside the rights and responsibilities of the population served and staff delivering the service within the constitution. These are clearly the "espoused" values of the service, but the extent to which those are evident "in action" in the organisations (Leavitt, 1988) is the profound issue of how it feels to be a staff member or a patient within the service. As Leavitt has pointed out, it is not that there won't be a "gap" between the "espoused" and "in action" values, but the size of that gap that needs careful scrutiny.

An attempt has been made, in the recent announcement by the Prime Minister (March 2025), to address the split organisational leadership at the top of the NHS. The decision is that over the next two years, NHSE will be abolished and the Department of Health and Social Care will become part of the organisation solely responsible for the organisational leadership of the NHS. This will put the politicians even more accountable for the NHS, and they will need to ensure that some of the functions crucial to the leadership of the NHS, which rest in NHSE in 2025, move to the newly formed Department. This would include the Chief Professional Officers, including the Psychological Professions Leadership Officer. It is hoped that this restructure will at least clarify the organisational leadership of the NHS.

At a national level, it is also important to mention two other organisations. First, the Care Quality Commission (CQC), which is intended to assess and report on the quality of care in the service delivery organisations and has recently been strongly criticised (Darzi, 2024). Second, the National Institute for Clinical Excellence (NICE), which evaluates treatments/interventions in terms of clinical and cost-effectiveness and decides whether these can be provided by the NHS. These are likely to be subject to some reform but are planned to continue in the post-2025 NHS restructure.

If, as the model indicates, there is to be a transformation in the services, it needs to be led and supported by the above structures. The call that Darzi (2024) has made for the transformation of service delivery away from the emphasis on hospital care to prevention, public health, and primary and community care potentially heralds a major shift in the operational focus of the NHS within the existing vision and values.

The mission/strategy is usually operationalised in plans for the NHS produced by NHSE, frequently called an NHS Long Term Plan, and subsequently supported by an NHS Workforce Plan. This usually covers a 10-year period, and such a plan is due in 2025. Underneath these national structures are the NHS organisations, funded by the NHS and responsible for ensuring the delivery of the national Plans. These are primarily the seven NHSE Regional Teams, the Integrated Care Systems (ICSs) and associated Partnerships and Boards, the Primary Care Networks, General Practices, Local Authorities (for Public Health), NHS Trusts, and other providers of services (voluntary, community, and private) (Powell, 2023; NHSE, 2024). This is a highly complex system, and each of these organisations can be understood by using the model, but it seems important to maintain an understanding of the whole NHS system when trying to make sense of the role of the constituent organisations.

Provider Organisations

The difficulty for the Ministerial and NHSE leaders is ensuring that the all the provider organisations deliver operationally the NHS's vision, values and strategic plan (DoH&SC, 2025). Darzi (2024) made the point that the NHS does not need to have another restructure, but the parts need to work together more coherently. This seems to have been taken on board in the current 10 Year Plan (DoH & SC, 2025). Many of these organisations, including the large NHS Trusts, attempt to develop their own vision, values, and strategies which are not necessarily well linked to the overall NHS vision, values and strategies. This problem was made worse by the creation of the purchaser-provider divide and the adoption of a market philosophy where these provider organisations were encouraged to see themselves as separate businesses competing with one another for NHS business. The recent changes under the latest Health and Social Care Act (2022), with the creation of ICSs, which have the responsibility to develop a delivery plan for the region for which they are responsible, are a move to enable the provider organisations to work together to deliver the NHS's vision, values, and strategy rather than competing with each other for NHS business.

The challenge for the NHS will be for the provider organisations, with their current leadership arrangements of the CEOs and Board level appointments to act less as separate businesses and more as organisations concerned with the operational delivery of a coherent NHS Strategy/Plan. In terms of the organisational model, their role is not in the setting of the vision, values and strategy but the delivery of the transformation of services, originally outlined in the Darzi report (2024), and now made concrete in the 10 Year Strategic Plan for England (DoH & SC, 2025). Essentially, it is their role amongst the transactional variables that will deliver the transformational vision/strategy.

Conclusions

When thinking about organisations and organisational change, it is helpful to have an organisational model to understand the whole system. It is also useful to understand how the "organisational leadership" is working and addressing the transformational variables in the model. The big picture of the whole system can be lost in the eyes of the public, many of the staff, and indeed the delivery organisations where the majority of staff work. For all staff, the most important work is acting in a way that is congruent with the NHS values, vision, and strategy. Darzi (2024) has produced a report with a thorough analysis of how well the NHS is working and has given some strategic pointers about what is required to improve matters. It is clear that the advice and recommendations need to be listened to and embedded in the 2025 NHS Plan if the NHS is to live up to the aspirations in its constitution.

Ideas in Brief

- Consider the whole organisation using the model and its boundaries.
- Understand the external influences on the organisation.
- Consider whether you are trying to understand the "organisational leadership" addressing "transformational variables" (external environment, stratagem, senior leadership group and culture) or the type of leadership and management shown by managers and staff in the delivery of the "transactional variables".
- When trying to change organisations, at any level, remember it requires a team or group of like-minded individuals.

Acknowledgement

Thanks to Assistant Professor Manu Melwyn Joy from the Ilihia School of Management Studies, Kerala, India, for his permission to use the figure of the model in this chapter.

References

Burke, W. W., & Litwin, G. H. (1992). A causal model of organisational performance and change. *Journal of Management, 18*(3), 523–545.

Darzi, (2024). Independent Investigation of the National Health Service in England. Department of Health and Social Care. London.

Department of Health. (2012). *The NHS constitution*. Department of Health.

Department of Health & Social Care. (2025). *Fit for the Future: The 10 Year Health Plan for England*. Crown Publications.

Leavitt, B., & March, J. G. (1988). Organisational learning. *Annual Review of Psychology, 14*, 319–340.

Mintzberg, H. (1989). *Mintzberg on management: Inside our strange world of organisations*. The Free Press.

Mintzberg, H. (2009). *Managing*. Financial Times Prentice Hall.

National Health Service England. (2024). *The structure of the NHS*. National Health Service England. https://www.england.nhs.uk/long-read/structure-of-the-nhs/

Powell, T. (2023). *The structure of the NHS in England*. House of Commons Library. https://researchbriefings.files.parliament.uk/documents/CBP-7206/CBP-7206.pdf

Psychological Professions Network. (2021). *Leadership and management in the psychological professions: Discussion paper*. Psychological Professions Network.

Psychological Professions Network. (2022). *Psychological professions representation on mental health trust boards: Discussion paper*. Psychological Professions Network.

Rao, A., Lavender, T., Bhutani, G., Farndon, H., Neal, A., & Waites, B. (2021). *Leadership development and support for clinical psychologists in health and social care*. DCP/BPS.

Roberts. V. G. (2019). The organisation at work: Contributions from open systems theory. In A. Obholtzer & V. G. Roberts (Eds.), *The unconscious at work: A Tavistock approach to making sense of organisations* (2nd ed.). Routledge.

Timmins, N. (1992). *The five giants: A biography of the welfare state*. Harper-Collins.

13 A View from the Inside

Leading as a Psychologist in Times of Conflict

Dr Adrian Neal and Dr Kathryn Walters

Introduction

This chapter has been written for personal and professional reasons. It is an opportunity to make sense of a number of connected and significantly challenging workplace experiences in the context of multi-layered organisational change and conflict. We aim to share our learning, which is ongoing, around how we all might navigate similar challenges. The chapter is centred on a *case study* of an organisation in a state of change and conflict, but specifically focuses on a series of workplace experiences including formal processes that felt atypical even for psychologists with decades of combined experience in senior leadership roles. We also draw on the Job-Demand Resource Model (JD-R) (Bakker & Demerouti, 2007) and Systems Leadership (Macdonald, Burke, & Stewart, 2024) for sense making.

Central to this chapter is a recognition that leadership roles within healthcare settings such as the NHS are commonly more psychosocially demanding than their job descriptions indicate. In our opinion, they often involve unacknowledged emotional load and labour, as well as cognitive and social demands. These demands rarely come with an adequate range of resources or preparation, and as such, the toll on personal wellbeing can be high. We will also reflect on the reality that, as a professional group, given that the pressure to adhere to organisational processes is ever present, we tend not to pause and ask what the *work* of leadership is, let alone understand its many demands and what resources

DOI: 10.4324/9781003492399-17

we may need to be both effective and sustain ourselves in often (intentionally and/or unintentionally) hostile organisational climates.

It seems that in the high-pressure and financially challenged organisations, the psychosocial work of leadership (i.e., that relating to people, social groups, and internal psychological processes) is often undervalued and possibly even rejected in favour of transactional processes and control. Yet, as psychologists it is this aspect of work (psychosocial) that we consider to be the priority. Direct experience of this dissonance can be a challenge for psychologists as leaders, as it can threaten our values, activate moral distress, trigger outrage, and/or leave us feeling lost and demoralised. We believe that this dissonance needs acknowledgement, and the imbalance addressed in order to mitigate risks posed to our organisations, ourselves, and the services we deliver. In an age where compassionate leadership is in the narrative of virtually every NHS organisation, there seems to be a marked risk of not talking about the elephant in the room; that is how NHS cultures are inherently psychosocially hostile, and that compassion is very difficult to embed and maintain.

This chapter will identify the key themes to emerge from the authors' lived experience of the issues outlined in the case study, and we will discuss how this relates to a deeper understanding of the work of psychologists as leaders.

Context

Set within a large NHS organisation, within a specialist clinical service of over 1000 people, over 18 months, the case study is mostly centred around a leadership team but expands to include the wider system and maps the impact of the implementation of a series of performance management processes. Historically, the clinical service had been performing well and was award-winning. It had a stable and consistent leadership team and well-established organisational structures.

Case Study

In response to concerns raised to senior organisational leadership, an entire service was required to undergo a rapid programme of service improvement. The clinical service leadership team was required to deliver on specific targets over a predetermined timeline. The clinical leaders were put under significant pressure for the duration of the process, making it difficult for them to feel valued or safe in their roles, and all were consistently overworked to the detriment of their health and wellbeing. In spite of this, improvement targets were met within the agreed timeline.

The impact of the improvement process was felt keenly by many members of the clinical service and was characterised by increased sick leave, feelings of occupational burnout, and demoralisation. Several staff left, citing the change process as the reason for leaving. For many, the experience was bewildering, and there was a strong sense that the intervention was not proportionate to the concerns. There was little direct acknowledgment of the impact on dozens of staff in the service, and this undoubtedly made the situation challenging for new members of the clinical leadership team.

Themes

"It's the How, as Much as the Why"

Formal corporate processes, be they disciplinary, performance, or organisational change in focus, are needed to support governance, standards, improvement, and patient safety. What we have seen in this instance is that it is *how* these processes are implemented that is fundamental. Moreover, the way processes are implemented can shape how they are experienced as well as how effective they are in achieving their intended aims. In our experience, the *how* can be critical in mitigating or exacerbating unintended negative impacts on both individuals and the wider system. The *"how"* can also be seen as a credible resource to mitigate some of the demands of formal processes.

As psychologists and leaders, it can be personally and professionally challenging, particularly if we are powerless to influence how these processes are implemented. Witnessing the many often small examples of what we might consider failures to understand social and emotional processes can trigger moral, values, relational, and emotional conflict. It can challenge the psychological contract (Cullinane & Dundon, 2006) we hold with our employer and even lead to questions about the purpose of our work and our own worth and identity. Unchecked, it can also trigger a deeper demoralisation and sow seeds of uncertainty relating to our own efficacy as a leader. What's more, bearing witness to these experiences can create a vicarious impact.

Imbalance, Power, and Control

All NHS organisations are complex, hierarchical, bureaucratic systems, with issues of power, politics, and control ever-present features of their landscapes. For the most part, these features however are just that and are taken for granted, even considered benign. The experiences outlined in the case study, however, put the reality of power and control (and lack of control) into stark focus, especially when they are experienced suddenly and an imbalance is created, whether intentional or not. For those directly involved, or even as bystanders, it can be hard not to experience this type of use of power in any way other than as threatening.

Of particular concern was how the power of a small group was quickly and consistently imposed over others within a system where the values of collaboration, equality, and fairness were held close. What's more, the experience of the sudden loss of power and control (or personal agency) was witnessed to be both confusing, destabilising, and again hard not to experience as a threat. In this situation, information (e.g. details as to why the improvement process was needed and the nature of the concerns raised about the leadership group) or the withholding of information appears to have exacerbated the experience and fostered a growing sense of powerlessness and lack of safety. Other factors that compounded the imbalance were the lack of clarity about the timeline, the outcome of the improvement process, whether there were capability issues that still needed to be investigated, and the struggle to have the voices of individuals heard without overt authorisation (i.e. invitation and permission) from the senior organisational leaders who initiated the process. One can imagine many of these failings were unintentional; however, the result was a deep suspicion that they were not. As psychologists, we know that once our threat centre is activated, we will see more evidence to support the idea that threat is present.

A central dilemma for psychologists who are leaders faced with this type of situation is how they might stay true to their values and the evidence base, with reduced capacity to influence (i.e.: soft power). Aside from the personal discomfort linked to bearing witness, there is again potential for experiencing a professional challenge that threatens self-efficacy and sense of purpose. For leaders who lead by empowering others to have ownership, autonomy, and control (all components of transformative leadership models such as compassionate leadership), to do rather than be done to, this experience may trigger acute conflict leading to the question: can we actually lead when there is an overt imbalance of power across the hierarchy of an organisation?

This experience also forces us as psychologists and leaders to ask, do we need to move away from our values to become more like those in authority to survive? Do we need to become more aggressive in our use of power and control to be effective in the NHS? Or put more succinctly, do we need to fight fire with fire? And if so, what does this mean for our finely tuned morals and values?

The Impact on Individuals

Experiencing psychological distress is not unusual while working as a clinician; the work exposes the professional to the extremes of the human condition, i.e., pain, suffering, loss, death, and disease. The work is demanding but can also be rewarding, and these demands or stressors are predictable, so by and large, they can be managed.

However, a major source of stress associated with working in the NHS is called "secondary stressors" (Williams et al., 2019) or factors not directly associated with clinical work. Secondary stressors take many forms but can include demands linked to organisational processes, including record keeping, bureaucracy, and formal processes such as formal HR investigations. We also know that such processes, if poorly carried out, will result in a range of psychosocial harms to both the individual investigated and the organisation (Neal et al., 2023).

The impact on key individuals at the centre of the case study has been significant. There has also been a marked impact across the wider service. Confidence has been damaged, and anxiety, fear, and suspiciousness have been activated. Those at the centre of the case study described this as a life-changing experience, where paths to recovery remain unclear. Looking more widely, we have seen harm to local culture and loss of trust across the service, including in the new leadership. Psychological Safety (Edmondson & Bransby, 2023) that has taken years to build has been damaged. For some, hope has been questioned and put into doubt. Morale and motivation have been impacted, and many have left the organisation, citing disillusionment and feeling unsafe. The *relational glue* helping to keep the many systems within the service connected seemed to be under immense stress. The psychologists working in this context are not immune to the impact. Psychologists whose work it is to lead again find themselves in conflict, observing the impact, feeling powerless to prevent it, yet still needing to lead by example. The work of leadership in this context becomes both unclear and in itself conflict-triggering, with the pull to survive, protect, and seek justice all competing. Moral distress (Morley, Ives, & Irvine, 2017) is inevitable and cannot but impact the wellbeing of the system.

Loss

In many cases, workplace change is framed as a logical process, one that focuses on strategy, numbers, and outcomes. However, for the recipients of such change, the experience is not purely rational. When the familiar structure and routines of a workplace are disrupted, it can feel like a loss of stability, identity, and sometimes purpose. It can also feel like a professional and relational loss. The professional loss speaks to our identities in work (and outside too), often honed over many years' service, and central to our definitions of who we are. Relational loss, in the context of organisational change, refers to the loss or disruption of interpersonal relationships, connections, and the sense of community that employees can experience within their workplace. These relationships are often the emotional glue that binds individuals to a particular organisational culture. Employees can build strong, sometimes even familial relationships with their colleagues over the years. When these emotional connections are disrupted or threatened, it can create feelings of loneliness, isolation, or anxiety, especially for those who relied on those bonds for support and professional growth. It is also upsetting to see those we value professionally being criticised and/or undermined.

At a personal level, there has been recognition of the gamut of negative emotions triggered during a change process, including anger, scepticism, despair, and paranoia/irrational fears – Am I next?

The psychological effects of organisational change can also be mapped onto the stages of grief; people do not simply "adjust" to change; they react to it. They mourn what has been lost, struggle with feelings of uncertainty, and, eventually, adapt to new realities. Elizabeth Kubler-Ross's five stages of grief model (1969) i.e., denial, anger, bargaining, depression, and acceptance, is a helpful model that largely captures the authors' personal experiences.

The concepts of status and identity in the context of organisational change are crucial to understanding how employees navigate such change. Status refers to the position or standing someone holds within a social group, like a workplace, while identity pertains to how an employee sees themselves in relation to their role, values, and the organisational culture. These factors are often at risk during times of significant change. If status and identity are threatened, it can lead to negative emotions already described, as well as feelings of insecurity, confusion, and catastrophic thinking (i.e., is the end of my career?) with an increased sense that one's role may become irrelevant, invisible, or devalued. There is also an impact on the future professional sense of self, with questions such as "What will others say about me?", "What will I do next?", and "Will I be credible?" becoming predictable sequelae.

For psychologists working within a corporate function, observing these processes and the impact can be distressing and, in extreme cases, trigger a sense of loss born out of the dissonance between personal and corporate values and expectations. Not dissimilar to the mechanisms underpinning moral distress, bearing witness can lead to a realisation that the organisation and its leaders may not be what or who they were assumed to be. This can lead to a loss of respect and, in some instances, a loss of hope, especially if there is a history of strong attachment and contribution to the organisation and its leadership.

The Legacy of Unresolved Issues

Following the experience of this form of organisational change (i.e., after the formal process has ended), there remains a strong sense of needing to "keep going" even when there remains little clarity as to why the initial change was initiated. The invitation, and sometimes the necessity, to return to business as usual while holding the unresolved is something all psychologists in senior leads will experience to varying degrees. Trying to function in a senior role while holding unanswered questions (e.g., Was this process necessary, or even deliberate? Was there due consideration of the impact it would have? And will there be any opportunity for reflection and learning?) can be demoralising and deeply frustrating. What's more, many of the strategies we know can help to manage uncertainty, such as focussing on one's own role, establishing relationships with allies, accessing mentors or sponsors, and trying to reinforce one's own values and skills, let alone consider one's future, all seem to be less effective when you are embroiled in layers of unresolved uncertainty.

Trust is the cornerstone of any workplace, and when there is a sense that it has eroded at a senior level, it can create a psychotoxic work environment and social climate. When trust in senior leaders diminishes, it's often because a change process was poorly communicated, misunderstood, or perceived as self-serving. In relation to communication around implementing organisational change, it is our view that specificity is crucial as it allows for greater clarity and focus, measurable outcomes, accountability, risk mitigation, and perhaps most importantly, collaborative employee buy-in. It is incumbent on those seeking to implement change to provide specificity, and also to listen to those who have to implement the change; not doing so can create a long and wasteful legacy.

Advocating for more transparency and open communication could be a way to create a bridge between senior leaders and staff, but it requires trust and a belief that the leaders will engage openly and have a willingness to learn. Without that, it can be a battle to maintain motivation and good faith. Given this, we find ourselves asking what it mean to "move on" and to find acceptance? We are also left asking what a restorative process for those caught up in the maelstrom of an imposed change process might look like when senior leaders are not motivated to reflect or learn.

Discussion

What Is the Work of Moving Forward?

Moving forward after trust and confidence in the organisation have been damaged is a complex and challenging process. We suggest that a helpful approach should include:

Recognition of impact and also of the work done during the organisational change is essential. Ideally, this requires open conversations where all parties are motivated to take responsibility for their actions and where it is safe to express feelings of anger, sadness, and disappointment.

Commitment to the people within the process. Too often in large organisations, change processes are implemented in a "firefighting" way, and the organisational lens quickly moves on to the next perceived problem. We must do what we can to maintain focus on the human experience of change. Bridge's Transitional model of change (1991) could help as it focuses on the internal psychological processes (transitions) needed to successfully engage in any external changes.

Restoration and rebuilding of expectations, relationships, and ultimately trust should centre on the acceptance that change for some has been negative. This will involve working together to create a shared vision and set of expectations. The need for *restoration* should be accepted as inevitable and embraced as soon as a change process is initiated.

Preparedness: As clinicians who have become leaders, senior psychologists will inevitably occupy spaces shared by colleagues with little or no or little clinical background, often with differing cultural (organisational) values, motivations and expectations. This will be exacerbated at times of extreme financial and political challenge. Importantly, there may also be differences in how these groups define leadership and management. Psychologists who are leaders will most likely be exposed to experiences that create both internal and external conflict. Navigating these experiences while keeping true to one's moral compass is potentially part of the work of leadership, though psychologists may find this an especially distinctive challenge and will need to find ways of preparing in advance and strategically choosing which resources will help.

Knowing we can leave. A relationship with an employer can be like any other relationship: powerful, containing, enriching, but it can also become hostile, dismissive, and even abusive. Given the power differential within large organisations, feeling powerless, without agency, and needing to be passive to survive is common. In these circumstances, it is important that we consider leaving the relationship as an active option in order to protect our own wellbeing (particularly our agency, self-worth, and identity) to limit further exposure to harm rather than see it as a retreat, a sign of weakness, or as shameful.

Ideas in Brief

- Our psychological contract with our employer is a powerful predictor of our engagement.
- Managing both inter- and intra personal conflict is a primary function of leadership.
- As leaders, psychologists may be exposed to corporate behaviour that creates moral distress.
- Unwanted changes in our working life can lead to strong emotions, including loss, grief, and hopelessness.

- The Job Demand-Resource model indicates that the psychosocial demands associated with organisational change are distinct from those linked to day-to-day occupational activity; as such the resources needed during times of conflict and change will also be different.
- Systems leadership indicates that work comprises social, commercial, and Technical activity. Corporate management may not automatically prioritise the social dimension of work as psychologists do.

References

Bakker, A. B., & Demerouti, E. (2007). The job demands-resources model: State of the art. *Journal of Managerial Psychology, 22*(3), 309–328. https://doi.org/10.1108/02683940710733115

Bridges, W. (1991). *Managing transitions: Making the most of change.* Addison Wesley.

Cullinane, N., & Dundon, T. (2006). The psychological contract: A critical review. *International Journal of Management Reviews.* July. https://doi.org/10.1111/j.1468–2370.2006.00123.x

Edmondson, A. C., & Bransby, D. P. (2023). Psychological safety comes of age: Observed themes in an established literature. *Annual Review of Organizational Psychology and Organisational Behavior, 10*, 55–78. https://doi.org/10.1146/annurev-orgpsych-120920-055217

Kubler-Ross, E. (1969). *On death and dying.* Macmillan.

Macdonald, I., Burke, C., & Stewart, K. (2024). *The work of management: A leader's guide to applying systems leadership* (1st ed.). Routledge.

Morley, G., Ives, J., & Irvine, F. (2017). What is 'moral distress'? A narrative synthesis of the literature. *Nursing Ethics, 26*(3). https://doi.org/10.1177/0969733017724354

Neal, A., Cooper, A., Waites, B., Bell, N., Race, A., & Collinson, M. (2023). The impact of poorly applied human resources policies on individuals and organisations. *British Journal of Healthcare Management, 29*(5), 112–121. https://doi.org/10.12968/bjhc.2022.0130.

Williams, R., & Kemp, V. (2019). Caring for healthcare practitioners. BJPsych Advances, 25(5), 334–343. https://doi.org/10.1192/bja.2019.66

14 Large Scale Change and Communities of Practice

Development of the Psychological Professions Network

Gita Bhutani, Liz Kell, and Clare Baguley

Introduction and Context

Historically, the Psychological Professions (PPs) have not had a single identity nor been recognised in service development nor workforce planning as a specific group significantly contributing to healthcare. This is despite the development of stepped models of care, such as NHS Talking Therapies, and the development of new practitioner roles, which have contributed to currently nineteen different roles within the PP taxonomy. In addition, the PP workforce has significantly expanded in size over the past 15 years (Health Education England, 2021; National NHS Talking Therapies Workforce Report, 2023) and patient/service users' surveys (Mind, 2024; NHS Digital, 2024) consistently highlight access to psychological therapies and interventions as an area of growing demand and need. This presents a challenge to the provision and development of health services alongside policies highlighting the need for 'parity of esteem' between physical and mental health (Department of Health, 2011; National Audit Office, 2023; National Audit Office Response to report, 2024). Traditional leadership and management structures do not routinely include PPs, and consistent leadership across PPs is often limited.

Prior to the development of the Psychological Professions Network (PPN), there were no fora for PPs to meet across professional or service setting boundaries. Professional bodies rarely acted in consort or with

DOI: 10.4324/9781003492399-18

a unified voice. Consequently, the voice for the PPs was fragmented and largely unheard. The challenge for the founders of the PPN and their allies was how to unify, grow and develop this voice. Initial conversations within the professional groups focused on 'how can we be heard?' which led to identifying a shared vision of why this is necessary. Subsequently, the aim identified for the PPN is how the benefits of the psychological professions can be maximised in the delivery of health and care to the public. Meeting this challenge has required change at many different levels within the public system of health and care. Leadership in this area requires a collaborative approach to bring this together. This chapter focuses on England only due to the devolved healthcare systems within the UK.

A Theoretical Approach

Key theoretical concepts underpinned the development of the PPN. These included the principles around Large Scale Change with the development of Driver Diagrams, Distributed Leadership and Communities of Practice. These support leadership enacted outside formal structures.

Large Scale Change

Large Scale Change (LSC) emerged conceptually from a recognition that health care has become increasingly more complex. Consequently, efforts to plan healthcare as a series of tasks that can be defined within a component, linear system will not work (Plsek & Greenhalgh, 2001). Instead, 'complex adaptive systems' are described that address the challenges of health care complexity. Several key features of complex adaptive systems are outlined. These include a recognition that participants in a system and the system itself are adaptive, and these systems are embedded within other systems and will co-evolve. This contributes to tensions that may not be resolved but can result in positive outcomes (e.g. variation in infection rates in hospitals can contribute to developing knowledge), as well as inherent non-linearity and unpredictability. All these features, alongside the interactions between 'agents' or participants in the system, will lead to emerging, novel behaviour (Plsek & Wilson, 2001).

Large scale change is the process of mobilising a large collection of individuals, groups and organisations towards a vision of a fundamentally new future state, by means of:

- *Key themes that can make a big difference*
- *A shift in power and a more distributed leadership*
- *Comprehensive and active engagement of stakeholders*
- *Mutually reinforcing changes in multiple systems and process*(NHS England, 2018)

Figure 14.1 Definition of large scale change in healthcare (NHS England, 2018).

The principles have been applied in healthcare, business, education and social movements (Best et al., 2012; Ganz, 2010; NHS England, 2018) (see Figure 14.1).

Implementation results in multiple activities across a range of settings, groups and individuals. The LSC model (Figure 14.2) shows the iterative processes required.

Typically, the outcomes are not precisely predictable due to the complexity of the programme. Repeated iterations may be required to

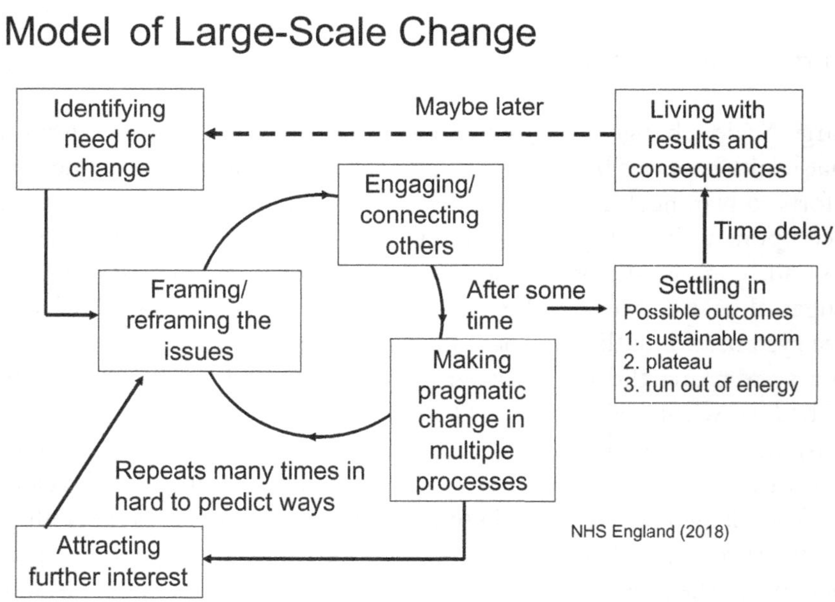

Figure 14.2 Model of large scale change (NHS England, 2018).

achieve change. The development of the change can be described using driver diagrams: a key feature in the implementation of LSC.

Driver Diagrams

Driver diagrams enable a visual description of the aim and the associated changes required. In their first iteration, they provide a theoretical approach to what changes are required. They are based on the initiators of change's ideas and thoughts around what could achieve the desired outcome. They have been used within a wide range of settings including retail, industry and healthcare (e.g. Langley et al., 2009). Driver diagrams are refined and updated over time, often increasing in complexity as more is learned about the changes in progress and the future requirements.

The use of driver diagrams can illustrate the theories and actions to support change. The implementation will result in a lot of activity. Detailed plans for each stage or process are beyond the capacity of the leaders of the change and will therefore require distributed leadership. This can enable wider engagement in the vision and often greater innovation and ownership of the change that is being proposed (NHS Institute for Innovation and Improvement, 2008).

Distributed Leadership

The concept of distributed leadership originated in the education sector but has been seen within the NHS as a mechanism to incorporate expert knowledge into leadership within the wider healthcare ecosystem (Mapani, 2023). It has been described as 'the distribution and allocation of leadership power to wherever expertise, capability and motivation sit within organisations' (Kings Fund, 2014).

Distributed leadership is focused on empowering people both within and across organisational boundaries. It differs from traditional forms of leadership: responsibilities are dispersed, and within healthcare, this offers a way forward to the clinical-managerial divide, requiring staff involvement at multiple levels. Time and preparedness are required to establish relationships, dialogue, and negotiations to achieve intended outcomes, including resource availability, decision-making, and objective setting (Mapani, 2023). The main intentions are engagement and empowerment, which subsequently result in a vertical flow of power from the centre through to the bottom (Brookes & Grint 2010). The evidence is clear, however, that it is *how* the leadership is distributed that matters most: purposeful, planned leadership distribution with careful design is more likely to impact positively (Harris, 2013; Harris et al., 2022). This lends itself to PPs given the breadth of practice.

Communities of Practice

Communities of Practice (CoP) are groups of people who share a concern or a passion for something they do and learn how to do it better as they interact regularly (Wenger-Traynor & Wenger-Traynor, 2015). Within this definition, three characteristics are crucial: a shared domain of interest enhancing commitment; community activities resulting in the development of relationships; and a shared practice that develops over time through sustained interaction.

CoP can be understood as a way for organisations to handle unstructured problems and share knowledge outside traditional structural boundaries, creating space for conversations with the value of connections and a sense of belonging. The practice of a community is dynamic and involves learning on the part of everyone (Wenger-Traynor & Wenger-Traynor, 2015). It enables coming together with a shared interest to fulfil both individual and group goals to do better.

Within a CoP there is a reliance on collaborative environments to enable systems of collective critical inquiry and reflection. There is not always consistency in the structure of CoPs, with some resembling informal networks with loosely defined goals and structures, and others having clearly defined goals and responsibilities (Li et al., 2009).

Although the initial concept developed by Wenger (1998) suggested CoPs emerge spontaneously, later work suggested organisations can engineer and cultivate CoPs (Wenger et al., 2002), often consisting of three different components: people, practice and capabilities (Saint-Onge & Wallace, 2003).

Implementation: Developing the PPN

From the identification of the need for change, a small group of PPs from a range of settings including clinical practice and education developed a vision. This was articulated as promoting excellence in psychological health and wellbeing to maximise the benefits of the psychological professions for the public. This vision was articulated and translated into achievable actions and goals that speak to the wider health system priorities and strategy.

The next stage (reflected in Figure 14.2 LSC model) included 'engaging', 'framing', and 'attracting further interest'. This included engagement with PPs to ensure all members of the psychological professions, across all grades and specialisms, can make a meaningful contribution to transformational change. Meaningful expert by experience (EBE) involvement and links to all aspects of the strategic workforce planning system supported this development. Routine representation of the network alongside all other professional groups (i.e. medicine and dentistry, nursing, allied health professionals (AHPs), health care scientists (HCS), pharmacy and public health professionals) contributed to 'pragmatic changes in multiple processes'. Further development of multiprofessional engagement with partner health professionals supported the examination of complex service delivery/development problems and consideration of novel solutions in an environment of enquiry and mutual respect. This is summarised within the PPN vision as 'Inform, Enable, Influence', providing a consistent overview descriptor of the key issues.

The driver diagrams that were initially developed aligned with the healthcare priorities at that time (2014). These became the primary drivers and included: Education, Clinical Excellence, Research and Innovation, and Promoting Psychological Wellbeing. Secondary drivers represented the groups' thinking about what would influence change in the primary drivers. Change ideas could then be developed as projects within the bigger programme and could be evaluated through the wide range of tools available. Figure 14.3 shows the initial driver diagram. This supported the development of multiple activities captured by the phrase 'lots of lots' provided by the change ideas (NHS Institute for Innovation and Improvement, 2011).

The complexity of the model required distributed leadership and the development of CoP supported this. The CoP provides a vehicle for the PPN to facilitate understanding and build a two-way dialogue to 'Inform, enable, and influence' the wider system and bring leadership to the PP workforce to enable confidence and agency in contributing to workforce development. The PPN can be seen as the bridge between practice and policy, planning and delivery within the health and care systems. This reciprocal relationship provides a unique source of grassroots understanding and professional expertise for the wider system. Figure 14.4 describes this.

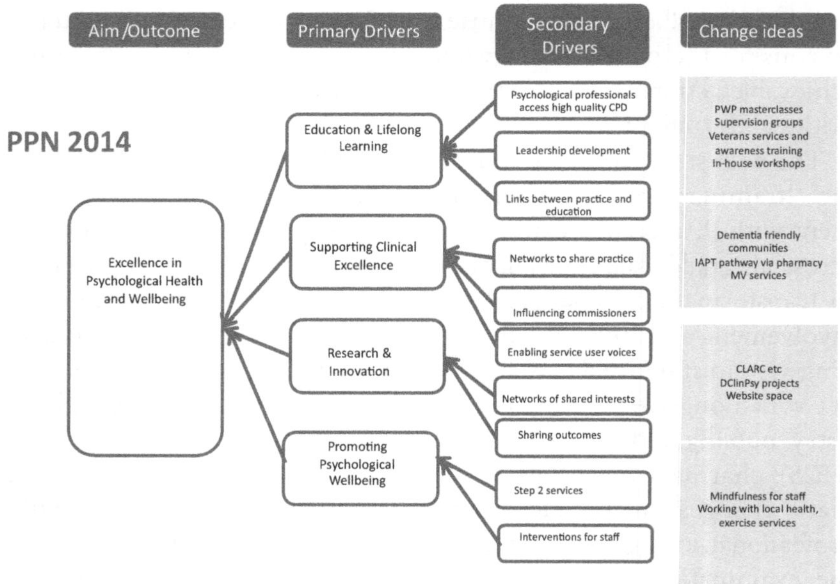

Figure 14.3 PPN driver diagram, 2014.

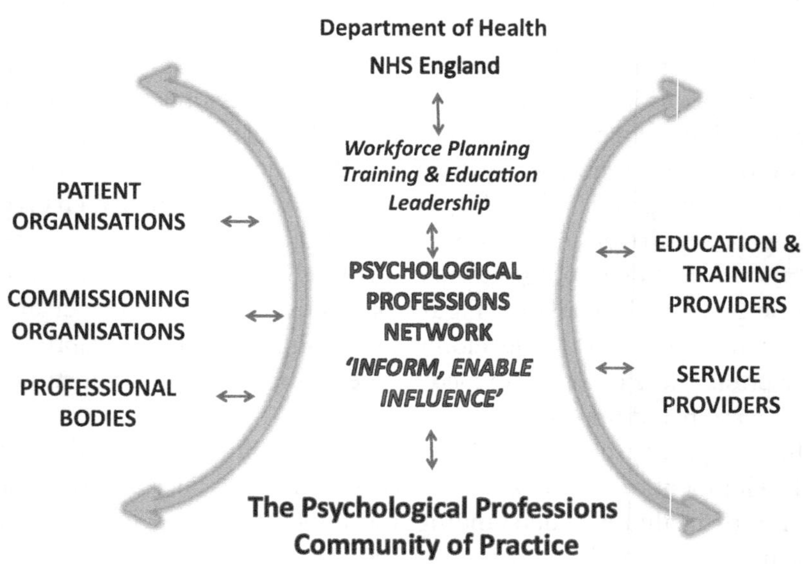

Figure 14.4 PPN 'inform, enable, influence' funnel.

Structural Change and Support

The importance of 'making pragmatic change in multiple processes' has been crucial. These include system support, dedicated leadership and governance structures, acceptance and support for change initiatives. Initial support was built by bringing together parallel planning and engagement fora and further support for staffing (programme lead, chair) and for the tools and actions required for engagement and the building of the network. These included communications (website, newsletter) and member events as well as CoP set-up support. Governance and accountability to the organisation were delivered through strategic workforce alignment and support for the implementation of transformational change initiatives, coupled with expectations of sharing learning and recommendations.

Where Are We Now? Using Our Tools

Driver diagrams have continued to be utilised with the PPN development. A revised driver diagram for 2024 (10 years later) is provided in Figure 14.5. There have been amendments to the vision. The primary

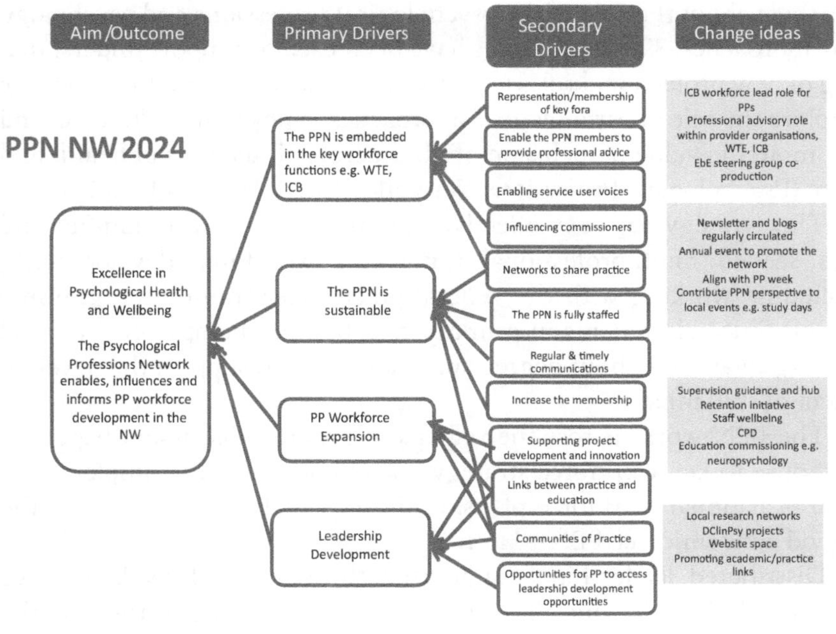

Figure 14.5 PPN driver diagram, 2024.

drivers are aligned to current priorities and policy drivers. A marked increase in the secondary drivers and change ideas reflects the maturity of the network and recognises that change has taken place.

A Multimedia Communication Strategy is central to the PPN work plan. This strategy supports:

- Share workforce development information to promote understanding and confidence
- Provide materials articulating the value of psychological approaches to the wider health and care system
- Host events to stimulate partnership thinking among health professionals and system planners about the roles psychological approaches and PPs can play

The PPN provides a weekly electronic newsletter, with administrative support for the convening of CoPs and an annual regional event aligned with the national PP week where PPs from all regions of England come together to share good practice, discuss key workforce development issues, and promote innovation.

One of the innovative features of the PPN work plan has been to co-produce educational materials and explanatory animations with the aim of promoting education and engagement of stakeholders and system partners about the role of the psychological professions and psychological approaches. These resources have been used to support understanding of new professional roles (e.g. Psychological Wellbeing Practitioner); explore the role of psychological approaches in physical health care; and promote the value of inclusion of EbEs across all sections of health and care (Psychological Professions Network – North West, 2013-2025).

This strategy has been effective in sparking interest in non-PPs and has seeded multi-professional innovative workforce developments, including working with the general practitioner training programme to introduce placements in primary care talking therapy services, and raising awareness about degree apprenticeships to support the development of skill mix.

The PPN works across the regions to produce discussion papers in response to key workforce strategy documents, including implementation of national workforce plans, leadership, and resources during the Covid pandemic (see PPN – Home).

Distributed leadership is supported through the PPN Workforce Council (PPNWC), which has been described as the 'engine room' of the PPN, providing a formal forum for ongoing dialogue about workforce development and innovation between representatives of the PP workforce. This supports the development of the annual workplan overseen by the Programme lead. This alignment supports the development of CoPs (see below) and also enables leadership development opportunities for members who can learn about wider NHS strategy and have the opportunity to become further involved in system-level work, e.g. bringing workforce intelligence from their own area into system reviews and workforce planning. Membership of the council can be advantageous to service providers by being part of Personal Development Plans in support of leadership development.

Representation within the PPNWC focuses on ensuring each PP professional grouping has a representative, usually through a role leading a CoP. The CoP taps into existing professional groupings but has also provided an important platform for the professional support and development of new roles, e.g. Psychological Wellbeing Practitioner (PWP). EbEs provide two representatives (from their CoP). In addition, members may be co-opted to provide representation in relation to a specific NHS strategic priority (e.g. perinatal mental health, physical health conditions).

Meaningful Service User involvement is included as a core objective within the PPN at all levels of its activity. EbEs are included in all aspects of the delivery of the PPN work plan. EbEs are encouraged to develop leadership roles in regional and national initiatives and are supported to take part by a clear system of remuneration that recognises the value of individual EbEs' time and expertise. They also contribute to interviewing for PPN appointments, developing conference programmes, contributing to position papers, and acting as critical friends to project and strategy development.

Engagement with other professional groups is key in developing 'a sustainable norm' in the promotion of PPs and psychological approaches to be embedded across health and care. The PPN proactively seeks and creates opportunities for multi-professional collaboration. Being embedded within NHSE workforce planning systems alongside fellow health care professional groupings, supported by a CoP ethos, creates unique opportunities to seed ideas and co-create solutions to complex clinical delivery problems. Additional examples include collaborating with local public health leads to develop a mental health awareness train-the-trainer education programme to upskill frontline workers to have the knowledge and skills to deliver an 'Every Contact Counts' conversation for mental health with people in their routine practice; developing resilience in practice workshops for dentists in their post-qualification foundation year of practice to help them and their clinical supervisors recognise and manage signs of workplace stress to support staff retention.

Living with the Results and Consequences

The PPN developed in the North West of England but has since spread to every part of England. There are seven PPNs in England aligned to NHS regional boundaries, each with a similar staffing and structural approach. There has been some variation in hosting arrangements, but the principles and aims have remained the same. This 'settling in' has supported the expansion of the membership from a few thousand regionally to nearly 16,000 in autumn 2024.

National workforce plans have developed alongside the PPN and include significant expansion targets for the psychological professions' workforce. In addition, there is more national structure and leadership than previously. While these cannot be causally attributed to the presence of the PPN, the amplification of the voice and its contribution to healthcare has no doubt contributed to system recognition.

Has the PPN Achieved Large Scale Change?

Kurt Lewin's three-step model of change (Lewin, 1947; Burnes, 2020) has been widely used to illustrate when Large Scale Change has been achieved (see Figure 14.6)

Considering this, the decision to change was taken by the village leaders, but the implementation would require engagement and action from a wide range of structures, groups, and individuals. This could include

Imagine a river flowing through the village where you were born. The river constantly changes in many small ways - higher or lower, muddier or clearer, and so on. But while it changes a bit every day, it remains recognisable as the river that flows through your village.

Now, imagine that village leaders change the course of the river, re-routing it around the village and paving over its old course for a new shopping street. That would be transformational change. If you left the village at an early age and now return years later, everything would seem very different. Transformational, or large-scale, change changes everything.

Figure 14.6 Large scale change description of achievement.

the planning permissions, the civil engineering plans, and actions to physically reroute a river, as well as individual retailers developing new shops on the new street. Encouraging the villagers to use the new shops could potentially be an example of 'lots of lots': a promotion from a bakery might engage some, and a promotion from a tool shop might engage others. However, both (and more) groups are necessary to achieve the vision of a new shopping street used by the villagers (and potentially beyond). Over time, the new shopping street is not seen as 'new' but becomes part of the day-to-day reality. Change will still continue as shops evolve in response to changing consumer preferences and wider socio-economic changes (e.g. population change, cost of living changes).

Within the context of the PPN, there has been achievement within the LSC model. The world of PPs looks different, and there is greater connectivity between the PP groupings. There is also greater interaction that supports 'inform, enable, influence' with the wider policy and workforce systems. Within the broader context, structural and policy changes (e.g. restructures, government changes), the PPN sits as one piece of a wider complex adaptive system. Structures that would represent parity with other healthcare groupings or system/provider delivery functions are not there. There is still more work to be done.

The PPN's establishment has provided and continues to provide a unique platform through which psychological professionals can be collectively supported to articulate and promote their specialist knowledge and skills, with the key aim of facilitating meaningful participation in the systems and processes underpinning workforce development and service transformation across health and care.

What Does This Mean for Leadership?

In the application of these models to the PPN, the leadership task has been to remain flexible, inclusive, and adaptable. Leaders have needed the ability to engage across the full range of settings with multiple stakeholders to develop and harness their voices in order to support shared goals. This requires leaders to be able to communicate the vision effectively communicate the vision but not attempt to micro-manage the components. This approach lends itself to the NHS and care system as a complex adaptive system.

Ideas in Brief

Change in complex adaptive systems such as healthcare requires a more innovative and non-linear approach to deliver a new vision

Principles of Large Scale Change support change requirements by recognising this complexity.

Distributed leadership and the development of communities of practice support implementation through multiple activities across a range of settings, groups and individuals.

The Psychological Professions are a diverse group of professions that have increased significantly in size but have not been routinely included in workforce planning, nor service or systems development in health and care.

The use of theoretical principles has supported the development of the Psychological Professions Networks, which has sought to maximise the benefits of the psychological professions in the delivery of health and care to the public.

References

Best, A., Greenhalgh, T., Lewis, S., Saul, J. E., Carroll, S., & Bitz, J. (2012). Large-system transformation in health care: A realist review. *The Millbank Quarterly*, *90*(3), 421–456.

Brookes, S., & Grint, K. (2010). *The new leadership challenge*. Palgrave MacMillan

Burnes, B. (2020). The origins of Lewin's three-step model of change. *The Journal of Applied Behavioral Science*, *56*(1), 32–59. https://doi.org/10.1177/0021886319892685

Department of Health. (2011). *No health without mental health: Gateway reference 14679*. Department of Health.

Ganz, M. (2010). Leading change: Leadership, organization, and social movements. In N. Nohria & R. Khurana (Eds.), Handbook of leadership theory and practice (pp. 509–550). HBS Press.

Harris, A. (2013). Distributed leadership: Friend or foe? *Educational Management Administration and Leadership*, *41*(5), 545–554. https://doi.org/10.1177/174143213497635

Harris, A., Jones, M., & Ismail, N. (2022). Distributed leadership: Taking a retrospective and contemporary view of the evidence base. *School Leadership and Management*, *42*(5), 438–356. https://doi.org/10.1080/13632434.2022.2109620

Health Education England. (2021). *Psychological* professions workforce plan for England 2020/21 to 2023/24 (Updated December 2021). Health Education England.

Kings Fund. (2014). *Developing collective leadership for health care*. Kings Fund.

Langley, G. J., Moen, R. D., Nolan, K. M., Norman, C. L., & Provost, L. P (2009). *The improvement guide: A practical approach to enhancing organizational performance*. John Wiley & Sons

Lewin, K. (1947). Frontiers in group dynamics. *Human Relations, 1*, 5–41. http://dx.doi.org/10.1177/001872674700100103

Li, L. C., Grimshaw, J. M., Nielsen, C., Judd, M., Coyte, P. C., & Graham, I. D. (2009). Evolution of Wenger's concept of community of practice. *Implementation Science, 4*(11). https://doi.org/10.1186/1748-5908-4-11

Mapani, A. (2023). Distributed leadership: A new perspective on leadership in driving innovation and transformation in healthcare? *Hospital Administration and Medical Practices, 2*. https://doi.org/10.54844/hamp.2022.0020

Mind. (2024). *The big mental health report*. Mind.

National Audit Office. (2023). *Progress in improving mental health services in England*. National Audit Office.

National Audit Office. (2024). *Response to 2023 report: Correspondence from Sir Chris Wormald, Permanent Secretary, Department for Health and Social Care, re Sixty-fifth report of Session 2022–23, Progress in improving mental health services, dated 5 February 2024*. https://committees.parliament.uk/publications/43339/documents/215812/default/

NHS Digital. (2024). *NHS -talking therapies, for anxiety and depression, Annual reports, 2022–23*. NHS England Digital.

NHS England. (2018). *Leading large scale change: A practical guide*. NHS England.

NHS Institute for Innovation and Improvement. (2008). *Quality improvement: Theory and practice in HEALTHCARE*. NHS Institute for Innovation and Improvement.

NHS Institute for Innovation and Improvement. (2011). *Part 1 Leading large scale change: A practical guide*. NHS Institute for Innovation and Improvement.

Plsek, P. E., & Greenhalgh, T. (2001). The importance of complexity in health care. *British Medical Journal, 323*, 6258.

Plsek, P. E., & Wilson, T. (2001). Complexity, leadership, and management in healthcare organisations. *British Medical Journal, 323*, 746–9.

Psychological Professions Network – North West (2013–2025). *PPN – North West*.https://ppn.nhs.uk/north-west.

Saint-Onge, H., & Wallace, D. (2003). *Leveraging communities of practice for strategic advantage*. Butterworth-Heinemann.

The National NHS Talking Therapies Workforce Report: England workforce data. (2022–23). An NHS Benchmarking Network (www.nhsbenchmarking.nhs.uk) project commissioned by NHS England, November 2023. The National NHS Talking Therapies Workforce Report: England workforce data (2022–23)

Wenger, E. (1998). *Communities of practice: Learning, meaning and identity.* Cambridge University Press.

Wenger, E., McDermott, R. A., & Snyder, W. (2002). *Cultivating communities of practice.* Harvard Business School Press.

Wenger-Traynor, E., & Wenger-Traynor, B. (2015). *Introduction to communities of practice: A brief overview of the concept and its uses.* Brief introduction to communities of practice.docx.

PART FOUR

A HEALTHY HIVE

Fostering Thriving Culture and Sustainability through the Tempest

15 Wellbeing as Leadership

From Paradox to Collective Practice

Dr Amra Saleem Rao, Gita Bhutani, Dr Adrian Neal, and Professor (Emeritus) Tony Lavender

At the heart of many healthcare and psychological professions lies a paradox: those responsible for delivering psychological care to others often struggle to safeguard their own wellbeing. This tension is particularly pronounced in emotionally demanding roles, where practitioners are expected to demonstrate resilience, empathy, and care, yet often receive insufficient support to attend to their own mental and emotional needs (Skovholt & Trotter-Mathison, 2016). Such discrepancies between organisational policies and practitioners' experiences can erode trust and diminish the impact of wellbeing initiatives.

Over a decade of research has shown that workplace psychosocial wellbeing is not a luxury, but a critical clinical, ethical, and organisational imperative. When healthcare professionals thrive, so too do the individuals and communities they serve (West & Dawson, 2012; Lundstrom et al., 2002). Yet, chronic stress and burnout remain widespread, contributing to medical errors, reduced patient trust, and high staff turnover (Miller, 2019; Panagioti et al., 2018; Hall et al., 2016). The economic burden of poor mental health in the UK remains significant, with Deloitte (2024) estimating the annual cost to employers at £51 billion, nearly half of which is attributed to presenteeism. Broader analyses by the Centre for Mental Health (2024) place the overall economic and social cost at £300.4 billion in England alone, reflecting both direct and indirect impacts. These statistics highlight the necessity for integrated policy responses that prioritise wellbeing, directly influencing workforce retention, service quality, and organisational resilience. Evidence

DOI 10.4324/9781003492399-20

suggests that organisational-level interventions, such as leadership engagement and systemic policy support, are more effective in promoting staff wellbeing than individual-level initiatives alone (Grawitch, Ballard, & Erb, 2024; WHO, 2023).

Despite the growing emphasis on wellbeing initiatives, such as mindfulness programmes, resilience training, flexible working policies, employee assistance programmes, and staff wellbeing services, many organisations continue to overlook the root causes of stress and burnout. Systemic issues, such as excessive workloads, unrealistic expectations, lack of autonomy, and unsupportive organisational cultures, remain prevalent (U.S. Surgeon General, 2022; Deloitte, 2024; Centre for Mental Health, 2024). In the UK, the relationship between managers and reportees has been identified as a key predictor of employee sickness absence and broader organisational Wellbeing (Black & Frost, 2011). Addressing these structural drivers is needed; otherwise, individual-focused initiatives may be perceived as superficial rather than effecting meaningful change.

The Work of Leadership

Addressing the paradox—where wellbeing initiatives overlook systemic causes of stress—requires leadership rooted in systemic awareness. Leaders need to go beyond surface-level solutions to tackle the root drivers of burnout, embedding wellbeing as a collective, cultural, and ethical responsibility. This shift demands reframing wellbeing not as an individual or organisational add-on, but as a shared, relational commitment. It also requires confronting structural stressors—such as discrimination, racism, and inequity—that contribute to burnout. As noted by others (Williams 2023; West et al., 2017), sustainable change depends on a willingness to engage with the systemic inequalities embedded in workplace culture.

To drive systemic change, leaders need to cultivate emotional intelligence, foster psychological safety, and critically reflect on how power, culture, and structural inequities fuel workplace stress (Edmondson, 2018; Goleman, Boyatzis & McKee, 2013). Emotionally intelligent leadership fosters trust and openness, enabling staff to voice their needs without fear. Systems-aware leaders also tackle root causes of chronic stress, such as excessive workloads, unclear roles, and under-resourcing (Obholzer & Roberts, 1994; Menzies-Lyth, 1988). Without such leadership, wellbeing risks becoming a superficial exercise rather than a core part of organisational culture.

Rather than engaging in performative responses, leaders are encouraged to adopt evidence-informed strategies, such as authentic leadership approaches that have been shown to reduce burnout and enhance workplace wellbeing (Spence Laschinger & Fida, 2014). As West and Dawson (2012) highlight, staff wellbeing is a strategic imperative tied to patient outcomes, team effectiveness, and organisational performance. Transformational leadership—centred on vision, support, and empowerment—has been shown to reduce burnout and increase engagement in healthcare settings (Bass & Riggio, 2006; Avolio, Walumbwa & Weber, 2009).

Stigma remains a barrier. Leaders may fear showing vulnerability, yet modelling it constructively fosters authenticity and connection (Brown, 2018). Cultures of care are shaped not only by policy but also by everyday leadership behaviours that either reinforce or disrupt fear-based norms. Psychological professionals face added complexity—trained to support others, they may suppress their distress, fuelling burnout and sustaining harmful norms (Skovholt & Trotter-Mathison, 2016). These dynamics highlight the importance of reflective spaces, supervision, and systemic support. Sustainable Wellbeing requires leadership that is emotionally attuned, reflective, and system-aware. Without it, initiatives risk being tokenistic rather than transformative.

Key Lessons in Restoring Balance for Psychological Professionals' Wellbeing

Healthcare systems have faced immense pressure in recent years, worsened by COVID-19, staffing shortages, and escalating burnout. Structural issues, such as rising mental health needs and health inequalities, alongside digital transformation and agile working challenges, have added to the strain. Ongoing policy reform and regulatory change have further contributed to a climate of uncertainty and heightened emotional labour. Reports highlight how shifting demands and unclear guidance have created frustration and anxiety among health leaders, undermining confidence and straining wellbeing (NHS Confederation, 2020). At the same time, the King's Fund (2021a, 2021b) emphasises that staff wellbeing depends on addressing the psychosocial aspects of work, including the hidden burden of emotional labour, within a long-term systemic approach rather than short-term fixes. The withdrawal of funding for wellbeing hubs in England represents a troubling rollback of hard-won progress, highlighting how uncertainty about the future of services can undermine commitment to staff wellbeing at precisely the time it is most needed (British Psychological Society, 2024; NHS Providers, 2024). Psychological professionals played a pivotal role during the pandemic, providing frontline support to traumatised staff, developing wellbeing assessment tools, and creating psychologically safe spaces (West et al., 2020). They also contributed to workforce development and implemented evidence-based wellbeing initiatives—ranging from digital support tools to peer programmes—that fostered compassionate and sustainable practices (Williams et al., 2022).

However, the paradox persists: those advocating for others' wellbeing often lack the resources to care for their own. Despite their critical role in recovery, concerns about burnout, moral injury, and vicarious trauma remain. The urgency of addressing the wellbeing of psychological professionals has never been more pressing, underscoring the need for systemic solutions.

To begin addressing this gap, the British Psychological Society (BPS) Leadership and Management Faculty, in partnership with the New Savoy Conference and the London School of Economics and Health Sciences, launched a UK-wide initiative. The aim was to reset the balance between staff wellbeing and service quality, developing tools to embed wellbeing across the psychological workforce.

Key initiatives include:

- **A Wellbeing Charter** promoting shared responsibility and embedding wellbeing as a collective organisational value (BPS, 2016; Hacker-Hughes et al., 2016).
- **The Psychological Practitioner Workplace Wellbeing Measure (PPWWM)** (Summers et al., 2019)- a validated tool that assesses six factors: Professional & Organisational Satisfaction, Support & Flexibility, Professional Role, Physical Environment, Clinical Supervision, and External Support.
- **Annual Wellbeing Surveys** to track trends and inform strategies
- **Collaborative networks and focus groups** fostering participatory co-production of solutions based on lived experience.

These efforts mark a shift from individualised wellbeing initiatives to a systemic, relational, leadership-engaged approach. Recognising professional wellbeing as an ethical, clinical, and organisational priority, this work sets a critical precedent: supporting those who support others is central to sustaining care.

What Does the Data Tell Us

The emotional labour and load inherent in psychological work have long been under-acknowledged, subsumed beneath narratives of individual resilience, mythologies about heroism, vocation, and duty. Yet, recent longitudinal data make these realities impossible to ignore. The UK-wide Wellbeing Survey of the psychological professions (2014–2021) involved 6,871 psychological professionals.[1]

- **Over two-thirds** of respondents reported persistently high levels of work-related stress.
- **Half of all staff teams** showed depressive symptoms—more than **10%** scoring in the severe range, with signs of burnout.
- Most starkly, **over 75%** of respondents indicated they would leave their roles if they could.

Harper et al. (2020) offer a sobering portrait of a workforce under significant and sustained strain. The 2021 survey further highlighted the profound impact of the pandemic, revealing that, while online work enhanced flexibility, 55.6% of respondents felt the overall effect was negative, citing increased discrimination and workplace bullying. These troubling findings highlight the urgent need for systemic change (Figure 15.1).

These findings align with concerns raised in the British Psychological Society (BPS) 2019 Membership Survey, NHS Staff Surveys (2023, 2024), and the Care Quality Commission (2021), highlighting systemic issues like emotional exhaustion and stress among professionals. They emphasise the need for structural changes and a holistic, systems-informed approach to wellbeing, driven by leadership and organisational alignment. Chronic underfunding, vacancies, and unsustainable workloads

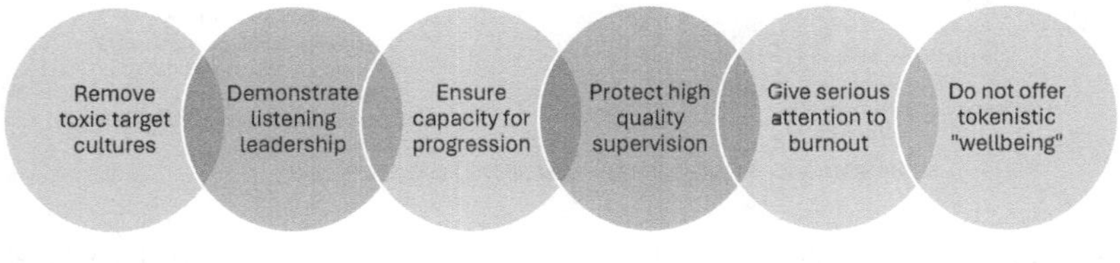

Figure 15.1 Psychological Professionals 2021 Survey themes.

impact clinical safety (West et al., 2020; Duffy et al., 2018). As one survey respondent noted: 'How can I offer psychological safety to others when I have none myself?'

From Divide to Dialogue: The Case for Systemic Transformation

The initiative underscores meaningful advocacy for psychological professionals' wellbeing while revealing deeper tensions within healthcare organisations. High stress, professional dissatisfaction, and workforce attrition indicate that individual solutions are insufficient. As Rao et al. (2021) argue, restoring sustainability in psychological services requires a whole-system shift. Their model outlines four critical domains for embedding wellbeing into professional culture: Organisational Culture, Leadership and Governance, Support and Learning, and Organisational Interventions (Figure 15.2). In light of the clear evidence and the persistent gaps in response, a fundamental shift in occupational wellbeing is needed—one that reconsiders not only the nature of support but also how services are led, structured, and experienced.

Effective leadership at all levels is crucial for the workforce's mental and occupational wellbeing. Our surveys indicate a disconnect between senior leaders and frontline clinicians. To explore this further, a series of focused groups were conducted with leaders and frontline workers

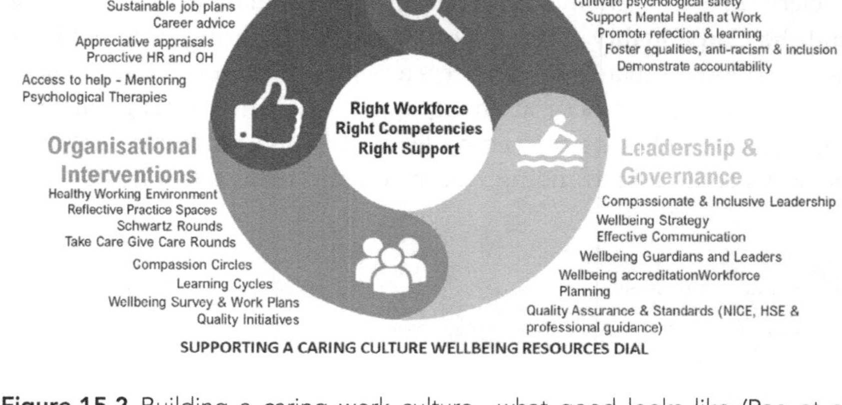
Support & Learning
Effective line management, supervision, CPD
Sustainable job plans
Career advice
Appreciative appraisals
Proactive HR and OH
Access to help - Mentoring
Psychological Therapies
Organisational Culture
Tackle stigma, discrimination and bullying
Cultivate psychological safety
Support Mental Health at Work
Promote refection & learning
Foster equalities, anti-racism & inclusion
Demonstrate accountability
Right Workforce
Right Competencies
Right Support
Organisational Interventions
Healthy Working Environment
Reflective Practice Spaces
Schwartz Rounds
Take Care Give Care Rounds
Compassion Circles
Learning Cycles
Wellbeing Survey & Work Plans
Quality Initiatives
Leadership & Governance
Compassionate & Inclusive Leadership
Wellbeing Strategy
Effective Communication
Wellbeing Guardians and Leaders
Wellbeing accreditationWorkforce Planning
Quality Assurance & Standards (NICE, HSE & professional guidance)
SUPPORTING A CARING CULTURE WELLBEING RESOURCES DIAL

Figure 15.2 Building a caring work culture—what good looks like (Rao et al., 2021).[2]

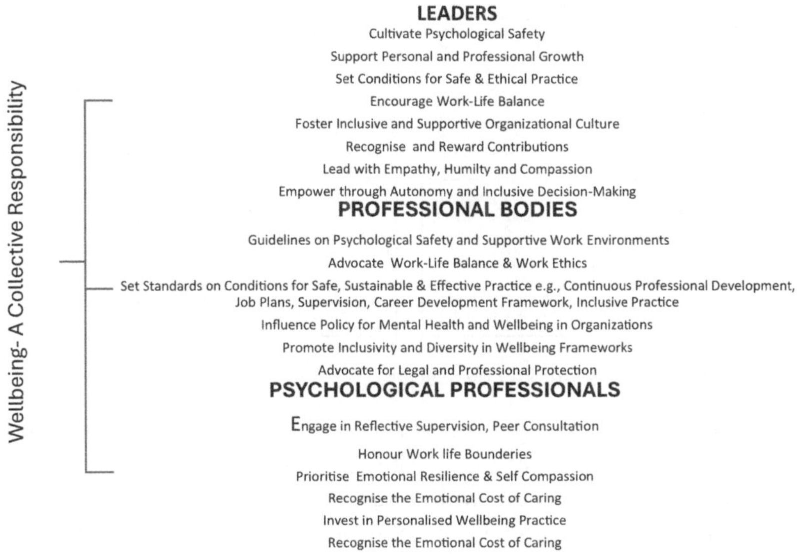

Figure 15.3 Focus groups key themes on wellbeing as collective responsibility.

separately and together, highlighting key themes: a return to 'command and control' leadership, the strain of productivity targets on staff support, and the need for genuine investment in workplace culture and supportive infrastructures to prevent harm and reduce attrition (Figure 15.3). A critical finding was the need to involve psychological professionals in decision-making, rather than sidelining them in policy development. However, fragmentation—such as divisions between medical and psychosocial models—remains a barrier to collaboration and service integration (Summers et al., 2021).

Both leaders and frontline professionals emphasised the need for a clear vision, sustainable workforce planning, and safe, thriving work environments. The King's Fund (2021) highlights the importance of resilient work cultures built on autonomy, belonging, and contribution, while the British Psychological Society (2024) draws on lessons from NHS staff wellbeing hubs to emphasise long-term investment in psychological support and leadership strategies that promote staff wellbeing. Such approaches are critical for mitigating workforce stress and sustaining effective, high-quality healthcare services, particularly under conditions of heightened demand.

In autumn 2024, a summit brought together professional bodies and clinical leads across the UK to address staff wellbeing challenges. Findings from the summit and wider professional dialogue suggest the

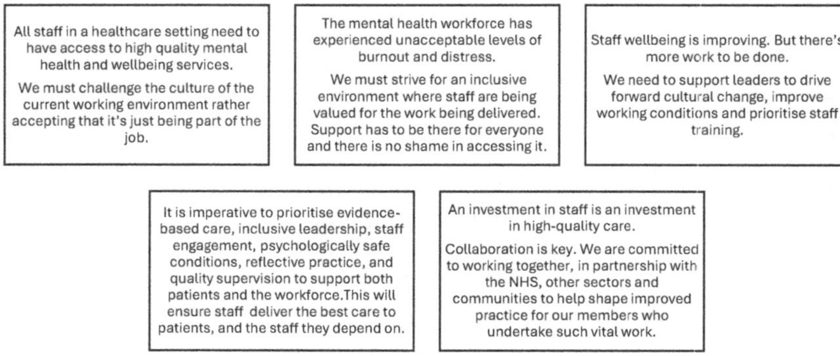

Figure 15.4 Legacy event key messages.

urgency of addressing emotional tolls, gaps in support, and the need for decisive action. See Figure 15.4 for key messages.

Addressing professional wellbeing requires more than structural reform or inter-professional cooperation—it calls for a cultural reset. Achieving genuine integration will require moving beyond operational interventions towards fostering environments grounded in care, relational connection, and psychological safety. Both individual and systemic perspectives are essential in this effort (Jackman & Steer, 2023), laying the foundation for a more sustainable, ethically grounded culture of care.

Psychological professionals' wellbeing demands ongoing inquiry. Key questions remain: Is burnout driven more by the emotional demands of clinical work, or by systemic failings like excessive caseloads, poor supervision, and weak leadership (Maslach & Leiter, 2016; Pines & Maslach, 2019)? Or is it a combination of both, varying by context (Shanafelt et al., 2021; West & Dawson, 2012)? Further research is needed to understand how emotional demands, resilience, and systemic factors interact to support sustainable wellbeing.

Closing Reflections: Is Wellbeing an Ethical Imperative for Leaders?

Is it not an ethical imperative to ask whether those delivering compassionate care should themselves work in environments that support their mental and occupational health? We cannot expect high-quality care from professionals who are unsupported, overburdened, and at risk of burnout. Supporting practitioner wellbeing is essential to the sustainability of healthcare systems.

Research consistently links staff wellbeing to patient safety, quality of care, and workforce retention (West et al., 2017; Hall et al., 2016). It also improves organisational performance through higher engagement, lower turnover, and better outcomes (Dixon-Woods et al., 2014; Shanafelt & Noseworthy, 2017). Prioritising staff wellbeing enables professionals to meet the complex needs of those they serve—especially in high-pressure, resource-stretched settings.

This is not a peripheral issue but central to clinical practice and moral responsibility. Leadership must move beyond performance metrics to ensure those who care for others are themselves supported to thrive—because care and wellbeing are inseparable.

Although this chapter focuses on psychological professionals, the wellbeing of all care providers is a cornerstone of ethical, sustainable practice. In roles centred on supporting others through distress and change, professionals must also attend to their own mental and emotional health. Self-care is not a luxury but a necessity for sustaining empathy, presence, and sound judgement (Skovholt & Trotter-Mathison, 2016). Without it, the ability to provide effective care suffers, harming both practitioner and recipient.

Wellbeing is a collective responsibility. While professional bodies play a key role in embedding it into standards and promoting psychologically safe workplaces (BPS, 2022), organisational cultures must reflect a genuine commitment—not just rhetoric. This means investing in wellbeing as a structural and relational priority (Bourke & Dillon, 2018; West et al., 2016), and shifting from traditional 'command-and-control' models to values-led, relational approaches (Leinwand et al., 2021).

Trust is built through consistent actions and decisions that demonstrate authentic care. Without systemic commitment, the burden of care becomes unsustainable, leading to burnout and compassion fatigue (Maslach & Leiter, 2016; West et al., 2016). Disconnected initiatives often fail to address the root causes of distress or foster systemic learning. As emphasised in other chapters, integrating wellbeing into professional expectations and organisational culture is essential for maintaining workforce mental and emotional health.

Leadership is the critical bridge between individual resilience and systemic sustainability. While psychological professionals bring compassion and expertise, the environments they work in are shaped by leadership quality. In under-resourced, target-driven systems, transactional leadership often prioritises compliance over care, yielding short-term gains at the expense of long-term trust and morale (Seddon, 2008). This erodes trust, amplifies stress, and undermines collective wellbeing.

To meet the demands of complex contexts, leaders are required to adopt transformational and adaptive approaches that foster psychological safety, meaning, and empowerment (Heifetz et al., 2009; Northouse, 2021). Balancing decisiveness with empathy and accountability with compassion, effective leadership builds trust through presence, relational intelligence, and systems thinking (Goleman, 2013).

Caring leadership creates the conditions for others to thrive through high-quality supervision (Kilminster & Jolly, 2000), sensitive pacing of change (Kotter, 2012), and embedding wellbeing into culture (Edmondson, 2018). By contrast, leadership focused solely on outcomes risks eroding morale in emotionally demanding settings. Addressing systemic issues, such as discrimination, inequity, racism, and the silencing of whistleblowers—is also essential to creating inclusive and truly supportive workplaces.

Ultimately, wellbeing is integral to the work itself. To build a profession and leadership practice that does not harm its healers, we must prioritise the wellbeing of those who provide care (Hacker et al., 2016). Caring for oneself while caring for others is an ethical stance that resists the normalisation of burnout and affirms the need for sustainability. If we fail to care for those who care, we risk eroding the very heart of psychological services and healthcare. Sustaining wellbeing demands a cultural shift—from self-sacrifice to self-awareness, from fragmented fixes to integrated practice, and from individual burden to shared accountability.

Ideas in Brief

- Psychological professionals often neglect their wellbeing despite caring for others, creating a workplace paradox.
- Wellbeing is a collective responsibility, embedded in organisational values and supported by leadership.
- Address the dynamics of burnout, moral injury, and vicarious trauma, particularly for psychological professionals.
- Leaders need to model authenticity, cultivate safety, and address systemic stressors such as excessive workloads and role ambiguity.
- Stigma surrounding vulnerability must be addressed.
- Wellbeing initiatives require systemic change, moving beyond superficial programmes to create sustainable, compassionate workplaces.

Reflective Exercise

Reflect on your leadership approach within your professional context, particularly in relation to the wellbeing of those you lead or work with. Consider the following questions:

- **Personal Reflection**:
  How do you currently balance the wellbeing of yourself and others in your leadership practice?
  Are there areas where you may be neglecting your wellbeing in the pursuit of organisational goals?
  What might be the reasons for this? What impact does it have on your leadership effectiveness? What support structures are available to you?

- **Leadership in Wellbeing**:
  How do you foster a culture of wellbeing within your team or organisation?
  Are wellbeing initiatives framed as individual or collective efforts?
  How can you shift the focus from individual responsibility to shared accountability in promoting wellbeing?

- **Systems Awareness**:
  What are the systemic factors in your organisation that contribute to stress, burnout, or disengagement?
  What underlying structures or cultural norms may need to be addressed to create a more supportive environment?
  A commitment to wellbeing requires addressing deep-rooted structural issues (privilege, discrimination, victimisation, inequity, racism, and turning a blind eye). How can you, as a leader, influence these changes to foster a genuinely inclusive and supportive environment?

- **Self-Awareness and Connection**:
  How do you show understanding and empathy in your leadership role?
  Are you comfortable acknowledging your challenges and struggles?
  In what ways could being open about your difficulties help build trust and create a safer, more supportive environment for your team?

Take a moment to jot down your thoughts, considering specific actions you can take to create a more supportive and sustainable leadership practise for both yourself and those you lead.

Notes

1 The details of the longitudinal data are discussed in the chapter on 'The composition and wellbeing of the psychological professions in the UK (2014 to 2021)' by Morris et al.

2 Acknowledgement—BPS Publication by Dr Amra Saleem Rao, Dr Natalie Kemp, Dr Gita Bhutani, Professor Reg Morris, Dr Elisabeth Summers, Katie Brown, Jeremy Clarke, Dr Adrian Neal

Bibliography

Avolio, B. J., Walumbwa, F. O., & Weber, T. J. (2009). Leadership: Current theories, research, and future directions. Annual Review of Psychology, 60, 421–449. https://doi.org/10.1146/annurev.psych.60.110707.163621

Bass, B. M., & Riggio, R. E. (2006). Transformational leadership (2nd ed.). Lawrence Erlbaum Associates.

Black, C., & Frost, D. (2011). Health at work – An independent review of sickness absence. Department for Work and Pensions. Available at: https://assets.publishing.service.gov.uk/media/5a7a1163e5274a319e7779eb/health-at-work.pdf

Bourke, J., & Dillon, B. (2018). The six signature traits of inclusive leadership: Thriving in a diverse new world. Deloitte University Press.

BPS. (2016). *Charter for psychological staff wellbeing and resilience.pdf* (accessed April 2025 https://cms.bps.org.uk/sites/default/files/2022-09/Charter%20for%20Psychological%20Staff%20Wellbeing%20and%20Resilience.pdf)

British Psychological Society. (2019). A damning picture of the challenges facing psychologists. The Psychologist. https://www.bps.org.uk/psychologist/damning-picture-challenges-facing-psychologists

British Psychological Society. (2022). White Paper – Psychological well-being at work. https://cms.bps.org.uk/sites/default/files/2022-06/White%20Paper%20%E2%80%93%20Psychological%20well-being%20at%20work%20.pdf

British Psychological Society. (2024, February 2). Learning from wellbeing hubs. https://www.bps.org.uk/psychologist/learning-wellbeing-hubs

British Psychological Society. (2024, March 27). *Government urged to reverse cuts to NHS staff wellbeing hubs*. Nursing Times. Retrieved on April 20, 2025, from https://www.nursingtimes.net/news/workforce/government-urged-to-reverse-cuts-to-nhs-staff-wellbeing-hubs-27-03-2024/

Brown, B. (2018). Dare to lead: Brave work. Tough conversations. Whole hearts. Random House.

Centre for Mental Health. (2024, March). The economic and social costs of mental ill-health. Centre for Mental Health. Retrieved from https://www.centreformentalhealth.org.uk/wp-content/uploads/2024/03/CentreforMH_TheEconomicSocialCostsofMentalIllHealth.pdf

Darzi, A. (2024). Independent investigation of the National Health Service in England. Department of Health and Social Care.

Deloitte. (2024, May 17). Poor mental health costs UK employers £51 billion a year for employees. Deloitte UK. Retrieved from https://www.deloitte.com/uk/en/about/press-room/poor-mental-health-costs-uk-employers-51-billion-a-year-for-employees.html

Dixon-Woods, M., Baker, R., Charles, K., Dawson, J., Jerzembek, G., Martin, G., ... & West, M. (2014). Culture and behaviour in the English National Health Service: Overview of lessons from a large multimethod study. *BMJ Quality & Safety*, *23*(2), 106–115.

Duffy, R. D., et al. (2018). Work as a calling: A theoretical model. *Journal of Counselling Psychology*, *65*(4), 423–439.

Edmondson, A. C. (2018). The fearless organization: Creating psychological safety in the workplace for learning, innovation, and growth. Hoboken, NJ: John Wiley & Sons.

Goleman, D. (2013). The focused leader. Harvard Business Review, 91(12), 50–60.

Goleman, D., Boyatzis, R., & McKee, A. (2013). Primal leadership: Unleashing the power of emotional intelligence (10th anniversary ed.). Boston, MA: Harvard Business Review Press.

Grawitch, M. J., Ballard, D. W., & Erb, K. R. (2024). Organizational-level interventions and employee Wellbeing: A meta-analytic review. *Journal of Occupational Health Psychology*, *29*(1), 1–20. https://doi.org/10.1037/ocp0000346(Also accessible via PMC: https://www.ncbi.nlm.nih.gov/pmc/articles/PMC10713995/)

Hacker Hughes, J., Rao, A. S., Dosanjh, N., Cohen-Tovée, E., Clarke, J., & Bhutani, G. (2016). Physician heal thyself (Luke 4:23). *The British Journal of Psychiatry*, *209*, 447–448. https://doi.org/10.1192/bjp.bp.116.185355

Hall, L. H., Johnson, J., Watt, I., Tsipa, A., & O'Connor, D. B. (2016). Healthcare staff Wellbeing, burnout, and patient safety: A systematic review. *BMJ Open*, *6*(2), e009837.

Harper, K., Bhutani, G., Rao, A. S., & Clarke, J. (2020). Wellbeing matters in IAPT practitioners: Identity vs system. *International Journal of Stress Prevention and Wellbeing*, 4(4), 1–12. http://www.stressprevention.net/volume/volume-4-2020/volume-4-article-4/

Heifetz, R. A., Grashow, A., & Linsky, M. (2009). The practice of adaptive leadership: Tools and tactics for changing your organization and the world. Harvard Business Press.

Jackman, L., & Steer, C. (2023). *Measuring mental wellbeing in Greater Manchester.* Greater Manchester Integrated Care.

Kaeding, A., et al. (2017). Professional burnout, early maladaptive schemas, and physical health in clinical and counselling psychology trainees. *Journal of Clinical Psychology, 73*(12), 1782–1796.

Kell, L., & Baguley, C. (2018). *What factors impact on the retention of psychological wellbeing practitioners?* Psychological Professions Network North West.

Kilminster, S. M., & Jolly, B. C. (2000). Effective supervision in clinical practice settings: A literature review. Medical Education, 34(12), 827–840. https://doi.org/10.1046/j.1365-2923.2000.00758.x

Kotter, J. P. (2012). Leading change. Harvard Business Review Press.

Leinwand, P., Kearney, R., & McGrath, M. (2021). The new CEO's guide to leading transformation. Harvard Business Review Press.

Lundstrom, T., Pugliese, G., Bartley, J., Cox, J., & Guither, C. (2002). Organizational and environmental factors that affect worker health and safety and patient outcomes. American Journal of Infection Control, 30(2), 93–106. https://doi.org/10.1067/mic.2002.119820

Maslach, C., & Leiter, M. P. (2016). Understanding the burnout experience: Recent research and its implications for psychiatry. World Psychiatry, 15(2), 103–111. https://doi.org/10.1002/wps.20311

Menzies-Lyth, I. (1988). Containing anxiety in institutions: Selected essays. London: Free Association Books.

Miller, S., Willard-Grace, R., Knox, M., Huang, B., Grumbach, K. (2019). Burnout and health care workforce turnover. Annals of Family Medicine, 17(Suppl 1), S1–S11. https://doi.org/10.1370/afm.2406

NHS Confederation. (2020). How do NHS leaders feel amid the crisis? NHS Confederation. https://www.nhsconfed.org/articles/how-do-nhs-leaders-feel-amid-crisis

NHS Leadership Academy. (2022). *Leading with clarity: Workforce planning and creating thriving work environments in healthcare.* NHS Leadership Academy Publications. Retrieved April 20, 2025, from https://www.leadershipacademy.nhs.uk

NHS Providers. (2024, April 12). *Funding cut to NHS staff mental health support services 'deeply concerning'.* Retrieved on April 20, 2025, from https://

nhsproviders.org/news-blogs/news/funding-cut-to-nhs-staff-mental-health-support-services-deeply-concerning

NHS Staff Survey. (2023). *Working together to improve NHS staff experiences*. Retrieved April 20, 2025, from https://www.nhsstaffsurveyresults.com

NHS Staff Survey. (2024). *National results across the NHS in England*. Retrieved April 20, 2025, from https://www.nhsstaffsurveys.com/results/national-results/

Northouse, P. G. (2021). Leadership: Theory and practice (9th ed.). Sage Publications.

Obholzer, A., & Roberts, V. Z. (Eds.). (1994). The unconscious at work: Individual and organizational stress in the human services. London: Routledge.

Office for National Statistics (ONS). (2024). *Labour force survey*. ONS.

Oxford Academic Health Science Network. (2023). Model NHS talking therapies staff wellbeing strategy. Oxford Academic Health Science Network.

Panagioti, M., Geraghty, K., Johnson, J., Zhou, A., Panagopoulou, E., Chew-Graham, C., Peters, D., Hodkinson, A., Riley, R., Esmail, A. (2018). Association between physician burnout and patient safety, professionalism, and patient satisfaction: A systematic review and meta-analysis. JAMA Internal Medicine, 178(10), 1317–1330. https://doi.org/10.1001/jamainternmed.2018.3713

Pereira, J-A., Barkham, M., Kellet, S., & Saxon, D. (2017). The role of practitioner resilience and mindfulness in effective practice: A practice-based feasibility study. *Administration and Policy in Mental Health, 44*, 691–704.

Pines, A., & Maslach, C. (2019). The burnout companion to study and practice: A critical analysis. Routledge.

Rao, A., Kemp, N., Bhutani, G., Morris, R., Summers, E., Brown, K., Clarke, J., & Neal, A. (2021). *Building a caring work culture – What good looks like*. British Psychological Society, Division of Clinical Psychology. Retrieved April 30, 2025, from https://cms.bps.org.uk/sites/default/files/2022-09/Building%20a%20Caring%20Work%20Culture.pdf

Seddon, J. (2008). *Systems thinking in the public sector: The failure of the reform regime... and a manifesto for a better way*. Triarchy Press.

Shanafelt, T. D., & Noseworthy, J. H. (2017). Executive leadership and physician Wellbeing: Nine organizational strategies to promote engagement and reduce burnout. *Mayo Clinic Proceedings, 92*(1), 129–146.

Shanafelt, T. D., West, C. P., Sinsky, C., Trockel, M., Tutty, M., Carlasare, L. E., ... & Dyrbye, L. N. (2021). Changes in burnout and satisfaction with work-life integration in physicians during the first year of the COVID-19 pandemic. JAMA Network Open, 4(7), e2113542. https://doi.org/10.1001/jamanetworkopen.2021.13542

Skovholt, T. M., & Trotter-Mathison, M. (2016). The resilient practitioner: Burnout and compassion fatigue prevention and self-care strategies for the helping professions (3rd ed.). Routledge. https://doi.org/10.4324/9781315737447

Spence Laschinger, H. K., & Fida, R. (2014). New nurses' burnout and workplace wellbeing: The influence of authentic leadership and psychological capital. Burnout Research, 1(1), 19–28. https://doi.org/10.1016/j.burn.2014.03.002

Summers, E. M. A., Morris, R. C., & Bhutani, G. E. (2019). A measure to assess the workplace wellbeing of psychological practitioners. *Clinical Psychology & Psychotherapy*, 27(1), 1–13.

Summers, E. M. A., Morris, R. C., Bhutani, G. E., Rao, A. S., & Clarke, J. C. (2021). A survey of psychological practitioner workplace well-being. Clinical Psychology & Psychotherapy, 28(2), 438–451.

The King's Fund. (2021a). *Building a sustainable workforce in healthcare: The importance of leadership and environment*. Retrieved April 20, 2025, from https://www.kingsfund.org.uk

The King's Fund. (2021b). Health care: Action needed on staff health and wellbeing. The King's Fund. https://www.kingsfund.org.uk/insight-and-analysis/articles/health-care-action-needed-staff-health-wellbeing

U.S. Department of Health and Human Services, Office of the Surgeon General. (2022). Surgeon General's Framework for Mental Health & Well-Being in the Workplace. U.S. Public Health Service.

West, M., & Dawson, J. (2012). Employee engagement and NHS performance. The King's Fund. https://www.kingsfund.org.uk/publications/employee-engagement-nhs-performance

West, M. A., Dawson, J. F., Admasachew, L., & Topakas, A. (2016). NHS staff management and health service quality: Results from the NHS staff survey and related data. The King's Fund. https://www.kingsfund.org.uk/publications/nhs-staff-management-and-health-service-quality

West, M. A., Dawson, J. F., & Kaur, M. (2017). *Making the difference: Diversity and inclusion in the NHS*. The King's Fund.

West, R., Michie, S., Rubin, G. J., & Amlôt, R. (2020). Applying principles of behaviour change to reduce SARS-CoV-2 transmission. Nature Human Behaviour, 4(5), 451–459. https://doi.org/10.1038/s41562-020-0887-9

Whittington, A. (2024). Next steps for the psychological professions workforce in England – Delivering the NHS Long Term Workforce Plan. Clinical Psychology Forum, 375, 29–38.

Williams, R., Jenkins, D. A., Ashcroft, D. M., Brown, B., Campbell, S., Carr, M. J., ··· Peek, N. (2022). Diagnosis of physical and mental health conditions in primary care during the COVID-19 pandemic: A retrospective cohort study. Lancet Public Health, 7(5), e366–e378. https://doi.org/10.1016/S2468-2667(22)00029-6

Williams, N. M. (2023, May 3). Effective DE&I strategies focus on systemic change. Forbes. Retrieved from https://www.forbes.com

World Health Organization. (2023). *Mental health at work: Policy brief.* World Health Organization and International Labour Organization. https://www.ncbi.nlm.nih.gov/pmc/articles/PMC10911318/

16 The Composition and Wellbeing of the Psychological Professions in the UK (2014 to 2021)

Professor (Emeritus) Reg Morris, Gita Bhutani, Dr Amra Saleem Rao, Jeremy C. Clarke, and Professor (Emeritus) Tony Lavender

Introduction

The poor workplace wellbeing and high rates of distress of staff working as psychological professionals have been amply attested in several countries over many decades (Pines & Maslach, 1978; Dorociak et al., 2017; Rupert & Morgan, 2005; Dattilio, 2015; Johnson,et al., 2012; Summers et al., 2021; Tay et al., 2018). These findings are especially significant because organisational factors that promote workplace wellbeing and the mitigation of distress are key factors in the effective delivery of services (Boorman, 2009; Salvagioni et al., 2017; Saddington, 2021; British Psychological Society, 2022b). They also influence staff intention to leave their posts (Lee et al., 2011). Despite intense interest in this area, there have been few attempts to assess changes in workplace wellbeing in the psychological professions over time. Such studies are necessary to assess the need for, and effectiveness of, initiatives to improve the wellbeing of the health workforce (NHSE, 2020a,b). To fill this gap, this article reports the findings of six successive surveys of the psychological workforce in the UK undertaken between 2014 and 2021.

In addition, there has been growing concern about the representativeness of the psychological workforce as the UK becomes increasingly

DOI: 10.4324/9781003492399-21

diverse in terms of ethnicity, gender, lifestyles and disability (Office for National Statistics, 2022a, 2022b; House of Commons Library, 2022). There have been recent moves to improve participation in psychological professions for under-represented groups (Health Education England, 2019) and the current surveys from 2014 to 2021 provide a yardstick against which to measure their impact.

A previous survey (Summers et al., 2021) found that disability is strongly linked to poor workplace wellbeing in the psychological professions. The association between health, disability and workplace wellbeing has been extensively studied, and a large-scale meta-analysis of 485 studies involving nearly 268,000 workers found that physical and mental health were exceptionally strongly associated with job satisfaction (Faragher et al., 2005). While earlier research focussed on the putative influence of workplace factors on health, some more recent research has considered the role of disability in determining workplace wellbeing and job satisfaction. This work has highlighted the importance of workplace adaptation to facilitate the inclusion of disabled people (Nevala et al., 2015; Addabbo & Sarti, 2022). The current surveys included questions that addressed the important question of how people with health conditions and disabilities experience their workplace.

Since the aim of the surveys was to provide census data about the composition and the workplace experiences of psychological professions at each time point, they did not employ a panel methodology which entails sampling the same individuals at each time point. Such an approach would not capture the prevalence of wellbeing and distress as the composition of the professions changed over time. Instead, the surveys were distributed as widely as possible to endeavour to obtain large and representative contemporary samples. Moreover, changes in the sample between time points were monitored by scrutinising the stability and variation in demographic data: age, profession, gender, ethnicity, specialty, etc.

Materials and Methods

Consent, Ethics and Data Management

The work is a secondary analysis of an anonymised database produced through the Division of Clinical Psychology Leadership and Management Faculty/New Savoy Partnership surveys of the UK psychological professions. The purpose of the surveys was to provide regular censuses of the profession, and they were not construed as research requiring research ethical approval. All surveys were conducted under the terms of the European General Data Protection Regulations (2016/679) or their predecessors and the ethical principles of the British Psychological Society. All data were anonymised, and no identifiable information was available to this study. Participation was voluntary, and consent for the use of the data was given within the surveys; participants agreeing for their anonymous data to be used in future reports or publications.

Sampling and Questionnaire Delivery

All the questionnaires were distributed by email through professional networks and social media groups. These groups served all parts of the UK and were chosen if the recipients were psychological/medical professionals working with psychological therapies. This included all branches of registered psychological wellbeing practioners, CBT therapists, psychological wellbeing practioners, child psychotherapists and any other professionals using psychological intervention methods. The surveys included only those who were currently employed by a UK health or social care organisation and were not designed for single-handed private practitioners.

From 2014 to 2016, the surveys were completed using the Questback® survey platform hosted by the British Psychological Society, and from 2017, all survey were conducted using the Qualtrics® survey platform.

Survey completion windows were as follows:

- 2014 December 2014 to January 2015
- 2015 November to December 2015
- 2016 November 2016 to February 2017
- 2017 December 2017 to February 2018
- 2019 January to March 2019
- 2021 May to July 2021

All questions required a response (forced choice).

Questions and Included Scales

All the surveys gathered demographic information. They also included several wellbeing items taken from the European Social Survey (2001) and workplace wellbeing items from the NHS staff survey (NHS staff survey, https://www.nhsstaffsurveys.com/). These encompassed questions about bullying, hours of unpaid work, discrimination, work stress, intention to resign, *etc.* From 2017, the surveys incorporated the PPWWM (Summers et al., 2020) and The Short Warwick-Edinburgh Mental Well-being Scale (Stewart-Brown et al., 2009).

Data Cleaning and Analysis

The forced choice nature of the questionnaire did not generate missing questions. Data were cleaned by removing any incomplete questionnaires, returns from participants who did not meet the inclusion criteria, and a very small number of questionnaires where the same option had been chosen for all questions.

Data analysis used IBM SPSS® version 25. All statistical analyses used bootstrapping (1000 iterations) to give a more robust test with respect to deviation from assumptions. All significant tests were two-tailed. Non-disclosure categories *'don't know'* and *'prefer not to say'* were excluded from percentage calculations.

With large samples such as these, statistical significance tests can demonstrate significance at conventional levels even when differences between groups are trivial. For this reason, indices of effect size (group differences) or shared variance (measures of association) indicate change and stability more appropriately.

Results

Samples and their Demographics

In all years, over 85% of respondents were from England, with Scotland having the next largest proportion (2.6% to 7.7%) and Northern Ireland the smallest (0.4% to 1.0%).

Table 16.1 shows the sample sizes and key demographic attributes of the samples in each year.

Table 16.1 Sample size and key demographic attributes of samples by year

Year	N	Female %	Male %	Hetero-sexual %	Other sexuality %	Disability or long-standing Illness %	White ethnicity %	Other ethnicity %	Median Age Category	Employed NHS %	Median Agenda for Change Band	Clinical psychologist %	CBT therapist %	Psychological Wellbeing Practitioners %	Counsellor %
2021	971	83.5	15.6	85.7	14.3	21.4	89.6	10.4	35–44 (29.8%)	85.0	8a (23.1%)	52.0	11.7	10.6	4.6
2019	1037	82.5	17.2	89.6	10.4	16.3	92.8	7.2	35–44 (28.8%)	91.2	8a (29.6%)	54.8	14.0	8.6	5.3
2017	1678	80.3	19.3	88.7	11.3	17.1	88.8	11.2	35–44 (28.7%)	87.7	7 (26.4%)	48.5	17.9	13.5	5.7
2016	1227	80.4	19.3	90.6	9.4	19.5	90.7	9.3	35–44 (28.0%)	89.1	7 (27.0%)	40.7	19.7	12.7	6.9
2015	1114	80.2	19.6	92.0	8.0	24.5	94.2	5.8	41–50 (27.2%)**	86.0	7 (32.0%)	† †	† †	† †	† †
2014	852	79.0	20.9	90.4	9.6	7.1*	96.4	3.6	41–50 (28.1%)**	93.7	7 (33.5%)	32.4	18.3	13.0	10.8
Total	6871														

* Question asked about disability only. In subsequent years longstanding illness was also included. † † Data not collected.

** Different categories used in 2014 and 2015.

Table 16.2 Variables relevant to workplace wellbeing

Year	Depressed ***		Job Stress ***		Bullied by Managers †		Accused of Bullying **		Unpaid Hours Worked ***		WEMWBS ***	PPWWM **	Discrimination by Patients and Public		Discrimination by Managers or Colleagues **		Sufficient Staffing		Wanting to Leave NHS *	
	Often %	All the Time %	Often %	All the Time %	Often %	All the Time %	Yes %	No %	Yes %	No %	Mean (SD)	Mean (SD)	Yes %	No %	Yes %	No %	Yes %	No %	Never %	Once a Year or More %
2021	11.6	2.1	33.3	10.0	2.2	1.9	4.5	95.5	77.7	22.3	21.20 (3.51)	89.65 (17.81)	6.5	93.5	16.1	83.9	12.5	76.2	20.3	79.7
2019	9.4	1.5	31.6	7.0	1.4	1.4	5.1	94.9	73.0	27.0	22.00 (3.77)	90.78 (17.51)	6.2	93.8	12.8	87.2	13.3	77.0	22.5	77.5
2017	9.9	1.4	† †		1.6	1.4	4.1	95.9	72.2	27.8	22.21 (3.92)	91.88 (17.55)	6.3	93.7	11.2	88.8	18.7	71.9	25.3	74.7
2016	14.3	1.5	43.8	17.7	† †		3.5	96.5	75.0	25.0	† †									
2015	10.4	1.6	50.3	18.9	† †		2.2	97.8	† †											
2014	8.1	0.4	43.9	14.9	† †		4.7	95.3	† †											

***p<.000; ** p<.01; * p<.05;

† Not analysed due to changes in questions over years. † † Data not collected.

Key Outcome Measures

Table 16.2 shows key outcome variables for each survey.

The PPWWM and the WEMWBS cover the three years that they were included in the survey. Both measures show a significant reduction over the years, although effect sizes are very small. For comparison WEMWBS general population mean was 23.7 for men and 23.2 for women (Ng Fat, Scholes, Boniface, Mindell, & Stewart-Brown, 2017). The means for the current three samples are all significantly lower.

For comparison with Carter et al. (2013) responses for any experience of bullying by managers, including the 'rarely' category, were collated. This was 19.6% for 2019 and 19.0% for 2017. For 2021, where the question included bullying by any staff, the figure was 21.1%.

Disability as Predictor of Issues/Distress

Table 16.3 shows how identifying as having a long-term illness or disability is associated with key wellbeing outcomes. The majority of the measures showed significant differences in the direction of poorer wellbeing for disabled people.

Table 16.3 The association of disability with key outcome variables

Question	2014	2015	2016	2017	2019	2021
Feeling depressed	ns	*	****	****	*	****
Job stress	ns	*	*	† †	ns	ns
Harassment/bullying at work †	****	**	****	****	ns	****
Treated with respect	***	**	*	† †	† †	† †
PPWWM score	† †	† †	† †	****	****	*
SWEMWBS score	† †	† †	† †	****	**	**
Percentage NOT receiving reasonable adjustments when perceived as necessary or perceived disability discrimination	† †	25.1%	† †	13.3%	11.6%	18.2%

**** = p <.000; *** = p =<.001; ** = p =<.01; * = p =<.05; ns = non-significant

† Bullying questions were differently worded over surveys but were the same for those with and without disability in each survey permitting comparison.

† † Data not collected.

Discussion

Over the six surveys, almost 7,000 responses were obtained. Demographic data for psychological professions as a whole has not been routinely compiled in the UK. The first comprehensive psychological professions workforce census only took place in 2023 (NHS Benchmarking, 2023). Therefore, the representativeness of the sample was assessed by comparisons with data for practitioner psychologists. The preponderance of females in all samples reflected the gender composition of the UK practitioner psychologist population, which was 81.2% in 2022 (Health and Care Professions Council, 2022). There was no evidence that the gender imbalance is declining over time. Indeed, the data suggest it may be increasing. However, two previous surveys (Summers et al., 2020; Summers et al., 2021) did not find gender differences in key workplace wellbeing indices. Ethnicity figures for recent years were also broadly similar to those of practitioner psychologists, with 87.1% white and 12.9% non-white (Health and Care Professions Council, 2022). In a previous survey (Summers et al., 2021), membership of ethnic groups did not show large associations with workplace or general wellbeing, apart from the finding that Asian psychological professionals had higher than average wellbeing.

Representativeness of the professional makeup of the sample can be assessed by comparison with a 2020 estimate of whole-time equivalents for psychological professions in England (Health Education England, 2021). In the most recent survey, clinical psychologists were overrepresented (52.0% compared with 39.2%), CBT practitioners were underrepresented (10.6% versus 15.2%), while psychological wellbeing practitioners and counsellors were equally represented (10.6% versus 10.4%; 4.6% versus 4.8%, respectively). The rank order of numbers in these professional groups for recent years was the same as in the Health Education England estimates of 2021. Although this survey reports numbers of respondents in each profession, the Health Education England estimates are based on whole-time equivalents. However, the two indices are highly correlated.

The percentage declaring sexuality as other than heterosexual increased over the years while the percentage identifying as heterosexual declined by about the same percentage, reflecting the national trend in the UK between 2014 and 2020 (Office for National Statistics, 2022). There was no clear trend in the percentage declaring as disabled or having a long-term illness; it remained between 17% and 25% for all the surveys where longstanding illness was included in the questionnaire. This is surprising since the proportion of disabled people in employment generally has increased markedly over the period of the surveys (Office for National Statistics, 2021). It appears that the psychological professions are not benefiting from the increasing numbers of disabled people active in the workforce. It is even more surprising in the context of a workforce that purports to value the participation and inclusion of disabled people as 'experts by experience' (British Psychological Society, 2022) or 'service users' (HCPC, 2024) who can bring lived experience into the workforce.

On the other hand, there was an indication that the psychological professions are becoming more ethnically diverse, with the proportion of those identifying as non-white increasing to closer to the overall UK percentage for NHS staff of 22.4% BME and 73.1% white (NHS Workforce Race Equality Standard 2021). This is a gratifying development that has been strongly promoted and encouraged by financial and policy support from the training commissioners in England (Health Education England, 2019). Meanwhile, the median age of samples appears to be stable, but interpretation is complicated by the use of different age band categories for the first two years of the survey.

Turning to the standardised outcome measures, the PPWWM and WEMWBS both showed significant changes over the four years in which they were administered in the survey. The change was demonstrated as a steady decline over this period. However, the depressed scores in 2021 may reflect the impact of COVID (Rose et al., 2021) but pre-COVID 2019 averages for both measures were lower than those in 2017, suggesting there may be other factors involved. The answer to the question of whether there is a long-term declining trend in the wellbeing of psychological professionals working in mental health requires a longer series of post-COVID surveys. The general wellbeing of mental health workers, as measured by the WEMWBS, is lower than the population average (Summers et al., 2021), so any further decline is a priority for workplace improvement measures.

Other indicators of workplace wellbeing showed a mixed picture. Feelings of depression combined across the categories of 'often' or 'all the time' remained under 16% during all six surveys, and there was no clear trend despite the differences between years. However, reports of frequent workplace stress have declined from their very high levels of around 60% or more in the first three surveys.

Responses to the question about having to work unpaid hours indicate that this is a problem area with rates of well over 70% in all years. This is much higher than the 57% reported in the most recent survey of all NHS staff (NHS Staff Survey, 2021) and suggests that it is a particular issue for the mental health workforce. Working long hours has serious implications for workplace wellbeing and work-life balance, with over 31% of NHS staff reporting not having enough energy for family, friends and leisure activities (NHS Staff Survey, 2021). This is a key finding since work-life balance is an important factor in career satisfaction for psychological professionals (Rupert, Miller, Hartman, & Bryant, 2012). It is probable that unpaid working hours are linked to reports of understaffing that affect performance. This was reported by between 70% and 80% of respondents in our three most recent surveys, suggesting that understaffing in mental health services is even more serious than in the NHS in general, where just over 52% of respondents reported understaffing (NHS Staff Survey, 2021). Similarly, the finding that around 75% of psychological professionals employed in the NHS regularly contemplate resigning compares with 30% for all NHS staff (NHS staff survey, 2021). Once again suggesting that psychological professionals have lower job satisfaction than the general NHS workforce. This is clearly an important issue for the NHS, and intention to resign is frequently converted into action, with one study in the USA showing 26% annual turnover in a community mental health service (Bukach et al., 2017), and turnover in the UK NHS mental health sector reported as 13.6% in 2015/16 compared with 8.6% for the NHS Acute Trusts (RoMHS, 2022). Such turnover rates have major implications for effective service delivery, training costs, continuity of care and diminished quality of service. It also increases the workload on remaining staff, engendering a negative cycle of longer hours, unpaid working and lowered job satisfaction leading to an increased likelihood of resignation. Much remains to be done to improve staff support and work satisfaction for psychological professionals to address the issue of high turnover. In England, there was temporary centralised funding for 40 regional well-being hubs in partnership with local Occupational Health providers (NHSE, 2020b) but this funding was largely withdrawn in 2023, with some limited additional funding made available until the end of March 2024 (NHSE England, 2024) . However, the impact on staff turnover is yet to be formally evaluated. Other suggestions are that turnover could be reduced by better rates of pay for mental health staff (Bukach et al., 2017). In the past, the UK operated an enhanced pension scheme for mental health workers, the mental health officer status (NHS Business Services Authority, 2022), that incentivised frontline workers to continue working in mental health until retirement. However, this was discontinued for new staff in 1995.

Experience of frequent bullying by managers ('often' or 'all the time') was not specifically asked about in the first three surveys and remained under 5% from 2017 to 2021. Bullying by leaders, managers, or colleagues was assessed as a single question in 2021, which accounts for the step increase from the two previous surveys that asked about bullying by managers only. However, the number reporting *any* bullying by managers in 2017 and 2019 (including the 'rarely' category) was just under 20%, which accords with the figure of 20% reported by Carter et al. (2013) for bullying by any staff (not only by managers) in an NHS sample. The bullying question in the most recent 2021 survey, which, like Carter et al., asked about bullying by any staff, produced a similar figure of 21.1% when the 'rarely' category was included. Similarly, being accused of bullying showed significant variation over the years but without any clear trend. Bullying is an important factor in workplace wellbeing. Carter et al. (2013) reported that bullying and witnessing bullying were associated with lower levels of psychological health and job satisfaction, and higher levels of intention to leave work. Even though rates of frequent bullying are low, vigilance and the development of workplace policy and its implementation are indicated.

Reported discrimination by patients and the public on any grounds, including ethnicity, religion and disability, appears to be stable at between 6% and 7%, approximately reflecting the rate of 7.8% reported by all NHS staff (NHS Staff Survey, 2021). However, discrimination by colleagues and managers is experienced at over double this frequency and exceeds the 9.1% found in the 2021 NHS staff survey. It is not clear which aspects of discrimination account for these elevated levels, but one possibility is that disability discrimination (discussed below) occurs because mental health managers in hard-pressed, understaffed services have less room for manoeuvre in making reasonable adjustments than their colleagues in other branches of the health service.

Disability was a variable of special interest since it has been shown to be linked to poor workplace wellbeing in psychological professionals, with higher effect size than other variables (Summers et al., 2021). Across the six surveys, the importance of disability was demonstrated by its relationship with poorer wellbeing scores in 21 out of the 26 separate analyses, demonstrating its importance. A major review and meta-analysis of the area identified disability as a major issue in workplace wellbeing (Faragher et al., 2003), and legal (Equality Act, 2010) and government guidance (Department for Work and Pensions, 2020) have been formulated to mitigate the disadvantage it engenders. However, it clearly remains a significant factor in reducing workplace and general wellbeing, and this survey demonstrates the perceptions of disabled people that the provisions of the Equality Act are not implemented in a significant proportion of cases.

Clinical and Organisational Implications

The psychological professions workforce has a lower than average participation of people with disabilities or long-standing illnesses. This limits the valuable contribution disabled people could make in terms of lived experience of health conditions (Byrne & Wykes, 2020). Moreover, those who are employed report lower workplace wellbeing than their healthy, able-bodied professional colleagues, with a sizeable proportion reporting that legally mandated workplace adjustments are not provided. There is a clear case for better auditing of the implementation of government guidance in relation to the Equality Act, (2010), as well as positive action when recruiting for training and employment to sustain the wellbeing and participation of disabled practitioners.

There is a suggestion in the data from the standardised measures that the workplace and general wellbeing of the psychological professions are declining. This is concerning since their general wellbeing was already below the national population average. This is echoed by the finding that several organisational and wellbeing indices for this professional group fell below those of the general NHS workforce. Current approaches to improving psychological wellbeing amongst NHS staff remain fragmented, with different organisations offering different approaches (e.g. van Agteren et al., 2018, Brand et al., 2017) despite NICE guidance (NICE, 2022) and a range of reports providing tools and resources to do so (e.g. Teoh et al., 2023).

While these approaches have the potential to improve resilience and bolster wellbeing, it is also vital to address the underlying problems of unrealistic expectations and targets, underfunding and understaffing and the vicious cycle of impaired workplace wellbeing and workforce turnover that they engender.

Strengths and Weaknesses

This paper reports the results of the only surveys of the psychological professions workforce in the UK and provides some insight into changes in its composition and the wellbeing of its members over a seven-year period.

The surveys relied on voluntary participation and distribution through organisations and professional networks. This could have induced sample bias. Also, changes in outcome measures over time could have been the result of changes in sample composition rather than the result of temporal influences. However, pragmatically, the surveys provide a snapshot of the state of the workforce as it was composed at each time point.

Ideas in Brief

- **Track trends to inform policy**: Six national surveys across seven years reveal evolving demographics and persistent challenges in wellbeing, diversity and inclusion among psychological professionals.
- **Recognise systemic inequalities**: Data highlights disproportionate experiences of workplace stress, discrimination and lack of accommodations – particularly for disabled professionals – calling for urgent, targeted action.
- **Support and retain the workforce**: High rates of unpaid hours, intention to resign and perceived understaffing reflect a sector under pressure, demanding system-level investment in workforce wellbeing and sustainability.
- **Promote inclusive participation**: Address the gap between policy commitments and practice by ensuring disabled and marginalised professionals are equitably supported, valued and represented across roles.

Acknowledgements

The authors gratefully acknowledge the contribution of Elisabeth Summers to the design and conduct of surveys in 2017 and 2019, and the contribution of members of the New Savoy Partnership and DCP Leadership and Management Faculty, Collaborative Learning Network (CLaN) Steering Group. They also acknowledge the Psychological Professions Network North West and the Association of Clinical Psychologists for facilitating the distribution of the questionnaires.

Disclosure/Declarations of Interest

The authors have no interests to declare.

Funding

This work was supported by funding from the British Psychological Society, Division of Clinical Psychology.

Data Availability Statement

The data that support the findings of this study are available from the corresponding author upon reasonable request.

References

Addabbo, T., & Sarti, E. (2022). Job satisfaction, work-related stress and disability. *Rivista Internazionale Di Scienze Sociali, 130*(2), 107–124.

Boorman, S. (2009). *NHS health and well-being: Final report*. Department of Health.

Brand, S. L., Thompson Coon, J., Fleming, L. E., Carroll, L., Bethel, A., & Wyatt, K. (2017). Whole-system approaches to improving the health and wellbeing of healthcare workers: A systematic review. *PLoS ONE, 12*(12), e0188418. https://doi.org/10.1371/journal.pone.0188418

British Psychological Society. (2022a). *Expert by experience*. Retrieved November 3, 2022, from https://www.bps.org.uk/expert-experience

British Psychological Society. (2022b). *Written evidence submitted by the British Psychological Society (RTR0135). Health and social care committee. The workforce: Recruitment, training and retention in health and social care report*. British Psychological Society. https://committees.parliament.uk/writtenevidence/43114/html/

Bukach, A. M., Ejaz, F. K., Dawson, N., & Gitter, R. J. (2017). Turnover among Community Mental Health Workers in Ohio. *Administration and Policy in Mental Health, 44*(1), 115–122. https://doi.org/10.1007/s10488-015-0706-1

Byrne, L., & Wykes, T. (2020). A role for lived experience mental health leadership in the age of Covid-19. *Journal of Mental Health, 29*(3), 243–246. http://dx.doi.org/10.1136/bmjopen-2013-002628

Carter, M., Thompson, N., Crampton, P., Morrow, G., Burford, B., Gray, C., & Illing. (2013). Workplace bullying in the UK NHS: A questionnaire and interview study on prevalence, impact and barriers to reporting. *BMJ Open, 3,* e002628. https://dx.doi.org/10.1136/bmjopen-013-002628

Dattilio, F. M. (2015). The self-care of psychologists and mental health professionals: A review and practitioner guide. *Australian Psychologist, 50*(6), 393–399. https://doi.org/10.1111/ap.12157

Department for Work and Pensions. (2020). *Recruiting, managing and developing people with a disability or health condition: A practical guide for line managers.* DfW&P. https://assets.publishing.service.gov.uk/government/uploads/system/uploads/attachment_data/file/938189/disability-confident-line-managers-guide.pdf

Dorociak, K. E., Rupert, P. A., & Zahniser, E. (2017). Work life, wellbeing, and self-care across the professional lifespan of psychologists. *Professional Psychology: Research and Practice, 48*(6), 429–437. https://dx.doi.org/10.1037/pro0000160

Equality Act. (2010). *The Equality Act 2010.* UK Government.

European Social Survey. (2001). *European Social Survey core questionnaire development – Overview.* Centre for Comparative Social Surveys, City University London.

Faragher, E. B., Cass, M., & Cooper, C. L. (2005). The relationship between job satisfaction and health: A meta-analysis. *Occupational and Environmental Medicine, 62*(2), 105–112. https://doi.org/10.1136/oem.2002.006734

Health and Care Professions Council. (2017). *Standards for education and training.* HCPC.

Health and Care Professions Council. (2022). *Response to request for demographic information for registered practitioner psychologists under the Freedom of Information Act 2000.* HCPC.

Health and Care Professions Council. (2024). Standards of conduct, performance and ethics (effective from 1 September 2024). Health and Care Professions Council. https://www.hcpc-uk.org/standards/standards-of-conduct-performance-and-ethics/

Health Education England. (2019). *Action plan to improve equity of access and inclusion for black, Asian and minority ethnic entrants to clinical psychology training.* Health Education England.

Health Education England. (2021). *Psychological professions workforce plan for England.* Health Education England.

House of Commons Library. (2022). *UK disability statistics: Prevalence and life experiences.* Retrieved November 30, 2022, from https://commonslibrary.parliament.uk/research-briefings/cbp-9602/#:~:text=How%20many%20people%20have%20a,22%25%20of%20the%20total%20population

Johnson, S., Osborn, D. P., Araya, R., Wearn, E., Paul, M., Stafford, M., Wellman, N., Nolan, F., Killaspy, H., Lloyd-Evans, B., Anderson, E., & Wood S. J. (2012). Morale in the English mental health workforce: Questionnaire survey. *The British Journal of Psychiatry, 201*(3), 239–246. https://doi.org/10.1192/bjp.bp.111.098970

Lee, J., Lim N., Yang, E., & Lee, S. M. (2011). Antecedents and consequences of three dimensions of burnout in psychotherapists: A meta-analysis. *Professional Psychology: Research and Practice, 42*(3), 252. https://psycnet.apa.org/doi/10.1037/a0023319

National Institute for Health and Care Excellence. (2022). Mental wellbeing at work (NICE guideline NG212). https://www.nice.org.uk/guidance/ng212/

Nevala, N., Pehkonen, I., Koskela, I., Ruusuvuori, J., & Anttila, H. (2015). Workplace accommodation among persons with disabilities: A systematic review of its effectiveness and barriers or facilitators. *Journal of Occupational Rehabilitation, 25*, 432–448. https://doi.org/10.1007/s10926-014-9548-z

Ng Fat, L., Scholes, S., Boniface, S., Mindell, J., & Stewart-Brown, S. (2017). Evaluating and establishing national norms for mental wellbeing using the short Warwick–Edinburgh Mental Well-being Scale (SWEMWBS): Findings from the Health Survey for England. Quality of Life Research, 26(5), 1129–1144. https://doi.org/10.1007/s11136-016-1454-8

NHS Benchmarking Network. (2023). *The National Psychological Professions Workforce Census: England workforce data 2022/23.* Commissioned by NHS England, Workforce, Training and Education Directorate

NHS Business Services Authority. (2022). *NHS Pensions – Mental health officer status (1995 Section only) member facts.* NHS Business Services Authority. Retrieved December 13, 2022, from https://www.nhsbsa.nhs.uk/sites/default/files/2022-03/Mental%20health%20officer%20status%20%2895%20only%29%20member%20factsheet-20220307-%28V1%29.pdf

NHS England. (2025). *Staff mental health and wellbeing hubs.* NHS England.

NHS Staff Survey. (2021). *National results.* Retrieved December 13, 2022, from https://www.nhsstaffsurveys.com/results/national-results/

NHS England. (2020a). *We are the NHS: People plan for 2020/2021 – Action for us all.* NHSe.

NHS England. (2020b). *Guidance for mental health and wellbeing hubs for health and social care staff.* NHSe.

NHS England. (2021). *NHS workforce race equality standard.* NHSe. Retrieved December 15, 2022, from https://www.england.nhs.uk/about/equality/equality-hub/workforce-equality-data-standards/equality-standard/

Office for National Statistics. (2021). *Disability and employment.* Retrieved November 3, 2022, from https://www.ons.gov.uk/peoplepopulationand

community/healthandsocialcare/disability/datasets/disabilityandemployment

Office for National Statistics. (2022a). *Ethnic group, England and Wales: Census 2021*. Retrieved November 30, 2022, from https://www.ons.gov.uk/peoplepopulationandcommunity/culturalidentity/ethnicity/bulletins/ethnicgroupenglandandwales/census2021#:~:text=the%20%22Asian%2C%20or%20Asian%20British,was%2081.0%25%20(45.8%20million)

Office for National Statistics. (2022b). *Sexual orientation, UK*. Retrieved November 30, 2022, from https://www.ons.gov.uk/peoplepopulationandcommunity/culturalidentity/sexuality/bulletins/sexualidentityuk/2020

Pines, A., & Maslach, C. (1978). Characteristics of staff burnout on mental health setting. *Hospital and Community Psychiatry, 29*, 233–237. https://doi.org/10.1176/ps.29.4.233

RoMHNS (Retention of Mental Health Staff). Retrieved December 6, 2022, from https://www.health.org.uk/funding-and-partnerships/programmes/romhs-retention-of-mental-health-staff#:~:text=Mental%20health%20care%20has%2C%20on,in%2010%20posts%20were%20vacant

Rose, S., Hartnett, J., & Pillai, S. (2021). Healthcare worker's emotions, perceived stressors and coping mechanisms during the COVID-19 pandemic. *PLoS ONE, 16*(7), e0254252. https://doi.org/10.1371/journal.pone.0254252

Rupert, P. A., & Morgan, D. J. (2005). Work setting and burnout among professional psychologists. *Professional Psychology: Research and Practice, 36*(5), 544–550. http://dx.doi.org/10.1037/0735–7028.36.5.544

Rupert, P. A., Miller, A. O., Hartman, E. R. T., & Bryant, F. B. (2012). Predictors of career satisfaction among practicing psychologists. *Professional Psychology: Research and Practice, 43*(5), 495–502. https://doi.org/10.1037/a0029420

Saddington, D. (2021). *How organisational factors influence clinical psychologists' decisions to leave the NHS*. [Unpublished doctoral dissertation]. Division of Health Research, Lancaster University.

Salvagioni, D. A. J., Melanda, F. N., Mesas, A. E., González, A. D., Gabani, F. L., & Andrade, S. M. D. (2017). Physical, psychological and occupational consequences of job burnout: A systematic review of prospective studies. *PloS one, 12*(10). https://doi.org/10.1371/journal.pone.0185781

Summers, E., Morris, R., & Bhutani, G. (2020). A measure to assess the workplace wellbeing of psychological practitioners. *Clinical Psychology and Psychotherapy, 27*(1), 11–23. https://doi.org/10.1002/cpp.2401

Summers, E. M. A., Morris, R. C., Bhutani, G. E., Rao, A. S., & Clarke, J. C. (2021). A survey of psychological practitioner workplace wellbeing. *Clinical Psychology & Psychotherapy, 28*(2), 438–451. https://doi.org/10.1002/cpp.2509

Stewart-Brown, S., Tennant, A., Tennant, R., Platt, S., Parkinson, J., & Weich, S. (2009). Internal construct validity of the Warwick-Edinburgh Mental

Well-being Scale (WEMWBS): A Rasch analysis using data from the Scottish Health Education Population Survey. *Health and Quality of Life Outcomes*, *7*(1), 1–8. https://dx.doi.org/10.1186/1477-7525-7-15

Tay, S., Alcock, K., & Scior, K. (2018). Mental health problems among clinical psychologists: Stigma and its impact on disclosure and help-seeking. *Journal of Clinical Psychology*, *74*, 1545–1555. https://doi.org/10.1002/jclp.22614

Teoh, K., Dhensa-Kahlon, R., Christensen, M., Frost, F., Hatton, E., & Nielsen, K. (2023). Organisational wellbeing interventions: Case studies from the NHS (Technical Report). School of Management (SOM) and Birkbeck, University of London.

Van Agteren, J., Iasiello, M., & Lo, L. (2018). Improving the wellbeing and resilience of health services staff via psychological skills training. *BMC Research Notes*, *11*(1), 1–5. https://doi.org/10.1186/s13104-018-4034-x

17 Workforce Wellbeing across Healthcare Partnerships

A Systemic and Relational Approach

Kerry Hinsby and Rajinder Dhanjal

A Changing Health and Care Landscape

Healthcare systems need to adapt to the increased complexity of presenting needs. With an ageing population, marked health inequalities, and financial pressures, services must transform to respond and improve outcomes. Whilst psychologists are increasingly innovating and delivering change in these areas, the current context requires an adaptive leadership style to embrace such challenges.

The chapter primarily focuses on healthcare in England, UK, where from July 2022, Integrated Care Systems (ICSs) became the legal framework for delivering health and social care. An ICS system includes a broad alliance of regional partners from the National Health Service (NHS), local authorities, and voluntary and community sectors (VCSE), emphasising locally determined services and cross-organisational collaboration to improve outcomes and reduce health inequalities. Occurring simultaneously, the COVID-19 pandemic created long-lasting impacts on the healthcare workforce's wellbeing.

Organisational structures and workforce relationships need to adapt to meet these aspirations and challenges. The importance of preventative and systemic approaches alongside treatment is demonstrated in workforce guidelines (NICE, 2022) and financial analysis (Deloitte, 2022). Systemic reviews (Taylor et al., 2024) highlight the incompatibility of some aspects of healthcare work with the psychological wellbeing

DOI: 10.4324/9781003492399-22

of the workforce. For sustainable workforce wellbeing, the individual distress should be considered within the context of the workplace, with the locus of change existing at multiple system levels (Neilson et al., 2018)

To deliver a coordinated response to workforce wellbeing in this context, NHS England funded 40 ICS regional wellbeing hubs (NHSE, 2021). These hubs were predominantly led by clinical psychologists and were novel in the scale and complexity of their remit, requiring rapid emerging evidence-based service mobilisation (Allsopp et al., 2023).

The chapter examines adopting a systemic and relational approach to establishing one such wellbeing hub. There is an emphasis on valuing different approaches. The first author brings the perspective of a white female clinical lead, whilst the other highlights the standpoint of a new leader from a marginalised background. We consider how our relative power has impacted our leadership individually and collectively.

Core psychological skills have been central to working with novel dilemmas, group dynamics, and organisational cultures. The following section offers our reflections on taking up leadership to improve workforce wellbeing, including our relational and systemic stance to naming, validating, and working with diversity.

Leadership in Novel Settings – How Psychological Models Help

Within complex systems, no one knows all the answers and solutions. Multiple skills, knowledge, and values need to be coordinated, heard, and integrated. Creating teams with rich networks and cultures, where such diversity thrives, allows more creative solutions to surface. However, unless attention is paid to the inherent differences and power positions among team members and partnerships that create this richness, the asset can quickly become conflictual. Tensions can develop, inhibiting collaboration and impacting negatively on individual wellbeing, team performance, and service provision. Figure 17.1 offers a visual representation of the interactions between strong leadership, diversity, and team performance over time.

Psychological literature has much to offer for managing complex leadership challenges and harnessing the richness of diverse perspectives and creativity in teams. This includes theoretical approaches describing broad principles and therapeutic models which can help navigate the relationships and power imbalances inherent in leadership roles. Social constructionism and cognitive analytical therapy frameworks are

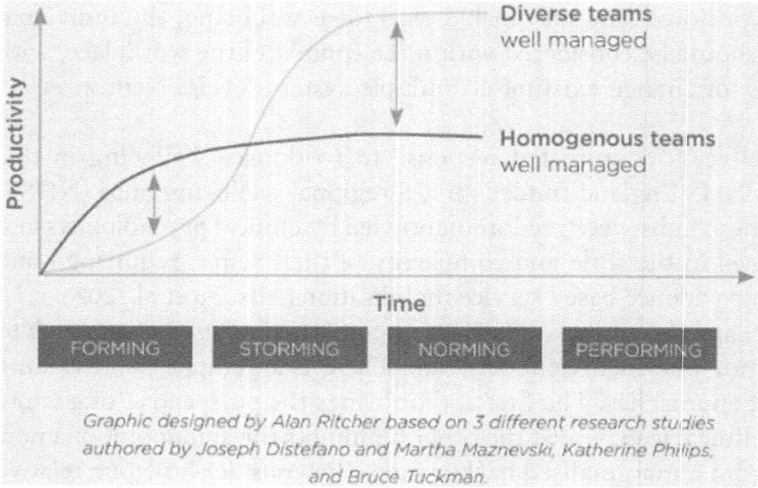

Figure 17.1 Impact of diversity and leadership on team performance.*

*This illustration by Alan Richter appeared with his permission in the Korn Ferry white paper, 'The Five Disciplines of Inclusive Leaders.' *(2019)*.

among such models that we adopted. Two service examples are offered as illustration.

Social Constructionism – A Collaborative Framework

Social constructionism offers an alternative critical lens towards taken-for-granted knowledge and processes. Its central tenets align with leadership demands in complex systems with a diverse workforce. It offers a value-driven approach, challenging traditional models and unquestioned dominant narratives, recognising the multiplicity of perspectives and addressing cultural and interpersonal power imbalances (Fairhurst & Grant, 2010).

The framework recognises the existence of multiple, equally valid ways of seeing any given situation, recognising that different understandings are often based within an individual's socio-cultural context. The fullest meaning of a situation, event or occurrence can only truly be derived through relationships and dialogues with others where multiple diverse perspectives are allowed to surface. In this context, language and conversation do not simply describe reality but serve to create reality (Gergen, 2005). If leadership only allows one perspective to be heard, then a rich diversity of solutions and options for future direction is lost.

In this context, leadership is not seen as vested in one person but is understood as 'how all members can co-create a future that maximises the team's effectiveness' (Roberts, 2007, p. 6). The focus of a team is to create the processes and relationships that allow the multiplicity of perspectives and options to surface rather than to aspire to find a unitary best solution.

This style of constructionist leadership also recognises the importance of power and inclusivity. Creating space to hear the perspectives that are less frequently heard is a critical skill for leaders. Replacing narratives of right and wrong with curiosity and inquiry is key. Emphasis is on co-creation and collaboration rather than formal hierarchies and leadership through positional power. Building a team underpinned by these concepts is more likely to deliver good quality outcomes, whilst also meeting the needs and well-being of team members.

Cognitive Analytical Therapy Framework (CAT)- A tool within Leadership

CAT is an integrative therapeutic model that is widely used with individuals and teams (Ryle & Kerr, 2020) and has much to offer to develop in a leadership role.

A central feature of CAT is to articulate the roles that people take up in relationships with one another. This is often termed Reciprocal Roles or Relationship Roles (RRs). In the early stages of a therapeutic process, RRs are represented as a diagram or a 'map' between two people. It can be useful to think of the top part of the role as the 'doing' position and the bottom part of the role as the 'feeling' position (Potter, 2020). Within a relationship, both parties learn the 'doing' and 'feeling' positions and this in turn elicits a response in reciprocation.

The CAT model can be used to look at roles that are highly likely to be 'in play' for those who are in the 'leading' and 'led' positions. Harvey (2024) offers a basic template that conceptualises the 'relationship dance' between both positions. They can both oscillate between the 'doing' and 'feeling' positions at any given point (Figure 17.2).

CAT focuses on early experiences in relationships that become internalised. However, it can overlook how relationships often take place against the backdrop of social inequality (Brown, 2019) an important consideration for leaders. CAT describes the difficulties that can often arise within relationships as 'dilemmas.' Recognising these within a leadership relationship can be the first step in changing the relational dynamic. For example, a common dilemma for marginalised groups

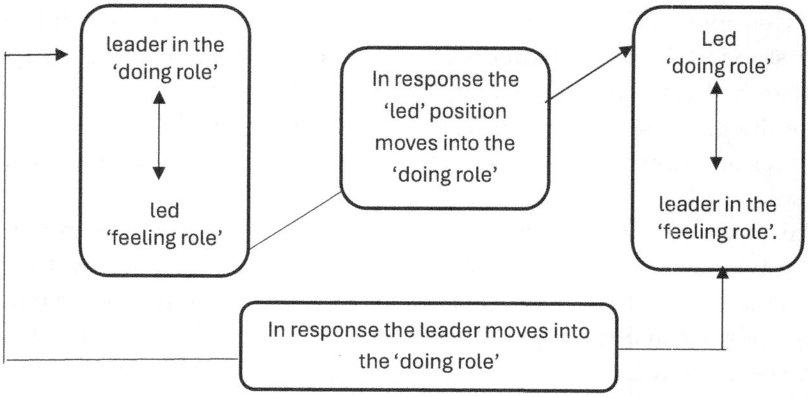

Figure 17.2 Leader and led reciprocal roles.

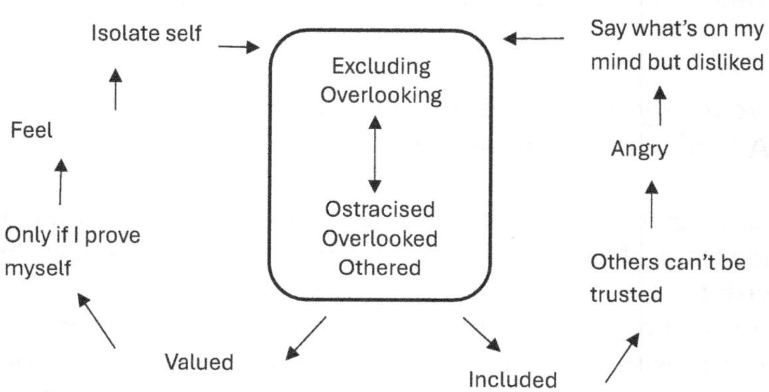

Figure 17.3 A dilemma in leadership.

when speaking up within the context of positionally unequal power relationships is:

> *'Either I speak up, but this means I am disliked and open to being excluded or I keep quiet, feel resentment and I am left feeling overlooked'* (see Figure 17.3).

The RRs that can occur are overlooking (doing) and overlooked (feeling). This may lead to one of two sequences of emotional and behavioural responses that lead back to the problematic RRs. This sequence can repeat itself with oneself (self to self), with others (self to others), and from others (others to self).

An awareness of the CAT framework enables a leader, or the person being led, to name the dynamics that arise in the relationship, which

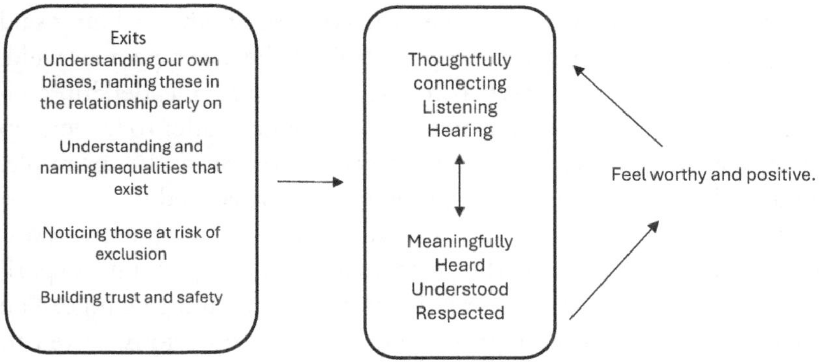

Figure 17.4 A healthy reciprocal role in leadership.

can be validating for both positions. Through this process, an opportunity is opened for a joint discussion and understanding of how such patterns may repeat themselves. Through dialogue, both the 'leader' and the 'led' become aware of the 'rupture' in their relationship. In doing so, a space is created to think through the experience and consider ways in which to repair the 'rupture' both in the moment and in anticipation of the future. Making the dynamic explicit creates a joint understanding and leads to new ways of working. In the above example, some of the 'ways out' of such patterns, often termed 'exits,' are shown in Figure 17.4. The use of these exits allows a 'healthier' RR.

When applied sensitively, the CAT framework can be useful for working with common difficulties experienced by a range of staff, including those from marginalised groups. It offers a psychologically informed and transparent way to improve the quality of professional relationships and, in turn, workforce wellbeing.

Use of Psychological Knowledge Base in Working with the Relational Thread

Systems leadership, as advocated by the British Psychological Society, p.7 (2022) requires 'moving at the speed of trust.' In our collaborative leadership, we were drawn to the importance of trust-building and effective relationships to strengthen workforce well-being and enhance care delivery.

Psychological research shows that regardless of modality, the therapeutic relationship is often the key indicator of outcome (Baier et al., 2020). The strength of the relationship is contained in the ability to shift dynamically and reflectively between the content of what is being said and the process of what is happening relationally between people (Held, 1991). The transfer of this asset from a therapeutic to a leadership context brings a unique perspective, which psychologists offer to leadership roles that may not be readily available to other professions. For example, one practical technique we adopt is the use of considered questions to maintain the dual focus on content and process. As in therapy, questions are asked not just to gather information but to generate experiences, direct attention, enhance relationships, and facilitate change. The box below illustrates some team-based leadership questions linked to process.

> **Use immediacy to ask about emotions in the moment:** 'I noticed the meeting went quiet with that suggestion – what was happening? Are we having the most important conversation?'
>
> **Model your internal thinking:** 'I am thinking of going two ways with the agenda at the moment; what are the thoughts of others?'
>
> **Focus on themes or patterns**: 'I am noticing that when we come together, we get stuck talking about the same issue without agreeing on actions. What's happening for us?'
>
> **Notice the themes that are not being talked about**: 'We have not mentioned how ethnicity impacts our service uptake. Can we pause and, for the next 10 minutes, exclusively focus on this aspect?'
>
> **Make the implicit explicit: '**I wonder if the team thinks that, as leader I have the answer to this dilemma?'
>
> **Review the process alongside the outcome:** 'How did we integrate all our ideas today?'

Such therapeutically informed questions offer new ways for teams and partner organisations to facilitate dialogue and enhance collaboration and trust. Explicitly contracting this approach with the team and partner organisations, alongside regular check-in reviews and experiential reflexivity, are complimentary psychologically informed leadership skills which can enhance team effective functioning (Rao & Mason, 2023).

Ideas in Practice: Systemic and Relational Approach to Supporting Workforce Well-Being

The case studies below illustrate the shift towards preventative and systemic ways of working to address lived experiences and health inequalities at work.

Case Study 1: Development of a Critical Incident Staff Support Pathway (CrISSP): A Regional System-Level Change Approach to Workplace Trauma

Trauma-Informed approaches are a framework for systems change intervention that recognises the high prevalence and impact of trauma (Emsley et al., 2022). Originally focused on patient experience (Harris & Fallout, 2001), increased understanding of the workforce's personal experience of trauma (Mercer et al., 2023), acknowledgement of trauma encountered at work (Hughes et al., 2012) and elevated levels of post-traumatic stress disorder amongst the workforce (Scott et al., 2023) have led to greater attention and resources being directed to support staff with workplace trauma.

The Hub's Critical Incident Staff Support Pathway addresses organisational, relational, and cultural elements of staff support for trauma whilst retaining the need for individual psychological therapy as required. The model offers bespoke training, supervision, consultation, and intervention based on critical incident stress management principles (Mitchel & Everly, 2003) and delivered within a trauma-informed care framework.

Whilst some organisations have developed their own critical incident response frameworks, the first author pioneered its implementation across multiple organisations with regional co-ordination.

Without any contractual agreement to rely on, the recognition of a mutual need and whole-systems approach formed the foundation for the work's development. We employed Myron's Maxims guiding framework noted below for implementing complex human-led change (Wheatley & Kellner-Rogers, 1996).

'People Own what they Create' was a driving force throughout the development of CrISSP. At the outset, a system-wide conference entitled 'Building the Vision' was hosted. We summarised the evidence base, workforce needs, and proposed service model. The model was designed

to balance sufficient content, direction, and scaffolding to avoid duplicating work across the system, but was flexible enough to allow individuals to own and adapt it within their organisational context.

'Start Anywhere but Follow Everywhere' was central to expansion. Rather than being driven by a fixed implementation strategy, we followed the readiness for change in the system and adapted the hub support to match organisational needs. Intensive collaboration and training were directed to early adopters, whilst a simultaneous connection with other organisations was maintained to explore their readiness. As the early adopters moved to model maintenance, the hub resources were redirected to organisations ready to implement the model. This dual approach allowed us to allocate a limited central resource for maximum impact.

'Keep Connecting the System to More of Itself' has been key to the model's sustainability. Developing a growing network of mutual aid and shared learning via peer supervision networks and partnership workstreams is integral. This approach consolidates learning, allows ongoing iteration of the model and affords the building of better understanding and relationships across the system. It has created the foundation for a coordinated and systemwide psycho-social response in the event of a large-scale critical incident.

Leading change across multiple organisations requires constant self-reflection on the pulls between vision, values and output pressures. Holding the CrISSP model afforded a great deal of knowledge and power both personally and systemically. Adopting a position of values-based change for long-term sustainability, with an emphasis on surfacing and scrutiny of our reactions, biases and needs, helped navigate these tensions. Returning to the question 'what's right for the system?' and consciously seeking the views or perspectives of those in the team and wider system that were actively different from our own helped work through the dilemmas as they arose.

Case Study 2: Schwartz Rounds on a System Level – Building Representation Reflective of the Workforce

Schwartz Rounds are a powerful forum where the sharing of perspectives through storytelling impacts positively on wellbeing (Maben et al., 2021). The hub's vision of breaking down barriers across healthcare and reducing inequality allowed an opportunity to take a whole system, inter-organisational approach to Schwartz Rounds, bringing together people across the ICS.

Our local evaluation of Schwartz Rounds aligned with national data. It indicated that Rounds often engage only a small proportion of the workforce and do not represent the diversity of staff, voices, and perspectives. Whilst there are many possible contributing factors, a consequence is the risk of system marginalisation being perpetuated.

One of the authors with an ethnically diverse background led the system change in this area. A commitment to share stories representative of the workforce with attention to a wider socio-societal context was both the vision and a challenge. The dilemma set out in Figure 1.2 can also be applied at a systems level to Schwartz Rounds. Driving change required naming the uncomfortable biases that occur within teams and systems. Working towards inclusivity involved active attention to building diversity at all levels in the Schwartz process. From creating diversity within leadership groups, steering groups, storytellers, and facilitators, we hoped a 'domino effect' would reach and engage a wider, more representative workforce.

This work has culminated in a regional delivery of regular Schwartz Rounds focusing on issues relating to racial inequalities and attention to creating diversity more broadly. Whilst further evaluation and research are required, this achievement has been an important milestone.

Such initiatives require careful attention to psychological safety and relational dynamics as there is still potential to cause further hurt in such spaces. Without attending to the psychological safety of all members, the reciprocal roles of 'overlooking and excluding' can readily be repeated within a round itself, either with storytellers, facilitators, or those attending.

Having an awareness of what we bring to work, including our identity, is important. The author leading the Schwartz Rounds project was one of the few ethnically diverse professionals in that setting. This can stir up a range of feelings. The use of psychological formulation at a system level can help integrate different theoretical approaches and multidisciplinary perspectives to enable a shared understanding, which in turn guides effective decision-making at a leadership level.

Reflections and Concluding Comments

Our personal and professional journey of leading in changing contexts has been marked by the dual roles and reciprocal learning of supporting the wellbeing of a newly formed team in an uncertain climate, whilst simultaneously leading the development of a wellbeing service for healthcare staff within a maturing ICS system.

The relational and organisational focus has been underpinned by the shared importance of attending to and managing difference and positional power as they emerge in work relations. Psychological models offer many principles and transferable skills to support the taking up of leadership. The focus on two models highlights their application to system-level change and service development through taking a critical view of accepted knowledge and structures and addressing relational dilemmas through dialogue.

As co-authors and joint leaders, harnessing our differences alongside our shared values has been central to our work and relationship. Understanding our own experiences of wellbeing required an analysis of our current and historical relationship to power. We found ourselves 'zooming in' (focusing on our own interpersonal relationship) and 'zooming out' (focusing on our relationship to the broader context and system). We recognised how powerful the social context (economic, political, cultural) is for all of us, despite it not always feeling visible in our daily lives. This led us to consider our own social positions, including class, age, gender, and professional status, and how this would impact upon the process of writing this chapter. At an individual level, we became more conscious, through dialogue, that we represented a microcosm of the workforce and the wider system.

We expect that the learning from our experiences will apply to a range of settings. No doubt, readers will find their own models and reflections of equal value but will draw upon a similar process of considered application and adaptation.

Ideas in Brief

- A considered application of existing psychological models and frameworks can help with emerging leadership challenges.
- 'Move at the speed of trust' when leading change. Adopt a focus on the relationships between individuals and organisations.
- Invest in relational, collaborative, and systemic change that respects diverse perspectives, invokes curiosity, and encourages thoughtful questions.

References

Allsopp, K., Varese, F., French, P., White, H., Chung, P., Hassan, A. A., ... & Hind, D. (2023). Implementing psychological support for health and social care staff affected by the COVID-19 pandemic: A qualitative exploration of staff well-being hubs ('Resilience Hubs') using normalisation process theory. *British Medical Journal open, 13*(8), e071826.

Baier, A. L., Kline, A. C., & Feeny, N. C. (2020). Therapeutic alliance as a mediator of change: A systematic review and evaluation of research. *Clinical Psychology Review, 82*, 101921. https://doi.org/10.1016/j.cpr.2020.101921

BPS Guidance. (2022). *Reducing the impact of social inequalities on mental health through the NHS community transformation agenda.* https://cms.bps.org.uk/sites/default/files/2022-07/Reducing the impact of social inequalities.pdf

Brown, H. (2019). Chapter 2 Reciprocal roles in an unequal world. In J. Lloyd & R. Pollard (Eds.), Cognitive analytic therapy and the politics of mental health (Chap. 2). Routledge.

Deloitte. (2022). *Mental health and employers – The case for investment.* Deloitte UK.

Emsley, E., Smith, J., Martin, D., & Lewis, N. V. (2022). Trauma-informed care in the UK: Where are we? A qualitative study of health policies and professional perspectives. *BMC Health Services Research, 22*(1164). https://doi.org/10.1186/s12913-022-08461-w

England NHS. (2021). Staff mental health and wellbeing hubs. https://www.england.nhs.uk/supporting-our-nhs-people/support-now/staff-mental-health-and-wellbeing-hubs

Fairhurst, G. T., & Grant, D. (2010). The social construction of leadership: A sailing guide. *Management Communication Quarterly, 24*(2), 171–210. https://doi.org/10.1177/0893318909359697

Gergen, K. (2005). *An invitation to social constructionism.* Sage Publications.

Harris, M., & Fallout, R. (2001). Using trauma theory to design service systems. *New Directions for Mental Health Services, 89*, 3–22.

Harvey, D. (2024). CAT-informed leadership: Navigating the emotional and relational pressures of the workplace. In L. Brummer, M. Cavieres, & R. Tan (Eds.), The Oxford handbook of cognitive analytic therapy (pp. 663–681). Oxford University Press.

Held, B. S. (1991). The process/ content distinction in psychotherapy revisited. *Psychotherapy, Theory, Research, Practice, Training, 28*(2), 207–217.

Hughes, R., Kinder, A., & Cooper, C. L. (2012). *International handbook of workplace trauma support.* Wiley-Blackwell.

Korn Ferry Institute. (2019). The inclusive leader. https://www.kornferry.com/insights/featured-topics/diversity-equity-inclusion/5-disciplines-of-inclusive-leaders

Maben, J., Taylor, C., Reynolds, E., McCarthy, I., & Leamy, M. (2021). Realist evaluation of Schwartz Rounds® for enhancing the delivery of Compassionate Healthcare: Understanding how they work, for whom, and in what contexts. *BMC Health Services Research*, *21*(1). https://doi.org/10.1186/s12913-021-06483-4

Mercer, L., Cookson, A., Simpson-Adkins, G., & Van Vuuren, J. (2023). Prevalence of adverse childhood experiences and associations with personal and professional factors in health and social care workers: A systematic review. *Psychological Trauma: Theory, Research, Practice, and Policy, 15*(2), S231–S245. https://doi.org/10.1037/tra0001506

Mitchell, J., & Everly, G. (2003). *Critical incident stress management: Group crisis intervention* (4th ed.). International Critical Incident Stress Foundation.

NICE. (2022). *Mental wellbeing at work.* https://www.nice.org.uk/guidance/ng212

Nielsen, K., Yarker, J., & Buitmann, U. (2018). IGLOO: An integrated framework for sustainable return to work in workers with common mental disorders. *Work & Stress*, *32*(4), 400–417.

Potter, S. (2020). *Therapy with a map: A cognitive analytic approach to helping relationships*. Pavillion.

Rao, A., & Mason, B. (2023). Examining leadership competencies. Are our Leadership skills future ready? *Clinical Psychology Forum*, *363*, 63–73. https://doi.org/10.53841/bpscpf.2023.1.363.63

Roberts, C. (2007). Leadership and Social Construction: Stereotype meets prototype. Conference paper. Leadership and Social Construction: (researchgate.net)

Ryle, A., & Kerr, I. (2020). *Introducing cognitive analytic therapy: Principles and practice of a relational approach to mental health*. Wiley.

Scott, H. R., Stevelink, S. A., Gafoor, R., Lamb, D., Carr, E., Bakolis, I., ... & Wessely, S. (2023). Prevalence of post-traumatic stress disorder and common mental disorders in health-care workers in England during the COVID-19 pandemic: A two-phase cross-sectional study. *The Lancet Psychiatry*, *10*(1), 40–49. https://doi.org/10.1016/S2215-0366(22)00375-3

Taylor, C., Maben, J., Jagosh, J., et al. (2024). Care under pressure 2: A realist synthesis of causes and interventions to mitigate psychological ill health in nurses, midwives and paramedics. *British Medical Journal Quality & Safety*, *33*, 523–538.

Wheatley, M., J., & Kellner-Rogers M. (1996). *A simpler way*. Berrett-Koehler Publishers.

18 Connections

Kalpita Kunde and Dr Lawrence Welch

Introduction

Leadership roles and expectations in today's diverse and dynamic working environment extend beyond traditional management and strategic planning. Adopting a trauma-informed practice is not just an option; it requires a deeper acknowledgement, understanding, and commitment to creating safe spaces where people feel respected, heard, supported, and empowered.

At the heart of trauma-informed leadership is the ability to forge genuine human connections. Leaders must prioritise the importance of self-regulation, mindful awareness, and dialogue for diverse perspectives based on empathy, respect, and mutual understanding. Leaders who embrace this practice are more likely to cultivate positive shifts in workplace cultures, which is an important bedrock for a productive, effective, and thriving working environment.

Importance of Trauma-Informed Care and Respecting Diverse Perspectives in a Complex System

A recent King's Fund paper highlighted that almost half of the adult population of England have experienced at least one Adverse Childhood Experience (ACE), while 9% have experienced four or more (Kings Fund 2019). Higher ACE counts are noted to be associated with being female. Such research highlights the importance of recognising the impact of

DOI: 10.4324/9781003492399-23

trauma on people's lives and has implications for leaders and organisations. They need to recognise and respond better to their workforce, as these figures indicate that their workforce is likely to have been likely to be exposed to traumatic experiences impacting their physical and mental health

Research has noted variations in response to adverse life experiences. For instance, the literature on gender-specific responses to trauma and trauma-informed care is now more established (Tabone et al., 2021). However, a particular gap remains around ethnicity and how services could become culturally informed (McCarthy et al., 2020). The origins and stories of trauma experienced by the workforce are important, be they brutal histories and influences of colonisation, slavery, partition, holocaust, war, or migration, as these have a significant impact on how people access treatment and services to support their wellbeing. It is imperative that we create safe spaces to allow these diverse stories to be heard and collaboratively use a needs-led and holistic approach to break down barriers and address the traumas.

A broader formulation may help us to understand how specific triggers of trauma can impact an individual's life, rather than using a one-size-fits-all approach. This may not always be feasible, but we must at the very least try by understanding individual factors. For instance, sensitive attention to cultural factors by utilising support from chaplaincy services or specialist evidence-based psychology services commissioned for the workforce to advise on cultural norms and practices is essential.

Trauma-informed approaches (TIAs) offer a way of working with people who have experienced trauma or who may be at risk of it to prevent re-traumatization and help people feel safe and empowered. They have only recently been included in the UK National Health Service (NHS) long-term plan and the NHS mental health implementation plan (NHS Long Term Plan, 2024). It is important to note that people's experiences indicate that trauma-informed approaches help in creating psychologically safer, more trusting, and generally more positive experiences for individuals accessing services and for the workforce (National Health Service England, 2024). Future research needs to focus on our diverse communities in terms of what trauma looks like from diverse perspectives and ensure services are needs-led and person-centred.

To make a significant impact on making workspaces safer, inclusive and more positive, trauma-informed leadership is key. Trauma-informed practices could encompass a variety of different models and settings. These may not only affect frontline practice but could also impact supervision, recruitment and human resource structures, policies and protocols (Covington S, 2018; Treisman K, 2024).

The challenge is about how leaders can find an honest way of reflecting on themselves before applying and adapting their learning within their work contexts in a meaningful way. It is in this context that it is worth reflecting on the importance of having an open and honest dialogue between health care providers, leaders, and the workforce as doing so becomes crucial to embedding open and transparent organisational structures, policies, and practices that are fully co-designed, co-produced, and trauma-informed.

Effectiveness in leadership to Foster Connections at Work

Speaking and listening to the workforce that feels genuine is important, as it allows leaders can convey to staff that they are noticing and observing in a non-blaming way. It may also be worth reflecting on the importance of acknowledging the sense of pressure that exists in workplace environments, which may result in painful feelings of 'I should be sorting all this out immediately so that I can fix it.' The toxic and almost compulsive need to display a strong, reactive, and forceful manner in constantly seeking solutions can take leaders away from being in an authentically reflective space. The real issue isn't just about the system and culture one works in; it is about how leaders can take some personal responsibility for stepping back and self-reflecting without resorting to simplifying the very complex impact workplace traumas and adverse experiences can have on practice and relationships (Treisman K, 2024).

We know from the research that kindness and our mental health are deeply connected. The research shows that kindness is an antidote to isolation and creates a sense of belonging (Kindness Research Briefing | Mental Health Foundation, May 2020). Empowering and enabling the workforce by relating to them in a respectful, open, kind and compassionate manner could have a transformative impact on them. We have a once-in-a-generation opportunity following the recent pandemic to learn from our experiences and reset and rethink what kind of society we want to emerge from the 'felt' crises.

From a relational perspective, it is essential to formulate a deeper understanding and awareness of the work cultures and nuances of the dynamics that staff have to navigate within, involving the self and the other. Working in a controlling and critical system that portrays a sense of power can often be experienced as punitive, critical, and dismissive, where individuals, communities, groups, and teams are left feeling silenced, inferior, attacked, disempowered, and helpless and hold the risk of re-traumatisation. A world where key performance indicators take precedence over one's health and wellness often creates cultures of perfectionism and threat. This then becomes the norm where there is no place for human fallibility, cannot be sustained, and leads to burnout, distress, and other mental health conditions.

Maintaining the flexibility, self-awareness and empathy that underlie effective leadership is no small feat in the context of an increasingly target-driven NHS . Self-awareness of leaders is crucial as effective self-regulation is associated with proactive and constructive leadership (Collins & Jackson, 2015) and is a prerequisite of servant leadership (Kerfoot, 2001; Porter-O'Grady, 2003, as cited in Howatson-Jones, 2004). It has been shown to assist with self-directed leadership development, ensuring integrity in empathy, containment and productivity whilst under pressure and exposed to significant stressors (Storey & Holti, 2013).

Mindfulness increases awareness of emotional experience in the moment and lengthens the time between this experience and its expression, facilitating a choice regarding emotional expression and reducing impulsive behaviours (Linehan, 1993; Raab, 2014). Taking a dialectical stance in opposition to rigid and/or dichotomous worldviews whilst being mindfully aware of the reactions of oneself and the other(s) without going into an attacking or reactive place is central to effective leadership (Mayer, Salovey, & Caruso (2004) ; Goleman et al., 2013). Effectiveness and positive impact in leadership occur when one is in true alignment with collaboration, co-production, delegating rather than micromanaging and working on "good enough" as opposed to a perfectionistic approach.

Building Dialogue and Connections – Respecting Diverse Perspectives

The other challenge is building dialogue and connections given the diversity of our views. One way of managing trauma is by having a dialogue about the experience with another person. However, dialogue is not as straightforward as the word implies. Dialogue is a central aspect of building connections with the 'other', finding a space in which it is possible to 'hear' what the other has to say rather than being triggered into the 'unconscious' reaction of dismissing the other. The word has been around for many centuries (originating from the Greek word 'dialegesthai' (New Oxford Dictionary of English)). The concept of creating a space for genuine dialogue has been widely discussed, yet its interpretation differs from person to person, influencing how we apply it in practice. Clearly, the relational space we create with patients is vital to our work, but gauging what will benefit the individual we are working with is not an easy process. It is recognised by a lot of research that this is the key place for helping the 'other'(e.g., Hovarth (2005).

As humans, we have a multitude of ways of interacting with the 'other'. We all seek generalisations that make sense to us and help us manage the complexity of the world. There are many times when the 'other' presents forms of understanding of different aspects of the world, which helps to clarify things for us. How we experience other people is a combination of our biological genes (Kandel, 2006) that we have inherited from our parents and also how our parents have treated us during our childhood. This is not to blame our parents because they have also inherited from their parents and were treated in certain ways as children.

It is important to be aware that our cognitive processing and ways of relating differ significantly despite the many ways in which we can come together. An example of this is that some people have the ability to talk a lot, whereas some tend to move more into the listening space rather than expressing themselves. It is easy to say that these are abilities that can be learned rather than recognising that we do not 'choose' our brains and how they operate. People can have very strong abilities but may have gaps in other areas.

It is hard to predict who we can interact with and build connections with. It is easy to have strong positive or negative reactions to others and to come up with 'reasons' for this without a deeper understanding of how we are drawn to what someone says or reject their point of view.

The awareness of the 'sinful' side of human beings has been around for centuries, as is demonstrated by religions which often highlight the need for kindness and love. Wikipedia provides an estimate of 10,000 religions – Christianity, Islam, Hinduism, and Buddhism "account for over 77% of the world's population." Each of these religions has many subdivisions indicating how people come together and then fall apart.

Managing dialogue is not straightforward in the workplace, which is dominated by managers who can be very fixed on asserting certain positions rather than 'understanding' the differences that exist in the workforce. Managers can assert that 'you need to treat everyone with equality and respect' without awareness of the forcefulness with which they express their views. One of the authors remembers when they were working in the NHS being told this, clearly a value they were in favour of, but the forcefulness with which it was stated ran in complete contradiction to the value it espoused. While these values are important, how they are understood individually can vary quite a lot. Creating real dialogue about it is not straightforward. At the same time, the workforce needs to develop an understanding of how leaders get into that place.

Breaking the Barriers – Working towards Authentic Engagement

Working in a capitalist system means that the structure of the working relationships is of a top-down nature, which the workforce gets drawn into a system where the instructions about how to do things come from above and people at the lower end can develop a deep internalised sense that they must follow commands rather than debating with others about how to do the work. Leaders can easily dismiss people in the workforce as 'lazy' rather than genuinely engaging with what has led the worker not to do what is required or to make a mistake. Discussion is often dismissed as a waste of time rather than recognising that coming to decisions and taking actions is a complex, ever-evolving process.

While clearly, we must take action on a wide range of issues rather than procrastinating, the part that is missing from this is the awareness that the 'correctness' of the decision may well change in the future. An example of this is the constantly evolving nature of science from which much can be learnt, but at the same time, the certainty that is expressed about the current state of science can easily change in the future when more research is done. Leaders with operational and management responsibilities can assert what needs to be done, such as filling in questionnaires to prove that one is getting good results in their work. They can have a powerful belief about the evidence the worker needs to show, taking a strongly judgemental position rather than treating the worker with "equality and respect." Of course, it is not just managers who are susceptible to this position. It is so easy to go into a powerful, dogmatic place where we dismiss the other's point of view and ask them the question, "How can you think that?" without realising that this is stated in a highly critical tone rather than genuinely asking the question. Of course, managers and leaders will have the same feelings towards those above them.

While we can come together in the work we do, at the same time we all have differences in what we 'see' and what catches our attention. Outside the workplace, we differ in what we cook, the exercise we do, the games we play, the films and music that we are drawn to, or our views on politics, for instance. While there is much that we can learn from 'experts' in these areas, there can also be times when we come up with 'new' perspectives about each area.

The most basic cultural 'change' is at the micro level of recognition that what is being done to the NHS has no democratic mandate – the people have not been asked to vote for this. It is also about being alert to the superficiality and double meanings espoused in many health and social care policies, which on the surface promote values that we are all committed to, but in practice are used to speak the wishes of management, not the workforce. Any change starts with forming a new awareness of reality as it presents itself to us. This requires fostering a sense that the views held at the workforce level have legitimacy and that the deep unconscious parent-child or teacher-pupil reciprocal roles, which can so easily be triggered by the latest management directive, need to be brought into conscious awareness in order to make possible a sense that the most effective service will be the product of adult-adult dialogue. Genuine Support, Respect, Active Listening/ Building Connections are some of the helpful exits from the traps and unhelpful patterns demonstrated in Figure 18.1.

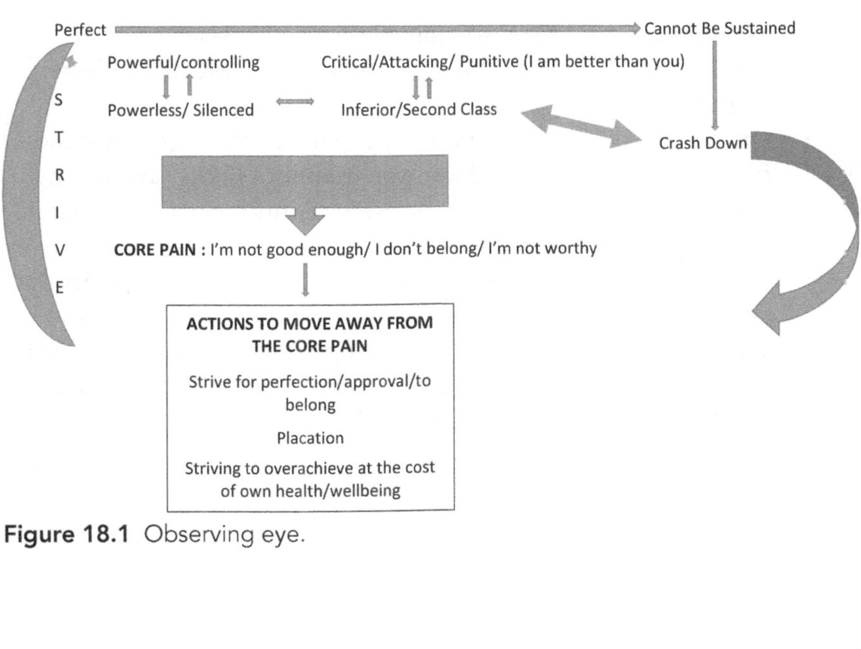

Figure 18.1 Observing eye.

The concept of reciprocal roles (Ryle, 1990;Leiman, 2002) could form a strong basis for the development of democracy through awareness that our fast emotional reactions to others can easily override our capacity to hear clearly what the other is saying. Our assumed knowledge of an area can make us super confident, so that we quickly dismiss another's differing viewpoint. Developing observing selves could open up space for dialogue between those who are working at a broadly equal level. While it is possible for those in authority to hear the views of those beneath them, the likelihood of this will be much less, particularly at middle management level, which is subject to powerful commands from above.

In conclusion, this chapter advocates for a paradigm shift in leadership, urging leaders to embrace trauma-informed approaches to foster authentic human connections and cultivate a thriving workplace culture. By doing so, leaders can create a more inclusive, empathetic, and productive work environment that supports the holistic wellbeing of all employees.

Ideas in Brief

- Importance of self-reflection amongst leaders, applying the learning to their working contexts and building real connections using honest dialogue by listening and speaking to the workforce. Moving away from the compulsive need to sort things out now to fix things immediately, whilst learning to 'tolerate' uncertainty
- Slowing things down so that we can let ourselves sit in an uncomfortable, vulnerable yet authentic, honest, and reflective learning space
- Discovering a way of noticing our painful feelings in a mindful, sensitive, and non-blaming manner. Being aware that while we have to make decisions, we cannot be certain that it is the right one.
- Being 'open' to the views of others rather than automatically going into the 'dismissive' space.
- We cannot use a one-size-fits-all approach; we must broaden our understanding of the layers of complexities of trauma and its triggers that remain live in an individual's life.

References

Boyle, M., & Johnstone, L. (2020). *A straight talking guide to the power threat meaning framework*. PCCS Books.

Collins, M. D., & Jackson, C. J. (2015). A process model of self-regulation and leadership: How attentional resource capacity and negative emotions influence constructive and destructive leadership. The Leadership Quarterly, 26(3), 386–401. https://doi.org/10.1016/j.leaqua.2015.02.005

Covington, S., & Bloom, S. (2018). Moving from trauma-informed to trauma-responsive: A training program for organizational change. Hazelden Publishing.

Goleman, D., Boyatzis, R. E., & McKee, A. (2013). *Primal leadership: Unleashing the power of emotional intelligence*. Harvard Business Review Press.

Hagan, T., & Smail, D. (1997). Power-mapping – 1. Background and basic methodology. *Journal of Community and Applied Social Psychology, 7*, 257–268.

Haslam, S. A., Steffens, N. K., Reicher, S. D., & Bentley, S. V. (2021). Identity leadership in a crisis: A 5R framework for learning from responses to COVID-19. Social Issues and Policy Review, 15(1), 35–83.

Howatson-Jones, L. (2004). The servant leader. Nursing Management, 11(3), 26–29.

Horvarth, A. O. (2005). The therapeutic relationship: Research and theory. An introduction to the Special Issue. *Psychotherapy Research, 15*(1–2), 3–7.

Linehan, M. M. (1993). Cognitive behavioral treatment ofborderline personality disorder. New York, NY: Guilford Press.

McCarthy, I.P. et al (2020). Confronting difference towards truth:Dealing with workplace bullhit. Business Horizons

Kandel, E. R. (2006). *In search of memory: The emergence of a new science of mind*. W. W. Norton & Company.

Leiman, M. (2002). Rigs, reciprocal roles, working models, and semiotic positions: Interpersonal approaches to early experience and therapy. *ACAT News*, 10–13.

Mayer, J. D., Salovey, P., & Caruso, D. R. (2004). Emotional intelligence: Theory, findings, and implications. Psychological Inquiry, 15(3), 197–215.

Mental Health Foundation. (2020, May). *Kindness research briefing*. Mental Health Foundation.

NHS Long Term Plan. (2024). Adult mental health services. https://www.longtermplan.nhs.uk/areas-of-work/mental-health/

NHS Health Education England. (2024). *Mental Wellbeing Commission Report*.

Ryle, A. (1990). *Cognitive-analytic therapy: Active participation in change*. Wiley.

Storey, J., & Holti, R. (2013). Towards a new model of leadership for the NHS. NHS Leadership Academy & The Open University Business School.

Raab, K. (2014). Mindfulness, self-compassion, and empathy among health care professionals: A review of the literature. Journal of Health Care Chaplaincy, 20(3), 95–108.

Tabone, J. K., Rishel, C. W., Hartnett, H. P., & Szafran, K. (2021). Trauma-informed intervention with children: Integrating the CANS assessment with the ARC framework in a clinical setting. *Journal of Child & Adolescent Trauma*. https://doi.org/10.1007/s40653-021-00357-x

The King's Fund. (2019). *Tackling poor health outcomes: The role of trauma-informed care*. The King's Fund. https://www.kingsfund.org.uk/publications/tackling-poor-health-outcomes-role-trauma-informed-care

Thirkle, S., Kennedy, A., Patel, P., & Sice, P. (2021). ROOTS: A reflective framework for mapping the implementation journey of trauma-informed care: User manual and forms. Northumbria University Newcastle & Tees, Esk and Wear Valleys NHS Foundation Trust.

Triesman, K. (2024). *Trauma-informed health care: A reflective guide for improving care and services*. Routledge.

19

Leading Wellbeing Practices in Prime Ministers' Offices

Jennifer Lees-Marshment

This chapter suggests a new direction for psychologists to explore: the leadership of wellbeing in a Prime Minister's Office, the most powerful workplace in a democracy. Prime Ministers hold the most powerful leadership position in a country and are tasked with governing millions of people. Despite such power, the decisions Prime Ministers need to make are immensely complex, and they require political advisers to inform and assist them. Advisers need to be high-functioning and healthy to support effective political leadership. However, political offices lack an appropriate human resource management (HRM) infrastructure.

This chapter makes a case for the role of leadership in setting out better wellbeing practices in political offices that managers in leadership positions over political advisers, including Chiefs of Staff, Directors, Team Leaders, Office Managers, Politicians and Civil Servants, should engage in. It argues that psychologists should champion their work in political offices, as the application of a psychological knowledge base has a vital role to play.

The Case for Better Wellbeing Practices in Prime Minister's Offices

All around the globe, political staff and advisers are busy working to help elected politicians, ministers, and Prime Ministers deliver on their policy promises. Despite their work being funded by the taxpayer, they have typically received little HRM and support to ensure they are

DOI: 10.4324/9781003492399-24

equipped to perform well. Parliamentary reviews have identified significant harassment, bullying, and mental health issues (Australian Human Rights Commission 2021; New Zealand Parliament, 2019; UK House of Commons, 2018). Yet there is little academic research on the wellbeing of political advisers. The exception is Weinberg et al. (2024). They report that an MPs' Staff Wellness Working Group (WWG) was established in the UK Parliament and has called for psychological support for staff. The group commissioned a staff survey of those who work for UK MPs in 2021 and 2023. Whilst there are good management practices amongst MPs and office managers, those working in these psychologically challenging jobs often face suboptimal conditions, including an "absence of universal and sufficient safeguards for physical and psychological wellbeing of MPs' staff."

The chapter focuses on political advisors working in Prime Ministers' Offices and analyses primary data collected through interviews with 67 advisers who worked in that top office in the UK, Canada, Australia, and New Zealand. 83% of those interviewed had also worked for other ministers, MPs, or in party headquarters, and thus their experiences provide a holistic insight into wellbeing in political offices at all levels. Another 20 practitioners, such as civil servants who worked in close association with advisers, were also interviewed. Interviewees gave informed consent for data from their interview to be used in research and publications, and for their name, role, and the Prime Minister they worked for to be identified. They were sent the transcript and allowed to make edits before it was approved for use in research.

An appreciative inquiry approach (Cooperrider et al., 2008) was taken to identify the best of existing behaviour to support the development of more positive behaviour in the future. Interview questions asked about what worked best in five areas: the nature of their role, recruitment and selection, orientation and training, performance, and future HRM. Data was first coded using the computer-assisted qualitative data analysis software NVivo. The topic of mental health was raised by participants. Out of a total of 253,000 words in interview transcripts, 9,000 words focused specifically on mental health. This data was then manually analysed for this chapter.

The data indicated that the job takes a toll on individual advisers' health until it burns people out, and they leave. One Canadian adviser who conducted surveys of staff reported that "burnout is just a huge, huge issue. It always has been." Other comments included that "there's just no opportunity to take a step back. You don't eat well because you're always on the go, and there's a lot of drinking because that's how you cope" and "it's relentless and you're constantly going···you've got that pressure in your brain going 'don't mess this up'." There is, therefore, a massive turnover rate in politics. People come in, work 24 hours a day, burn out, and go on to their next job."

Historically, there has been little support on offer in a Prime Minister's office. An Australian adviser talked about how, during covid, they were working at home and doing 14–16 hour days "we did not get one check-in call from the Chief of Staff, no 'are you okay?', nothing, let alone a thank you at the end for handling it. It's appallingly bad··· in terms of duty of care." But even without such a crisis, support was lacking. A UK adviser recalled how initial communication from the Cabinet Office came "from the propriety and ethics team. And that was just to make sure basically you weren't doing anything naughty. There was no element of 'we are here to support you and make sure that you're comfortable and happy in your role'."

Traditionally, there has been a 'hero' culture in politics, and people just don't really talk about struggling because it's "seen as being weak, or you're not as tough as everyone else." Unhealthy attitudes such as "what are you complaining about, you're one of the lucky ones, you get to be here and be part of this team" or "pull up your sleeves, put your wellington boots on and leap in" can persist.

The push for extreme hard work above all else can develop in any organisation, including political offices, regardless of the ideology of the party or leader in power. One striking example is how New Zealand Prime Minister Jacinda Ardern talked of the need for kindness, supporting mental health and young people. Yet this did not prevent her advisers from experiencing the same challenges, as one explained:

> *I had quite a number of really ironic moments where I was asked to stay late to work on mental health blogs and collateral and really sacrificed my own mental health in doing so...*
>
> *We all believe the cause is really important but the only way we're going to get there is if we look after our people too. I think there are better ways of doing it, and it doesn't necessarily have to come at the sacrifice of people's well-being. Especially when you're working for a government that talks quite openly about promoting mental health and well-being.*

Overall, the political adviser workplace has traditionally and typically been a very unhealthy one. The lack of support to maintain mental health causes burnout, which in turn increases turnover, which then increases the usual pressures of a high-level job, making them impossible to manage for many. Instead of taking people and draining them to the last drop, we need to implement measures to support long-term high performance.

Best Practices to Support Mental Health in Political Offices

This section looks at suggestions from advisors interviewed for what actions can support mental health in political offices. Figure 19.1 outlines core practices. These are derived directly from the data collected, asking interviewees to share positive practices they experienced, observed, or

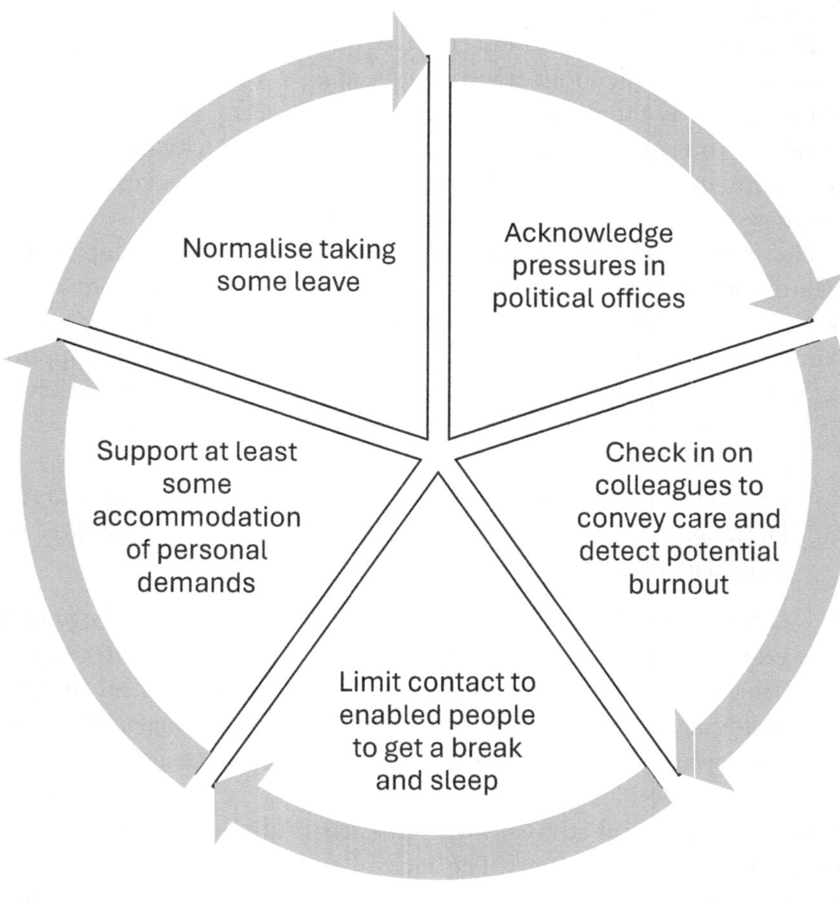

Figure 19.1 Key practices to support political advisers' wellbeing.

developed on the job, which made them grounded within this specific workplace. Political advisor roles have no job security because advisors lose their jobs if the politician they work for loses theirs; restricted or no access to standard workplace protections and rights because political offices are often legally exempt from standard workplace legislation, a disjointed if not non-existent line management and HRM infrastructure; and there is rarely any handover as those previously in the role were typically from a competing party or leader. The suggestions come from those who have worked in these offices, which means they are 'soldered in the ring of fire', so to speak, making them more viable for others to implement in other political offices. Whilst it will never be feasible to reduce the pressures of working in politics, advisors are not asking for this. But it is possible for political managers who hold leadership positions over political advisers, including Chiefs of Staff, Directors, Team Leaders, Office Managers, Politicians and Civil Servants, to engage in practices that help staff manage and navigate pressures in a way that prevents them from being so overwhelmed they fall down.

Acknowledge Pressures in Political Offices

One of the simplest things political managers can do is create an environment where people feel comfortable voicing their concerns about the pressure from working in politics so that advisers then feel more supported and able to discuss it. Just recognising the challenges everyone faces is important and helps office wellness, and then employees' wellness, and it ultimately leads to better functioning offices and better output.

If it is talked about, it also helps avoid individuals feeling they are alone in finding it hard, and colleagues can feel comfortable discussing how to balance and maintain their mental health. Advisors also need to be able to go to their managers and say, "I'm struggling here," so that where possible, support can be provided before they reach the burnout stage. One advisor explained that they would have an hour-long one-on-one conversation with their director every few weeks, which gave them the chance to discuss how to deal with pressures or issues in the workplace. It almost sounds too simple, but just being able to talk about it helps significantly.

Check in on Colleagues to Convey Care and Detect Potential Burnout

More empathetic management and proactive questions can help identify unhealthy behaviours as well as convey care, which helps staff feel supported. Advisors suggested that performance reviews should include check-ins about their mental health and whether they are looking after themselves. They explained that advisors "are a bit like an elite athlete and operating at a very high performance level" and are working under an extraordinary amount of stress to deliver "solutions to complex problems that affect a lot of people." Political managers need to take the time to chat informally with colleagues, walk around the office, and proactively watch for signs of burnout. Compassionate conversations at an early stage can help prevent unhealthy behaviours from developing into problems requiring disciplinary meetings. A UK advisor also suggested politicians need to care about their advisors:

> *There is also a responsibility from the Prime Minister and his or her Chief of Staff that they should take a strong interest in these individuals. Because we did never really have any. There was no sort of random but clearly thoughtful tap on the shoulder "how is it going?" when wandering around the office on a Friday afternoon…It comes back to that point about not just HR leadership, but also just general leadership.*

Limit Contact to Enable People to Get a Break and Sleep

Political advisors need to be supported in setting boundaries on their availability and demands on each other. Whilst political offices will never adhere to anything near 9–5 Monday to Friday, and there will always be exceptions due to events or crises, it is important to ensure people get breaks from work to enable them to make better, more strategic decisions. Rules and norms need to be established to limit contact by stating that people can't be called or emailed at certain times – for example from 9pm in the evening to 6am in the morning – unless it's a crisis. This helps staff feel able to put their phones away at night and discourages a 'hero mentality' of working later than needed and being constantly available. Australian PM Anthony Albanese's Chief of Staff

Tim Gartrell reported that they actively advised staff to avoid contact overnight:

> *We're all pretty good at not messaging each other through the night. And trying to have a cut off....usually by 9/9.30pm people are getting to bed and using technology options such as 'do not disturb with exceptions.' So having the phone enabled so that if there's any crises, you know who's going to call you, and you'll take the call, and then the rest can wait. The PM is very good at that, we only get rung when we really need to be and he's quite disciplined about that, so that helps.*

Another advisor recalled that one of their offices had rules that they couldn't email each other after 7.30 pm, or if they did, they had to do a delayed response that would be delivered in the morning. If it was urgent, they had to call, which "made you think critically, 'is this thing important enough for me to call this person?'." Such rules help build healthier cultures where advisors do not "feel anxiety if they haven't checked their phone every thirty minutes" or that they need to respond at "ten o'clock at night." This also applies to weekends. Yes, it's a 24–7 hour workplace but there need to be some boundaries to ensure advisors think, "is something going to happen on a Saturday afternoon that is going to make a difference, or could you save that call until Monday?" Political work will always be demanding, but advisors need to be supported to manage disconnecting from it.

Support at Least Some Accommodation of Personal Demands

Complete work-life balance in political advisor roles is mostly impossible. However, there still needs to be action taken to tip the scales so there is some degree of time for personal lives, because socialisation outside work helps staff cope with the job. Political managers need to create cultures where it is acceptable and indeed encouraged to have a life outside work. "It's an ongoing effort – but normalizing that it's okay and actually necessary and important to their success that they be able to have some outside life." It's not easy because, as those interviewed acknowledged, "when you work in politics it is your life," so there has to be direct intent from those in leadership positions to showcase taking some time for their personal lives. But it is essential.

Political managers who were parents of young children tried to model taking time to attend to them. One noted that they "made sure to lead by example, and set some boundaries," whilst another talked of "modelling reasonableness about work-life balance and what was required. And that face time, as in being in the office for the sake of being in the office, was never required or helpful."

Other managers suggested small but significant ways of carving out time for family from the long working day. They suggested to parents of young children, "it's okay to turn off your phone, so long as you tell people 'so and so is now the person to contact every day between 4 and 6 or 5 and 7' because you've got to go pick them up from childcare, you've got to make food, and you've got to have a little playtime." Another advisor would tell their colleagues, "right, take your kids to school tomorrow morning···go and do that and then come in," or when it was quiet, "go and get them from school because they're not going to be at school forever." Or they might encourage staff to go home in the evening when it was not 100% essential they were needed.

Politicians who manage staff can also be accommodating. When a minister forgot it was Halloween and asked for a discussion at 7.30pm, reminding him of the event was all it took to cancel the request. In another instance, an advisor recalled the Prime Minister was comfortable having children around:

> *If I had jobs at the weekend at Chequers, which is the PM's country retreat, and they were staying with me at the weekend and I had to go over there, they would come with me and [the PM] was lovely. And the same with Downing Street; I've got pictures of them running around Downing Street. He was really good like that and that helped. It did help. I was very lucky that he and the staff didn't find children an issue.*

Such an approach requires being conscious to avoid a "mission comes before anything else" culture. This is not easy in partisan politics, especially when it is normal for people to volunteer long hours during election campaigns to get their party over the line and into power. But whilst that can work for the short-term spell of elections, it won't for government. And not only is it crucial to support individuals, it also helps their professional "perspective and judgement" if they get out of the office and talk "to people who are outside of this environment who can tell them what's on their mind."

Normalise Taking Some Leave

Whilst it is unlikely that political advisers will ever take as much annual leave as civil/public servants or other professionals, there is increasing awareness that they do need to be supported, if not instructed, to take some leave for their own personal benefit but also their performance. Even short breaks help maintain mental health. In one case, a Chief of Staff gave advisers a mental health day each month, encouraging coordination between colleagues to manage that, which promoted the idea that it was appropriate to check out and take leave. Other political managers talked of insisting that staff take leave, discussing how they need to police people on taking holiday and insist, mandate or force advisers to go on leave. It helps them work more effectively when they get back from leave, as they can "recharge and come back better."

There are always going to be periods of excessive work, so to mitigate that, political offices need to insist on taking time to recuperate when it is somewhat less manic. Getting the Prime Minister to tell cabinet ministers to ensure their advisers take leave is also valuable because "people turn to the Prime Minister for guidance on this sort of stuff" and it "can lead to a cultural shift overnight." They need to remind them that whilst a forthcoming event or project is important, such opportunities will come again, and they will do better work if they take leave.

Implementing such innovations is crucial if we want to not only support individuals in these roles but also good government. Positive wellbeing practices will have multiple benefits for democracy by recruiting the best people into the roles, enabling them to perform at the highest level, supporting the Prime Minister to make the best decisions, staying in post and retaining institutional knowledge.

New space for Leadership: Thriving and Driving Wellbeing from the Top

Just as mental health has become an issue in many workplaces, attention needs to be paid to support wellbeing in politics, including within the highest and most powerful office of the Prime Minister. Those in leadership roles are required to reflect on the sustainability of work practices for themselves and those they manage to ensure that we enable thriving conditions in all workplaces.

This applies equally to political offices where talking about wellbeing and mental health may be even more challenging given the pressures and level of responsibility. More recognition and permission are needed for attention to be paid to the wellbeing situation-specific needs of political advisors working in the background, enabling our elected politicians, including the Prime Minister, to do their job. Whilst political offices have unique characteristics that mean standard practices such as 9–5 working hours and 4–5 weeks of annual leave are not feasible, analysis of data grounded in the experiences and reflections of those who have done the job identifies key effective and achievable practices that leaders can use to support the wellbeing of political advisors.

Given the need to have a system-wide approach to bring a shift to workplace culture, inter-disciplinary collaboration across different branches of applied psychology and other relevant fields such as political management can have a profound impact on a hitherto neglected area of practice. Psychological professionals and academics in organisational work and political psychology have a great deal to offer by bringing in psychological and organisational thinking to work together with leaders in politics to advocate for awareness raising and 'why' and 'how' of bringing change in this very important area in government and politics. We cannot leave it to political advisors to do this work alone to develop and preserve good practices. The innovations developed under one leader and party are at risk of disappearing when they lose power to another in the next election.

Psychologists can also integrate their psychological knowledge and understanding of wellbeing practices and organisational change processes from other workplaces that have volatile and atypical workplace characteristics. Above all, they need to shout loud and clear that wellbeing is important in every workplace and matters to all, even in the most powerful of institutions.

Although public discourse commonly dismisses politicians and their advisers as the worst of the professions, it is no wonder we see problematic behaviour when they work in such underdeveloped workplaces. You get the best out of employees when you treat them well. It is time to research and advocate for more consistent good practices in political offices, including training and support for political managers in leadership positions to employ more creative approaches to support wellbeing amongst their colleagues.

Prime Ministers make decisions that affect millions of people and thus supporting those who advise them helps improve their judgement and overall capacity to solve problems, spend public money fairly, legislate appropriately and represent us in international relations. All of this fundamentally affects the well-being of a society. Raising awareness of this hidden yet profoundly important professional group is not just about taking care of the wellbeing of political advisors but the wellbeing of us all.

Ideas in Brief

1. Political practitioners in leadership positions over political advisors need to support the mental health of advisors to avoid burnout and high turnover if they want them to perform well
2. A systemic lens and responsible leadership are important, including acknowledging pressures in political offices, checking in on colleagues, enabling breaks and sleep, supporting the accommodation of personal demands, and normalising taking leave.
3. Psychological and organisational thinking can help to improve workplace wellbeing.
4. Psychologists need to become engaged in helping to initiate and implement sustainable improvements in the functioning of political offices, as this will improve the wellbeing of us all.

References

Australian Human Rights Commission. (2021). *Set the standard: Report on the independent review into commonwealth parliamentary workplaces*. Australian Human Rights Commission.

Cooperrider, D. L., Whitney, D., & Stavros, J. M. (2008). *Appreciative inquiry handbook: For leaders of change*. Berret-Koehler Publishers, p. 3.

New Zealand Parliament. (2019). *Bullying and harassment in the New Zealand parliamentary workplace. External independent review.* New Zealand Parliament.

UK House of Commons. (2018). *The Bullying and Harassment of House of Commons Staff Independent Inquiry Report by Dame Laura Cox*. UK House of Commons.

Weinberg, A., Warhurst, E., & Fairweather, T. (2024). Mental health and well-being of MPs' staff. In C. Leston-Bandeira & S. Sage (Eds.), Political management in practice: Lessons from around the globe (pp. 73–90). Routledge.

20

Hope in the Dark

Compassionate Leadership for High-Quality Care

Interview with *Michael West* by *Dr Amra Saleem Rao*

Amra Rao: The work of leadership is becoming more challenging across settings and organisations. The book focuses on Rethinking Leadership for Clinical and Applied Psychologists in a complex world, where things are often volatile, uncertain, and ambiguous. The book looks at how best to manage complexity and embrace required change to foster thriving cultures and high-quality care.

What would you most like to share for this book regarding the role of leaders in developing thriving workplaces in today's world?

Michael West: We are currently facing the biggest crisis in health and social care, with large numbers of vacancies and increasing levels of staff stress, so much so that more than one in three staff now report being burned out at work, either often or all of the time. We're seeing more and more staff quitting our health and care services because of the pressures that they're under. They're exhausted and tired of being exhausted. Others talk about feeling ineffective in their work. This is not what they signed up for. They signed up to deliver high-quality, compassionate care. They find themselves engaged in many activities which don't seem centrally focused on delivering high-quality care.

We're seeing huge demands on our healthcare services, particularly in mental health and intellectual disability services, with very long waiting lists. All of this is undermining the well-being and effectiveness of those clinical and applied psychologists working within healthcare services. There is greater complexity in terms of the demands—an ageing population with multimorbidities.

DOI: 10.4324/9781003492399-25

This tells us that the approaches we've been taking to leadership generally in our health services are ineffective. We've got the largest workforce in Europe in the NHS, with 1.4 million people focused on promoting the health and well-being of the population. What we're doing in the process is damaging the health and well-being of a large proportion of that huge workforce. This clearly indicates that our approaches to leadership in healthcare services are ineffective or inappropriate.

It is a time for transformation of leadership. But what and how? The work of psychologists is firmly based on evidence.

In England, in particular, we have a source of evidence that is unparalleled in the world. We've been running a national staff survey in the National Health Service (NHS) for 21 years. It's the biggest, longest-running annual staff survey anywhere in the world in any sector. We have responses from more than 650,000 people a year. I have been synthesising all of the learning from the staff survey and from the work of academics, policymakers, and so on. The staff survey data demonstrates the factors that are most important in predicting the performance of NHS Trusts.[1] Nothing comes close to comparing with the staff survey in terms of its predictive validity.

What emerges is that the most important predictor of Trust performance in the subsequent three years concerning care quality, patient satisfaction, staff retention, financial performance, and avoidable patient mortality is staff engagement, particularly staff involvement in decision-making.

There is an important leadership clue. The data also tells us about the factors that predict staff engagement. Number one is compassionate, supportive leadership. Other factors are an appreciative environment, a non-hierarchical culture, good teamwork, and supportive colleagues.

The most important predictors of patient satisfaction are the extent to which there are cultures of equity and inclusion in trusts and staff workload. The more overloaded the staff are, the lower the levels of patient satisfaction. The more we have cultures of equity and inclusion, the more satisfied patients are because in trusts that have cultures of equity and inclusion, patients are treated with greater civility and compassion. These factors translate into care quality and financial performance of the trusts.

Then comes teamwork as a predictor of all these outcomes. We know that the quality of teamwork is critical to the performance of Trusts. We think only about 40% of NHS staff work in real teams. The more staff who do, the better the quality of care, much lower levels of staff stress, higher levels of patient satisfaction, better financial performance and again much lower levels of avoidable patient mortality.

Burnout, workload, and morale are critical factors that emerge from the staff survey. Therefore, the more staff are burned out, the more they have chronic excessive workloads; the worse is care quality, financial performance, and patient satisfaction are, the higher levels of staff turnover and errors will be.

The point of a very long answer to your question is that we have an evidence base about the importance of compassionate leadership involving staff in decision-making, creating cultures of equity and inclusion, ensuring effective teamwork and addressing the issues of chronic work overload and burnout. This evidence base is so robust that it clearly tells us clearly, where leaders should be putting their efforts. Compassionate leadership has to be at the core.

Amra Rao: What you have said about burnout, stress levels, and workloads reminds me of the results of the BPS/DCP Leadership and Management Faculty and New Savoy Conference Annual Wellbeing Surveys between 2014 and 2018. The results have highlighted concerns about the well-being of psychological professionals.

Such findings are worrying. However, they tell us what the key barriers and what can be done to overcome them to improve workforce wellbeing.[2] What do you think are the threats to leadership in the current context?

Michael West: I think the biggest threat is a sense of hopelessness. Many leaders are finding themselves in positions where the demands on them are exceeding their resources. I talk to many NHS leaders, who I think are experiencing moral distress. They feel they want to support their staff to deliver effective and compassionate services, but they often don't have enough staff and resources. The buildings they're working in may be inappropriate for purpose. They don't see the light at the end of the tunnel. We are in the health service, which is currently understaffed. Resources are insufficient to respond to the demands. There's a danger that leaders begin to feel isolated, hopeless, and ineffective. They develop a sense of learned helplessness in the context of leadership. This is a real threat.

I read last year Rebecca Solnit's wonderful book 'Hope in the Dark: Untold Histories, Wild Possibilities,[3] which argues that hope comes from us taking collective action together as leaders. One of the aspects that leaders in clinical and applied psychology and many other areas should focus on is taking collective action as leaders. Rather than just being victims of the complex, difficult, and challenging aversive environment, we need to come together as leaders and articulate a vision of the kind of change and transformation we want to see, be clear about what our four or five clear goals are as a leadership group, and work together to bring about those changes.

The problem is that if leaders are isolated and working individually, they can develop a sense of hopelessness and helplessness and are much less effective. When we work together, taking collective action both in terms of influencing upward and changing our workplaces, then we can be profoundly more effective.

Amra Rao: Looking at these threats to leadership, do you think there is anything unique or different about leadership in health-specific settings?

Michael West: The most remarkable thing about healthcare in our research over the last 40 years in the NHS particularly and healthcare organisations generally is that you find pretty much universal commitment to the principle of delivering high-quality compassionate care. It is extraordinary. There may be 0.01% of people working in healthcare who don't share that value of compassionate care, but that is the core work value of the vast numbers of people. In what other industry would you find a workforce united around a shared purpose and value in such a profound and powerful way?

The opportunity we have as leaders is to harness this positive energy, creativity, innovation, and motivation around this core commitment and recognise that our leadership will be successful to the extent that it is aligned around this core value. Leaders lead to ensure the delivery of high-quality, continually improving compassionate care. If our vision and values are explicitly and overtly aligned around this vision, we will be much more effective as leaders.

Amra Rao: You have led the way in promoting compassionate and inclusive leadership in healthcare settings. I want to hear about your personal experiences of leadership, both in terms of taking up leadership and followership. What would you most like to share with us for this chapter that you feel is significant and groundbreaking, and why?

Michael West: Certainly, my leadership journey has evolved. When I was first was in leadership positions, I was not a good leader at all. I was focused on achieving goals rather than on building relationships.

I made all of the mistakes associated with that approach. Over time, through being led by inspiring leaders and with the evolving knowledge that came from our research, it became clearer to me that being compassionate, developing humility as a leader, and recognising that leadership was also about teamwork were the key themes.

One of the hallmarks of good leadership is humility, the recognition that we don't know what to do as leaders in many circumstances. The role of leaders isn't necessarily to have solutions to problems. The role of leaders is to bring attention to bear on the most difficult issues we face. For me, what's been particularly remarkable is the experience of working in teams. Leadership is about leading teams, which is about ensuring that we have clear direction as a team and that we have a shared vision of what we want to achieve that is translated into four or five clearly agreed challenging goals with investment in creating a positive environment where people listen deeply to each other.

I've led some extraordinary teams. One was a big research project team for the Policy Research programme in the Department of Health looking at the extent to which there were cultures of high-quality care across the NHS in England. This combined a diverse group of professionals - sociologists, political scientists, statisticians, anthropologists, patient representatives, and psychologists. It was the most wonderful, extraordinary, brilliant, and creative time for me.

What we did was create an environment where we had a clear direction, where we came together regularly to meet, listen to each other, and share ideas. My role as a leader was really to facilitate everybody's input and help integrate them to ensure that we had a climate that was positive, supportive, and respectful, in which we could have vigorous, enjoyable explorations about different perspectives. It was a hugely successful project that made a real difference to our understanding of cultures of high-quality care in the NHS. We underestimate the importance of leading teams and recognise that leading teams isn't necessarily about necessarily driving the speedboat. For me, it was often about feeling like I was hanging on at the back and enjoying the journey rather than feeling that I had to be the one in charge.

Amra Rao: That's helpful. Leadership happens with people and alongside people rather than alone. It is important to stay connected with where your team is and to facilitate working conditions for a thriving work culture.

Michael West: I did a PhD on the psychology of meditation back in the 1970s. Meditation practice has always been part of my life since my first year at university. I continue to write about it and contemplative traditions. As part of that work, I was privileged to explore different philosophies, religions, and cultures around the world to try to understand the place of contemplative practices in different traditions, in prayer, and in meditation. Of course, in all of the major philosophies and religions of the world, compassion is a fundamental component.

The research I was doing from 1984 onwards, when I was first appointed as a research fellow in the Medical Research Council unit in Sheffield, was about seeking to understand the conditions in teams and organisations, particularly healthcare, that enabled us to achieve our goals of being effective. We conducted a very big study of manufacturing organisations in the UK and found that the most important predictor of productivity and profitability was how people were managed. We did a similar study in the NHS and found that the most important predictor of patient mortality was the sophistication of people management practices. We designed the national staff survey, which told a similar story. We saw increasingly how the quality with which people were led, managed, and supported was turned out to be the key predictor of the performance of NHS organisations.

For me, these areas of research and interests running in parallel became increasingly integrated. I suppose if there was a moment that crystallised it all for me, it was when I looked at a copy of what is probably the most prestigious theoretical management journal in the world. The Academy of Management Review published a special issue in 2011 (REFERENCE) on compassionate leadership and cultures, with wonderful articles that articulated and synthesised a lot of the themes that I've been exploring. I was also very aware of Paul Gilbert's work on the compassionate mind[4] & foundation of compassion.[5] It crystallised for me that pretty much everything we were talking about in healthcare was about the importance of compassionate leadership and cultures to achieve high-quality compassionate care and the need to continually improve the support for staff if we were to deliver that care.

It has been an exciting journey. Since I first started writing and talking about compassionate leadership and presenting this model, I have felt incredibly privileged and inspired by all of the places that are seeking to apply this thinking and knowledge, and not necessarily because of the work that I've done. For example, Deborah Lee, consultant clinical psychologist in Berkshire Health, was central in the decision by the trust to retrain all its staff in compassionate leadership.[6] They've been doing that for six or seven years now. The Trust has the lowest levels of staff stress and the highest levels of engagement. They are rated outstanding for care quality.

Compassionate and inclusive leadership is the first principle in the NHS People Plan. Health Education and Improvement Wales, with the support of the Welsh Government, has decided to ensure that there is compassionate and inclusive leadership across all of health and social care. This is the programme over 10 years. They are in their third year now. In Northern Ireland, the commitment to creating collective and compassionate leadership across healthcare has been in place for six years. I am doing work in the Republic of Ireland where compassionate leadership is part of the national strategy called 'Sláintecare', focused on delegating responsibility for decision-making around healthcare to regions, building multidisciplinary team working with compassionate leadership at the core. The Royal College of Surgeons of Ireland has compassionate leadership as part of all its undergraduate and postgraduate medical and nursing education programmes.

I'm also working with the Global Compassion Coalition[7] on developing compassion in healthcare around the world. We have over 130,000 members within a year with a very strong social movement to develop compassion in health and social care. I hope that in a world that is very dark at the moment, this movement will continue to grow and touch the lives of not only populations but also all of those who work in healthcare.

Amra Rao: Thanks for sharing this incredible journey. It is a story of hope, dedication, hard work, and learning from experience with humility. Could you shed further light on the key behaviours and critical dimensions of compassionate, inclusive, and collective leadership?

Michael West: Paul Gilbert is the guru of compassion among psychologists in the UK. He defines compassion as a sensitivity to suffering in oneself and others with a commitment to prevent or alleviate it. As a way of simply operationalising this, Paul would specify more behaviours, but I feel it will be helpful to specify four key behaviours. If I am to be compassionate towards you if you're in pain or distress, I must *attend*, *understand*, *empathise* and have the *intention to help*.

Attending has two elements. The first element is being present with the other. That enables me then to 'listen with fascination', to use Nancy Klein's[8] wonderful phrase. Attending comprises being present and listening with fascination. This provides the platform for seeking to understand the causes of the pain and distress through having a dialogue. That, in turn enables to have an empathic response to feel the pain or distress but hopefully have enough presence not to turn it into my drama. This gives me then the motivation for the fourth element, which is having the intention to help in some way.

Compassionate leadership involves enacting those behaviours in the context of leadership. Leaders need to have courage to be present with those they lead and listen to them with fascination. Let's take an example: if you're a leader in maternity services where a midwifery matron says to you, 'We cannot deliver safe services for women and their families because we don't have enough qualified midwives to provide safe care. What are we to do?'. Leaders with the courage to understand the challenges that those they lead face do not work not by imposing an understanding from a remote hierarchical position, but through dialogue. They can empathise with what it's like to be a nurse on your third hour night shift in a row, where you haven't had time to take a rest break, where you feel bad because you didn't spend sufficient time with an elderly distressed lady, and where you've got to drive home feeling so exhausted that you're afraid that you'll not be able to drive safely. In the context of leadership, this means helping those we lead by ensuring that they are clear about what they are required to do, helping them to perform their jobs more effectively, removing the obstacles that are getting in the way, and offering the resources they need to do their jobs effectively: the right number of staff, the right training, and the right equipment.

This is not some new fancy model of leadership. We've known this for 60 or 70 years that those four behaviours—listening, understanding, empathising, and helping—are critical to effective leadership. The most important skill of a leader is listening to those we lead, and the most important task of a leader is helping those we lead to do their jobs more effectively.

If leadership is not inclusive, then by definition it's not compassionate. In our research from the 1980s onwards when we first started looking at healthcare teams, we have always included diversity as a variable in terms of professional background and demographic background. Research including ours has shown that more diverse teams with clear direction and a positive climate are much more innovative and therefore more productive and effective than more homogeneous teams. So compassionate leadership is inclusive leadership, which means that we are attending, understanding, empathising and helping everybody at least equally, but particularly with those who are other than us in some way.

Diversity is the basis of creativity and innovation. We need transformation and innovation in our health services, making sure that we're creating an environment where we listen to everybody, and where we're curious about differences, whether it's different professional backgrounds, different experiences, or different demographic backgrounds.

Curiosity is the basis of inclusion. I have talked about how creating cultures of equity and inclusion is important to compassion and civility in our organisations and in our interactions with patients. If we create environments where everybody feels valued, respected, supported, and included, then we make maximum use of the huge wealth of knowledge skills and abilities within our teams and organisations. Currently, because of our discriminatory cultures, we are wasting vast amounts of resources in terms of knowledge, skills, and abilities. We are damaging people in the process because discrimination, exclusion, favouritism, secrecy, fear, and blame are impacting the cultures of our organisations.

Compassionate leadership is about being collective because it's not about me becoming more powerful; it's about helping everybody have agency. We have the largest, most skilled, most motivated workforce in the whole of the healthcare industry. We manage them through command and control; it makes absolutely no sense. It's absurd. We know that the most effective organisations in the world usually have no more than three or four reporting levels. In the typical NHS organisation, reporting levels are in double figures. It is estimated that for every reporting level, you add about 10% to bureaucracy. The more hierarchy we have hierarchy the more we suppress innovation; people give up trying to make change because they have to get permission. Moving towards more collective leadership is absolutely critical. I was talking with colleagues in Tyne and Wear and Esk Valleys recently. They've just reduced the number of hierarchical levels in their trust from 10 to 5. At Esbjerg Hospital in Denmark, they have four and a half thousand staff, and they have only three levels of hierarchy in the organisation. There's an executive team, a middle management team, and then the frontline staff. In the Netherlands, community health organisations in Buurtzorg[9]have 10,000 staff, but they have just one level.

Amra Rao: Psychologists need to demonstrate good leadership in various roles they take across their career trajectory. What can help them to take leadership at all levels irrespective of the role they are in?

Michael West: We must call out the damage that hierarchical command and control cultures are doing in terms of suppressing innovation, increasing stress, and inefficiency. Second, it's recognising that the only way we're going to be able to care for the population's health is, if we work in integrated ways across boundaries. A lot of the work that clinical and applied psychologists do involves linking with different agencies. This requires working together between health, social care, local councils, the voluntary sector, schools, etc.

We can do this, and so much research supports this by building more effective teamwork. Teamwork is about horizontal working, which is antithetical to hierarchical command-and-control working. As I said earlier, we know that only about 40% of staff in the NHS work in teams that have clear goals and meet regularly to review their performance. There's a huge amount of work to do to build effective team working.

Psychologists have a good knowledge of how to do that because the research on the psychology of teamwork is very sophisticated and well-developed. In places like North Bristol Trust, psychologists are providing team coaching across the organisation. One of the things that we can do is draw attention to the need to start managing teams effectively in healthcare. We should be training leaders to lead teams. Healthcare is about teamwork not about individual work; it's about how we work together in teams to deliver healthcare. Yet we are so focused on doing individual appraisals. Why aren't we doing team appraisals? Why don't we provide team coaching? Why aren't we training leaders to lead teams? We need to train all of our staff in the NHS to work in teams because the more we build teamwork, the more we create innovation, and the better our care outcomes.

Staff survey data show how important teamwork is for care quality and staff wellbeing. Effective teams release creativity and innovation. I think the best barometer of the team's functioning is the extent to which it is developing and implementing new and improved ways of doing things. Team working across relevant agencies is the key to how we can do this. We have good intelligence in psychology about the key elements of effective team working. One of the five or six key goals of every team in the NHS should always be improving the effectiveness with which we work with other teams and departments in the organisation.

Amra Rao: I have been talking to people lately about their experiences and struggles with organisational cultures. One of the themes that emerged is centred on the challenges of holding compassion. What might be the factors that make holding compassion difficult? I want to share real-life examples and questions emerging from my conversations with others.

- *What is the role of Compassionate Leadership for a ward manager struggling to manage 60 people?*
- The thread of technology in the form of digitalisation and artificial intelligence is expanding. This dynamism of human interactions and technical systems adds to the complexities in the post-pandemic era. Organisations are stretched by targets and business priorities. One particular example is of a director who is struggling with reporting systems, pressures to meet targets, high demand, staff sickness and staff turnover and recruitment challenges. He ends up saying in a meeting that he does not have the headspace and time to be compassionate.

What are your thoughts? What are your three key messages to manage such situations?

Michael West: Well, the first key element of compassionate leadership is being present with and listening to staff. I speak with a lot of leaders under pressure who spend their time in Zoom or Teams meetings, going from one meeting to the next, trying to manage targets, priorities, and key performance indicators. What we've found is that in any NHS organisation, often there are so many targets, key performance indicators, and priorities that people are simply overwhelmed. No one knows what's important anymore. In the best-performing places, we find that leaders ensure that there is a clear direction. There's a vision of what we're there to do as a team, or as a ward or an organisation, and that's translated into five or six clear agreed challenging goals, not fifty-six.

There are challenges because that's the nature of goal setting. It's listening, ensuring clear direction and that people's efforts are aligned around that direction, recognising that as leaders we need to get together and push back against those conditions and circumstances that are creating such traumatised and pathologised organisations. I think leaders in the health service seem to be often afraid to push back and rightly so because individuals who push back often get chewed up and spat out by the organisation. But when we do that collectively, we are much more likely to have an impact.

Certainly post-pandemic, the UK is second in the league table of organisations relying on hybrid working. At the top is Canada. The least hybrid working is found in France, Greece, and South Korea. In the UK, we seem to err on the side of using technologies rather than face-to-face interactions, and yet the evidence we have suggests that being together face-to-face is a very different experience psychologically and neurophysiologically from working remotely.

We need to have a much more intelligent approach to managing how we use technologies to help us work effectively and to recognise that to work creatively, to manage conflicts, to develop new and improved ways of doing things, and to build relationships, we need to be face to face. There are times when it's helpful to work remotely. It can help with personal non-work lives, but we need to find an intelligent balance and have these discussions about how we can do that. My three key points are: listening, ensuring clear direction, and working collectively together as leaders.

Amra Rao: What are your thoughts on managing the dissonance and lack of acknowledgement that may be seen and experienced between the espoused values and leadership approach of an organisation and the actual behaviours of senior leaders? For example, transparency versus secrecy, inclusion versus exclusion, the value of all perspectives versus the privileging of specific roles or professions, vision versus actual behaviour. Why the gap? What do you think are the paradoxical tensions? What is required to deeply embed compassion in the operation?

Michael West: Why is this gap? I think there are three things that will explain that gap.

One is that we place people in leadership positions without training them to work as leaders effectively. What happens to people who are put in leadership positions in such a way is that they lack confidence. They are insecure about their leadership, and they tend to be a bit afraid. I think in these circumstances, and the research evidence supports this, they tend to revert to command and control.

The *second* is the culture that we're creating in our organisations when we look at the UK national organisations, particularly in England, less so in Wales and, I would say, less so I would say in Scotland, Northern Ireland, and the Republic of Ireland. We have a very top-down system of national oversight, regulation, and inspection. I think in England, especially compared with other countries, Denmark & Netherlands, for example, it's very top-down, heavy-handed regulation and oversight. I think that transmits itself down through organisations and creates the *third* element that I believe is responsible, which is a culture of fear. I think many leaders feel afraid because of the somewhat punitive culture that this top-down, command and control KPI culture creates. The combination of not having well-trained leaders and managers, a hierarchical top-down culture, and creating a mixture of fear and blame rather than learning and innovation are responsible for creating this dissonance.

What we need to do is, first of all, repeat the evidence about what does work again and again and again. It's not about presenting the evidence once, as I talked with you about. You know the evidence we've got from this extraordinary treasure trove of data which is the national staff survey over 20 odd years. The evidence tells us very clearly what kind of culture, management and leadership practices we need to develop. We have to present that again and again and again. We also have to monitor leadership within our organisations. I think every leader in a position of responsibility should be seeking feedback from those they lead about the extent to which their leadership is enabling and the extent to which they are experienced as compassionate leaders. We need to monitor the extent to which their teams are working effectively. We need to monitor much more effectively the extent to which every team and every department is embodying an inclusive environment in order to support leadership and team development.

We have well-developed technologies in psychology for enabling us to do that: monitor leadership. In many organisations in the UK, like Northumbria Healthcare, which is one of the most outstanding Trusts over the last 10–15 years. They are very good at conducting Pulse surveys to identify where the dark spots and light spots are in the organisation so they can intervene. Wrightington, Wigan and Leigh have been doing the same in terms of staff engagement for 10–15 years now and they offer good models for how we can monitor and intervene to support development.

Amra Rao: Thanks, Michael. Let me briefly touch upon ethics and politics in leadership. You have spoken about courage, confidence, and the capacity for collaborative work to shape a culture of compassion, safety, and inclusivity at work. What are your thoughts on how leaders should manage controversial topics that intersect between health, science, ethics and politics? An example of this in recent years is related to the Cass Review. This has created tensions in the profession (especially related to disagreements, psychological safety, users' voices, and inclusion). What are your thoughts on how leaders navigate this fairly, compassionately, and effectively?

Michael West: Leadership is about creating the conditions where we ensure that we promote the well-being and engagement of others and that we ensure innovation and effectiveness in the teams and organisations we lead. That's about creating conditions of psychological safety. Leadership is not necessarily about having solutions to problems. It is about ensuring that we are modelling compassionate leadership and building effective teamwork.

In addition to that, I think there are five key elements that are required for psychological safety, within which we can then navigate some of these difficult waters.

One is that we need to have an overall vision as a team or department of what we're here for. That might sound somewhat trivial and obvious. Very often I come across departments and teams in the NHS where they've lost sight of the vision. It is part of a leader's responsibility to continually reinforce or repaint that shared vision, what we're here to do around delivering, ensuring the delivery of high-quality, continually improving compassionate care and the associated values.

The *second* element is ensuring that we're creating cultures of reflection, innovation and learning rather than fear and blame, because when we create cultures of fear and blame, we are much less able to navigate these difficult waters. If we have a culture that is open and reflective, where we take the time to meet regularly to reflect on what it is we're trying to do, how we're going about it, and what we need to change, we are much more likely to be innovating and learning. It's about creating a learning environment where the role of leaders is to acknowledge, 'I don't know what to do.' This is part of being a good leader. When we don't know what to do, it's the role of the leader to trust others by coming together repeatedly and sharing our collective knowledge, skills and abilities. This can help in navigating ways forward.

Third, we have frequent contact with each other. You alluded to this before in your question about technologies. It becomes very difficult to manage tricky issues when we're not spending sufficient time face-to-face. If we're going to have difficult conversations, we must spend sufficient time being face-to-face. We need frequent contact with each other to be able to work through difficulties and differences.

Fourth, we need to have a culture within our teams and departments—a commitment to valuing difference, whether it's a difference of opinion, professional background, or demographic background. It's easy to say we need to be curious about differences, but we need to have the presence and the awareness to say, 'Oh, that's interesting that's different. I wonder what that's about; let me explore and learn more.' We need to create an environment where we're curious about differences rather than shutting down. That also means that we must be intolerant of chronic interpersonal conflict in teams. Chronic interpersonal conflict is a disaster for teamwork. It also makes it virtually impossible to make good, open decisions or to listen to each other deeply. We need to value differences of opinion about what we should be doing, how we should be doing it, and who's responsible.

Finally, cultures of humility, mutual support and recognition of our interconnectedness are critical to us being able to navigate our way through these difficult waters. Arrogance, 'I'm right you're wrong', 'I'm in a senior position to you'—that kind of arrogance does not create psychological safety. Mutual support and understanding are the basis for creating psychological safety and a recognition of our interconnectedness.

AR- Fabulous, you have found a way to respond to a very complex question on managing the intersection between health, science, ethics and politics and the associated conflicts. I would like to pick one particular area further. In our conversation, you have spoken about curiosity, embracing difference rather than adopting a defensive stance, and avoiding discomfort and conflicts inherent in such conversations.

How do you think leaders can deal with race, identity and equality in today's organisations? This is an area where we see the dissonance in the espoused values, policies, practices and experiences of people at the ground level. What do you see as leader's responsibilities in working with the gap between policies and practice?

Michael West: The way these issues are currently dealt with in NHS organisations is primarily through having organisational policies and procedures around promotions and appointments. There are practices and policies, for example, supporting the creation of black and minority ethnic staff networks or LGBTQ+ staff networks. A lot of processes and practices are being implemented, but the reality is that since the introduction of the Workforce Race Equality Standard back in 2015, the lived experience, for example, of staff from minority ethnic groups has continued to deteriorate. I wouldn't argue against it because we have evidence that having these policies and practices in place is helpful, but it is not enough.

What we need to do is ensure that inclusion, respect and civility are part of the responsibility of every individual member of staff. We need to monitor it in teams and departments to intervene. Until we have inclusion, respect and valuing people as part of the fine texture of the way we operate in our organisations, we're using blunt instruments to bring about change through policies, practices and networks. I'm not wanting to dismiss or argue against those, but they are not sufficient on their own. We need to get to the level of individual and team behaviours in today's organisations.

It's just so fundamentally important because the NHS is the most important institution in our society. It's the institution that has the most influence on compassion across our society. It's the biggest employer by far. If all of those 1.4 million people who come to work every day encounter compassionate, inclusive, and respectful cultures, they will take that back out into their families and communities. If the million people who use NHS services every 36 hours encounter compassionate care regardless of their demographic background, then they take that back out into their families and communities.

So, it's incumbent on us as an institution and society to model what an inclusive, equal, positively diverse culture looks like. That means that this should be one of the key objectives of every leader, every team, and every department. We need to monitor that regularly; just as I talked about monitoring the behaviour of leaders, it's a core element. I indicated earlier that the data we have from the staff survey over the last 20 years tells us that creating an inclusive, positively diverse environment is core to patient satisfaction, care quality, and even financial performance. So we need to move beyond policies and practices to focus on individual team and departmental cultures and behaviours. I don't think we are there yet.

Amra Rao: A helpful proposition, a community of inclusive practice within the NHS can have an impact on wider society. Once you have a good experience of being taken care of, you are more likely to take it away and offer the same to others.

What are your thoughts on compassion fatigue? Do professionals working in caring professions face risks? Staff in healthcare are continuously challenged by the high relational content and emotional demands of caring. Psychological professionals are no different. There are concerns about their well-being. What do you think might be the limits around compassion? How best can we deal with these challenges?

Michael West: All the evidence that has been gathered thus far tells us that when you are compassionate to somebody else, you benefit. In randomised control trials, GPs and nurses were asked to be extra compassionate in their interactions with patients over two weeks. That has a significant impact on their mental health, with lower levels of anxiety, stress, and depression.[10]

Compassion is not the problem. The problem is empathy fatigue. It's when we are continually empathising with people and we're not able to help. I see it with two of my children who are clinical psychologists; when they feel that they're not able to provide the care and support they should be providing, it is morally distressing. It is stressful when we are continually exposed to situations where we empathise with others who are in pain or distress, but we don't feel we're able to make any difference. We are evoking an empathic response repeatedly. We see this in neuroscience studies,[11] when we ask people to be empathic towards others in pain or distress; that's associated with the activation of pain centres in the brain. When we ask people to be compassionate, that's associated with the activation of the reward centre in the brain, which is completely different. So continually evoking those empathic responses rather than compassionate responses is very damaging to health and well-being.

We must develop amongst healthcare professionals, clinical and applied psychologists of course, the knowledge associated with self-compassion—the courage to be present with ourselves, to be curious about our reactions, to be aware of when we're feeling bad, and to bring a nurturing attitude towards ourselves. After all, each of us is as deserving of love as every other human being on the planet, and caring for ourselves is not simply a leadership skill. As a way of being, it is critical for our ability to be compassionate to others. Also, we know that when leaders practise self-compassion, those they lead are more compassionate towards those they provide care for.

It's also putting into practice what we know about the factors that affect staff stress and well-being. In particular, staff stress results from our failure to meet the core needs of staff—the need for autonomy and control, involvement in decision-making, and working in cultures of learning and innovation rather than fear and blame. We need to meet the core needs for belonging, contributing to a positive difference, and working in well-functioning supportive teams and compassionate cultures. This requires addressing the issue of chronic excessive workload, which is the number one factor in staff stress and the number one reason why staff are so likely to quit the NHS.

Amra Rao: This also highlights for me the need for collective responsibility of the leadership chain across the organisation. This requires engagement with the followership to listen to their experiences to foster a culture of care and compassion. It can be challenging for individuals to have compassion when the culture is contradictory and does not have the fabric you have spoken about.

Micheal, you have given us many nuggets of wisdom on how to embrace those challenges in response to complex questions. What are the key headlines and standout messages that you would like to get across to applied psychologists to lead and influence?

Michael West: I've talked about compassionate leadership generally, but the most important skill for our leaders is listening to those we lead. I also think also about the importance of practising self-compassion as a leader and developing effective teamwork. Additionally, I would say that working together with other leaders to bring about change in what can often be a toxic and hostile environment is crucial. I believe these four messages are important.

Amra Rao: Excellent, grateful for an inspiring discussion. We could have spent more time unpicking the complex tasks of leadership. You have given readers a lot of food for thought to reflect on their context and consider what they need to rethink in their leadership practice to bring hope in tough times and show compassionate leadership for high-quality care. Thank you.

Ideas in Brief

- The quality with which people are led, managed, and supported is the key predictor of the performance of NHS organisations.
- Leadership is about creating the conditions of psychological safety to ensure well-being and engagement for innovation and effectiveness in teams and organisations.
- The most important skills for leaders are listening and engaging those they lead, with compassion, and developing effective teamwork and collective action.
- Leaders can't work in isolation. They need to come together to articulate a vision of high-quality compassionate care, change and transformation, and take collective action, influencing upward and changing workplaces to be profoundly more effective.
- Compassionate leadership is core to cultivating thriving workplaces. This requires involving staff in decision-making, creating cultures of equity and inclusion, ensuring effective

teamwork and addressing the issues of chronic work overload and burnout.

- When leaders practise self-compassion, those they lead are more compassionate towards those they provide care for.
- Humility is the hallmarks of good leadership , the recognition that we don't know what to do as leaders in many circumstances. Type the Paragraph Text
- The role of leaders isn't necessarily to have solutions to problems. It is to bring attention to bear on the most difficult issues and develop teamwork—*attend, understand, empathise* and have the *intention to help.*
- Healthcare is about teamwork, not about individual work. We need to train staff to work in teams because the more we build teamwork, the more we create innovation,care quality and staff wellbeing.
- Diversity is the basis of creativity and innovation. Curiosity cultivates inclusion. Diverse teams with clear direction and a positive climate are much more innovative, productive, and effective than homogeneous teams.
- Leadership's task is to create environments where everybody feels valued, respected, supported, and included, to maximise the use of the huge wealth of knowledge skills and abilities within teams and organisations.

Interview—September 2024

Notes

1 An NHS trust is an organisational unit within the National Health Service of England and Wales, generally serving either a geographical area or a specialised function.

2 Rao et al. (2021), Building a caring work culture—what good looks like, The British Psychological Society.

3 Rebecca Solnit (2016) Hope in the Dark: Untold Histories, Wild Possibilities, Haymarket Books.

4 Gilbert, P. (2009). The Compassionate Mind: A New Approach to Life's Challenges. London: Constable and Robinson Ltd.
5 https://www.compassionatemind.co.uk
6 Creating a compassionate culture in organisations, NHS Leadership Academy, https://learninghub.leadershipacademy.nhs.uk/leadership/leadership-listens-3/
7 https://www.globalcompassioncoalition.org
8 Nancy Kline (2015). More Time to Think: The power of independent thinking: Cassell
9 https://www.buurtzorg.com/about-us/buurtzorgmodel/
10 Conversano C, Ciacchini R, Orrù G, Di Giuseppe M, Gemignani A, Poli A. Mindfulness, Compassion, and Self-Compassion Among Health Care Professionals: What's New? A Systematic Review. Front Psychol. 2020 Jul 31;11:1683. doi: 10.3389/fpsyg.2020.01683. PMID: 32849021; PMCID: PMC7412718.
https://doi.org/10.1016/j.neuropsychologia.2021.107925
11 Singer, T., & Klimecki, O. M. (2014). Empathy and compassion. *Current biology*, *24*(18), R875-R878.
https://doi.org/10.1016/B978-0-12-805308-9.00020-8

21 Psychological Safety and Leadership

A Conversation with Amy Edmondson

Dr Amra Saleem Rao

> *"Psychological safety means an absence of interpersonal fear. When psychological safety is present, people are able to speak up with work-relevant content."*
>
> **Amy Edmondson**

> "For knowledge work to flourish, the workplace must be one where people feel able to share their knowledge! This means sharing concerns, questions, mistakes, and half-formed ideas."
>
> **Amy Edmondson**

Amra Rao: The book examines how best to take up leadership in this complex world and foster change to develop a thriving workplace to ensure high-quality care. Considering your work on organisational learning, psychological safety and leadership, and 'The right kind of wrong', what would you most like to share for this book that can help us critically appraise leadership?

Amy Edmondson: This is a big question – one that isn't conducive to a simple answer. I hope we can tease this out in our conversation. I wrote a whole book on psychological safety.[1] More recently, I wrote a book on failure[2] and its role in bringing progress and success in facing uncertainty. I have another book on teaming.[3] All of them speak to the role of leadership in these very challenging times.

DOI: 10.4324/9781003492399-26

Amra Rao: Many elements of your writings are relevant to consider when rethinking leadership. Let's start with your own experiences of leadership and followership. What would you most like to share with us that you feel is significant, and why?

Amy Edmondson: I don't have a lot of personal experience in either leading or following. I've been a writer, teacher and researcher for most of my career. I had an early career as an engineer, another period doing consultancy, and a period writing, followed by the last 30 years as a researcher and teacher. I don't have a great answer.

Amra Rao: It is a humble position to take. You have been a champion of psychological safety and are known for your insights about management, valuing teamwork and the importance of an enabling learning environment to help organisations stay ahead of change. You have helped germinate a large body of academic research in management, healthcare and education. You have shown leadership in several ways, including putting forward new ideas.

Amy Edmondson: Yes, as a thought leader but not as an actual people leader.

Amra Rao: You highlight an important point: there are different ways to lead and influence. It could be through formal and informal roles. Leadership is about bringing new ideas and vision, setting up direction, and taking people alongside you. This is not the same as transactional and operational skills, which are mainly focused on management. Leadership skills overlap with management, but they have some distinct dimensions. What are your thoughts?

Amy Edmondson: That's true. All managers need to lead, and all leaders need to manage. I see leadership as the art of engaging the efforts of others to achieve something, generally something very challenging. A leader will consider what to do to have a positive influence on others. Management is enabling the coordination of actions to ensure the execution of work to achieve results. They are both important, but have a different focus. It is hard to imagine that you can be a good leader if you can't manage. It's also hard to be a good manager if you can't lead.

Amra Rao: What do you consider to be the key areas to address in rethinking leadership?

Amy Edmondson: I always come back to the idea that our mental models, which are taken for granted, encompass ideas about leadership and management that are remnants of the industrial era or at least remnants of a time and situation where things were more predictable and certain.

More often than not, people fail to revisit those ideas to assess their applicability for the current moment. Industrial-era theories of managing and leading are not a good fit for the current era, for times of hyper-uncertainty, high interdependence and low predictability. These times require us to think differently. People in positions of leadership need to think differently about the changing reality and what they must do to enable others to work together well and do their best at work.

Amra Rao: You are highlighting that a leader needs to enable and engage with people. This requires a collaborative and distributed approach to leadership. US healthcare leadership approaches are viewed as very individualised. What are your comments on that?

Amy Edmondson: I completely agree. The work that needs to be done in healthcare, especially, requires collaborative effort, certainly in a hospital setting, which is one area of healthcare. Hospitals' 24/7 operations require difficult decisions, complex diagnoses, and challenging delivery of protocols and tasks.

Inherent interdependence in such settings means that the role of the manager is to enable collaborative work to happen as well as possible. It's not about "doing what you are told," because each case is different. In operations management, this kind of work is closer to a job shop than an assembly line. However, it's not a job shop where individual workers do individual tasks; rather, it's complex collaborative work that calls for teaming to get it done. This kind of work means never facing a replica of the prior day. We're still learning about what managers and leaders can do to increase the chances that this kind of work goes well.

Amra Rao: There is increased interdependence in today's global world where things are often uncertain, ambiguous, volatile, and complex, requiring a new way of engaging and thinking. What do you consider to be the key opportunities and threats for leadership right now?

Amy Edmondson: I don't know what you mean by opportunities and threats. Could you be more specific?

Amra Rao: I'm thinking about the wider social-political contexts within which organisations and, more specifically, health and social care organisations operate. The post-COVID world is faced with many new challenges, such as long-term financial and health impacts, Long Covid, and hybrid working. Many countries are faced with cost-of-living crises. Political and social unrest is on the increase. The application of AI and socio-technological advances offers new options, but today's world is becoming increasingly brittle, non-linear, and at times incomprehensible. In my view, it presents us with both opportunities and threats.

Amy Edmondson: I see. I guess one way is to say that there are many changes in the broader context that are making work that was already very difficult, even more so. Unfortunately, there is no easy answer to this. I think all the things you just said about technology, societal social unrest, expectations, and ever-present smartphone cameras – such that we are working with an audience 24/7 – are certainly not helping and, in fact are making the job, the work, more difficult.

Amra Rao: We have an example here. Meeting online to think about psychological safety and leadership allowed us to meet rather than travel across the globe. It has saved us time and money. However, it is not the same as face-to-face contact, being in the presence of another human. The quality of conversation and engagement is altered, more so when one is both an onlooker and gazed at on a screen. Post-COVID, online work has become a new normal. Whilst it has benefits, it is worrying when one does not consider what might get lost in virtual contacts.

I found it helpful when you stopped us earlier and said that 'it doesn't work for me,' allowing us to look at what options we can consider to have this conversation. Most people are not able to challenge in this way.

Amy Edmondson: Perhaps there are as many risks as advantages. There's certainly the convenience of virtual visits, where we can connect without travelling. There are also risks, including the possibility of missing something important that would have been picked up in person. In healthcare, there is a lot that virtual visits cannot do.

Amra Rao: I want to talk about some of your key contributions. You coined the term psychological safety, exploring its relationship to team learning and performance. The term is often used to describe people's perceptions of the consequences of taking interpersonal risks in a particular context, such as a workplace. From your perspective, what role can leaders play in creating psychological safety and fearless organisations, and why? What are the leadership behaviours that foster this?

Amy Edmondson: Behaviours that come from a mindset of humility, curiosity and empathy are the behaviours that create psychological safety. Psychological safety describes a learning environment, and learning environments are created by attitudes and behaviours of genuine learning. More specifically, something very important for leaders to do is expectation setting, in particular by repeatedly emphasising the uncertainty and customisation of complexity that exists in healthcare delivery, which you and I have been talking about.

Explicitly setting expectations in this way highlights the need for voice, for speaking up when something goes wrong, or when you are not sure of something. That is what psychological safety means. It is the belief that you can speak up without fear of humiliation. Psychological safety and speaking up are important for obvious reasons in healthcare, and yet people will spontaneously hold back rather than speak up, especially when they're not 100% sure of what they have to say or whether their questions will be well received. It's quite natural to hold back. To wait and see.

The first step in trying to prevent that is to repeatedly emphasise the nature of the work as the kind of work where things can go wrong, not because people are incompetent, but because it's uncertain and interdependent. This helps people recognise that their voice must be offered freely so patients receive safe care. This is the first step in setting of the stage.

Then, with genuine curiosity, noting that any of us can miss things, it's helpful to ask good questions – saying things like, 'I want to hear from you', 'what did you see', 'how do you think the patient is doing'. Whatever the appropriate context or question you have, inquiry is a vital skill and behaviour.

This, of course, must go with listening and responding productively, being appreciative of what you hear, and engaging with it in a learning-oriented way. If you approach work with a learning mindset, these behaviours will happen naturally. A learning mindset naturally leads to the behaviours that build psychological safety.

Amra Rao: A mindset of humility, curiosity and empathy to engage in a learning-oriented way seems important to enable psychological safety and effective teamwork. Are there any situations or particular contexts where psychological safety is not possible to achieve?

Amy Edmondson: There are many. Psychological safety is not the norm. It is hard to build. It is unusual. And so, I think it is helpful to assume it is *not* present because this will encourage you to work hard to build it. By working hard to build it, I mean showing up with curiosity and interest in what others know and see, and listening appreciatively to what they say. Listening to learn.

Amra Rao: This requires leaders to be aware of the need to invest in fostering a work culture that recognises the importance of psychological safety and trust.

Amy Edmondson: It is required not because it is such hard work but rather because it is naturally difficult for people to speak up. It is natural to hold back, especially in a hierarchy. It is natural because self-protection is spontaneous – and a more powerful instinct than the instinct to contribute. But you can flip that; you can turn it upside down. You can make a desire to contribute more powerful than the instinct to self-protect; but you have to do it on purpose. It takes effort.

Amra Rao: Psychological safety is seen as crucial for the performance of teams. Many leaders and managers believe in the importance of psychological safety as the lack of it impacts the engagement of the workforce and the expression of their views and unique perspectives.

An environment of fear inhibits constructive feedback and learning from mistakes. Stress and anxiety in the workplace affect well-being, which we know is linked with decreased job satisfaction and high staff turnover rates. Despite many benefits of psychological safety, many feel frustrated whilst attempting to create safety in systems. What do you think are the obstacles that can come in the way of enhancing psychological safety?

Amy Edmondson: It's the automatic processes that give rise to coming across as an 'I know it all' – a form of arrogance. If people think you believe you've got all the answers, then why would they bother trying to contribute? They may fear they will not be heard or that their views will be rejected.

Amra Rao: Let's look at a few scenarios which I have come across in my consultancy work and conversations with colleagues. 'How would you respond to a colleague who claims they are feeling unsafe when you (as a leader/manager) are simply trying to hold them to account?'

Amy Edmondson: The most important question is to ask for more information, such as to request a concrete illustration of what they mean by the statement, 'I feel unsafe.' That statement is abstract. Increasingly, I've been hearing stories of this from around the world. Such comments can be used as a weapon. 'You can't give me feedback because it makes me unsafe.'

So, let's get clear on what psychological safety means. It means a learning environment – an environment where candour is expected and welcomed. It doesn't mean things are easy or comfortable. Learning is uncomfortable! Imagine that you're in the shoes of someone who's just heard, 'I'm the person trying to hold you accountable'; that's also very abstract. We don't get very far if we stay at the top of the ladder of inference. We need to learn the skills of learning from each other and getting clear on what we see and need to do a good job.

In short, I'd want first to understand as much as possible what that person really means. If it turns out that they mean they're not comfortable hearing that they didn't do a good job on something, then gently help them see that – and see the importance of welcoming feedback as an essential part of work and life. It is the job of the manager to help them see where they did well and where they came up short, to help them do tasks to a certain level, whether it's quality, timeliness, or something else.

What we are talking about now is the skills of having a high-quality conversation. Most of us lack training in this. High-quality conversations happen at the lowest level of concreteness possible, with data, with evidence – 'I saw X. I inferred Y; how did you see it?' It's important to reflect together on shared data and shared observations, not opinions. We need to understand each other's discomfort or unhappiness about something. And we need to be clear and compelling as to why it's in everyone's best interest to follow through on commitments. We're talking about learning and about the necessity (and the difficulty) of high-quality, honest, data-driven conversations. Many people lack well-developed skills and require support.

Amra Rao: Let's look at another one. The psychological paradigm is often disregarded in health care with a focus on the bio-medical model. Psychological professionals are often the sole members of their discipline within their (clinical) teams, which can contribute to an environment that does not feel psychologically safe for them to offer alternative views. How can this be changed?

Amy Edmondson: Setting the stage, inviting input, and responding productively are three categories of leadership activities that I think are very important. These are sets of behaviours that anyone can do and would be well advised to do in the service of being a good leader and enabling others to do a good job.

If you have lost confidence, say so. I know it seems counterintuitive because that's the very thing you're saying it is hard to do. There's something wrong in any world or any organisation where people believe that their days are supposed to be easy and effortless, especially in healthcare. It's a misunderstanding about what work is about. Work is about doing hard things well with other people.

People can be reinvigorated in one of many ways. There is not one best way to reinvigorate or re-inspire someone to do good work. One way is reconnecting with a sense of purpose. Another is rethinking and recalibrating the importance of one's role – realising that if you don't speak up about a concern or raise a question, that could very well lead to bad outcomes in safety or quality.

What is needed is helping people think clearly about what is needed. So, it's helpful to start with the goal: What is the goal of this team? Is it a patient-facing team? Is it the delivery of safe, high-quality care that is our goal? If that's the goal, then what do we need to do? Every one of us needs to work together to make that happen – that is the first principle. This is basic but still necessary, and it is not always done.

Secondly, consider what we need to do to increase the chances of reaching that goal. I don't think people respond as well to advice in a vacuum as they do to contextualised thinking about *what it's going to take and why*. Nobody likes to be uncomfortable, nobody really loves to work hard, and nobody really likes the discomfort of speaking up. But when they are fully aware of how important it is to achieve the goals they have signed up to achieve, then it gets a little easier.

Amra Rao: There is often tension in the debate around whether to avoid failure at all costs or take risks and learn from mistakes. I want to switch to failing well to grow. In your book, 'The Right Kind of Wrong – The Science of Failing Well', you offer a framework to think, discuss, and practise failure wisely. Is there a link with psychological safety?

Amy Edmondson: An environment where people feel able to speak up about mistakes or other things that can lead to failures is called psychological safety. There are two aspects of the relationship between psychological safety and failing well: First, preventing preventable failures. Second, the willingness to experiment in new territory to innovate and discover something new to make progress.

Amra Rao: Failure is not always an option when you are faced with a threatening environment filled with many negative experiences. Discrimination, prejudice, and racism are common experiences for people from minority and underprivileged backgrounds. I have often had conversations with professionals, including psychologists from minority backgrounds, who say that they do not have the freedom to fail without consequences.

Amy Edmondson: In the book, I have written about 'unequal licence to fail'. This makes the point that your question is making. You know that if you are from an underrepresented group, either by your race, gender, sexual orientation, or nationality, you feel anxious about failing as it can be attributed to your identity group. It is hard not to feel responsible at times as you are representing your identity group. We all need to be more cognizant of these issues to level the playing field.

There's no magic wand to erase the prejudice, stereotyping the automatic psychological responses of attributing a failure to the group when an individual is underrepresented in a particular role. The only answer when something doesn't have a magic wand is to make it discussable. Once it's made discussable, then we are required, like it or not, to confront it directly and realise how unhelpful our spontaneous thinking really is! It is much harder to make spontaneous inferences when they're out in the open and you see how unhelpful they are, even how illogical they are.

Let's do the thought experiment: a white man from a privileged background is hired into an executive role and it turns out to have been a bad hire. The person fails miserably in the role. Nobody – and I really mean nobody – would say, 'well it's because we hired a white man of a privileged background, we should never do that again'. Right? It would be nonsensical. We know that minorities are underrepresented in executive/senior leadership roles. And if an individual from an underrepresented group is hired, and it turns out for whatever reason to be a failure, a bad hire, then the first thing people will think involves an attribution to the group category. It's a given. We know that happens.

Once we start making this a topic of inquiry, however, we are likely to conclude that we should stop doing that. It's a bad thing to do; it's illogical. It doesn't help us achieve our goals. If our goal is to ensure that everyone has equal access to climb whatever ladders, it can't be just on paper. That is a stated societal goal in both of our countries (UK, US). It is important to know that sociological and psychological forces will make it hard. But I want to be part of the group that fights against that and fights hard to make it discussable.

Amra Rao: Let's take this further and link this to the role of leaders. How do you think leaders can work with racism, identity, and equality, and address power dynamics in organisations?

Amy Edmondson: My thoughts are simply that that is part of their responsibility.

Amra Rao: What does that look like in practice? Leaders are in a position of influence. However, we know that sometimes it is difficult to change organisational culture. It can be tempting to turn a blind eye. Stereotyping, power struggles, and discrimination are quite prevalent in organisations. What do you think leaders need to be doing, as you say they're responsible?

Amy Edmondson: They need to call attention to it. Leaders in higher-level positions have more visibility; more people are looking to them for cues about what is valued around here, what is acceptable, and what we care about. It is the job of leaders to articulate what they care about and to have their behaviour line up with what they say.

That does not mean that people won't make attributions – people may conclude that you are not walking the talk, for example, even when you may be, in your heart and soul, walking the talk. It will not necessarily be seen that way. Psychological research has shown that making unflattering attributions about others is a natural human response. Don't take a leadership role if you are not happy to have people criticising you or thinking things about you that you believe are unfair!

You still have an opportunity and a responsibility to call attention to the things that you're trying to do. Leadership is about change. Part of your job is to call attention to the things that you would like to see changed and how and why this change will require the efforts of everyone. You must name it. You must invite them to help bring change about change, and you must create ways of holding yourself and others accountable for progress or lack thereof. I don't see any shortcuts.

Amra Rao: Psychologists work in the domain of reflecting and integrating experiences – connecting thinking, feeling, and action helping individuals, teams, and organisations to foster change. Contexts of intergenerational trauma, discrimination, stereotypes, and socio-economic pressures are not uncommon in people's personal and professional lives. Those in the caring profession are impacted by the nature of the work. What would you consider to be the key aspects of working with these challenges?

Amy Edmondson: I don't really believe I have anything new or particularly relevant or helpful. It is a complex topic, and others have commented thoughtfully with expertise about it, so I had better stick to what I know.

Amra Rao: You have put a lot of focus on psychological safety and soft teaming, on how to lead in a certain way by bringing your voice and taking responsibility. From my perspective, this can be best done when there is collaboration. When you are working in an environment where interprofessional rivalries are rife, people feel insecure speaking openly, as you spoke earlier; this is not an easy task. Nevertheless, knowing and voicing our vulnerabilities enables connections. I see many nuggets in your writings, provoking thought and considering how to deal with tough realities at work. I am interested in how you see someone managing interprofessional rivalries in such an environment.

Amy Edmondson: I have written about three practices.

The first two are most important for answering this question, but the third one might matter too. First, the practice of self-awareness. Second is the practice of managing conversations, which we discussed earlier. Third is the practice of building relationships.

Self-awareness (or self-management) is the capacity to pause and become aware of your thinking, so it's possible to reframe it more productively. Managing conversations is about having high-quality conversations that are data-driven, deeply learning-oriented, and curious. These conversations have a balance of questions and answers. High-quality conversations help us make progress on challenging issues, where there is no easy answer. Few people have truly well-developed skills in this area, and we can all improve both our self-awareness and our conversation skills.

The third practice is about taking the time in an ongoing way to build meaningful relationships at work, where we understand where others are coming from. In meaningful relationships, we don't superficially blame others for our frustrations. When we build strong relationships, we have an appreciation for what others are up against, what they're trying to do, and what they bring.

With attention to these three practices, we're less likely to make unflattering or negative attributions about others when we are experiencing frustration in a conversation related to an issue. It's natural to be frustrated if you're in a work environment and people disagree strongly on an issue that you feel passionately about. You will feel frustrated, and you will momentarily not like or appreciate them. You are likely to see *them* as the problem, but they're not. Nobody else is the problem; the problem lies in the very thorny nature of the issue itself. These interpersonal skills are rare and need space to be developed; they are the skills of wisdom and maturity.

Amra Rao: Thank you. This offers a useful framework to deal with interpersonal challenges at work.

What are your key headlines and standout messages that you would like to get across to psychologists?

Amy Edmondson: We find ourselves in times of great uncertainty and challenge. Nobody chose this, but that's where we are, and this reality calls for a different way of being, a different way of leading, different levels of humility, curiosity, and empathy. They are hard to embrace and internalise, but they are enormously powerful and helpful when we do.

Thank you very much, Amy. Anything else you would like to highlight?

Amy Edmondson: The only thing I'd add is that I believe that everything that you and I have been talking about is fundamentally an issue of skill building. These are not issues of personality. Anyone can, if they want to put the effort into it, develop the skills you need to be a good leader and a good manager. The skills of self-awareness and facilitating high-quality conversations are invaluable but challenging. We shouldn't underestimate the challenge that this entails. I think a lot of people are looking for easy answers – you know the sort of one-minute answers, but I don't have those.

Amra Rao: That is a humble way of holding a powerful position. You have led in marvellous ways. Your work has influenced many people's thinking. I want to acknowledge that. In our attempt to address difficult areas, I appreciate how you responded to my line of inquiry by saying, 'I can't answer this' and 'I don't know'. You made us pause, clarified the question taking up an enquiring stance with humility to open up the way for mutual exploration. Well, that's an important skill.

Amy Edmondson: – Thank you. I agree! And thank you for including me.

Amra Rao: Thank you for the work you do and for taking the time to have this conversation to discuss your excellent thought-provoking contributions.

> *"What I hope is clear at this point is that you don't have to be the boss to be a leader. The leader's job is to create and nurture the culture we all need to do our best work. And so anytime you play a role in doing that, you are exercising leadership."*
>
> Amy C. Edmondson: *The Fearless Organization: Creating Psychological Safety in the Workplace for Learning, Innovation, and Growth*

Notes

1 Edmondson, Amy C. The Fearless Organization: Creating Psychological Safety in the Workplace for Learning, Innovation, and Growth. Hoboken, NJ: John Wiley & Sons, 2018.
2 Edmondson, Amy. Right Kind of Wrong: The Science of Failing Well. New York, NY: Atria Books, 2023.
3 Edmondson, Amy C. Teaming: How Organizations Learn, Innovate, and Compete in the Knowledge Economy. Jossey-Bass, 2012.

PART FIVE

BREAKING THE MOULD

Race, Culture, and Identity—Can Leadership Truly Transform without Confronting Power Dynamics?

22 How Can Psychologists Lead Well?

Anti-Oppressive Leadership Principles and Practices for Practitioner Psychologists

Dr Charlotte O'Brien, King-Yin Chan, and Dr Laura Anne Winter

The chapter shares our thinking on how to develop and grow authentically as anti-oppressive leaders across the many varied and commonly confronting contexts in which we work as practitioner psychologists. Upon qualification, psychologists and psychological professionals are frequently thrust into professional leadership positions while holding little knowledge about what a leader is or how to lead well. Leadership is also not always formally addressed by psychological training programmes (Fassinger & Shullman, 2017), despite regulatory bodies such as the Health and Care Professions Council (HCPC) requiring us to demonstrate leadership competencies in our roles and understand leadership qualities, benefits, and behaviours (HCPC, 2023).

Definitions of leadership are, in contrast, extensively available (see e.g., 'Our Leadership Way' by the National Health Service [NHS, 2024] which sets out six principles of inclusive and compassionate leadership). However, we aim to highlight in this chapter that we hold a unique opportunity as practitioner psychologists to collaboratively reimagine the concept of leadership by decolonising our minds, moving beyond white, westernised, patriarchal, and hierarchical ideas of leadership, and perhaps finding solidarity together in anti-oppressive practices of love and social justice (Liu, 2020).

DOI: 10.4324/9781003492399-28

We start by situating ourselves as Counselling Psychologists, valuing humanism and relationships, aiming to facilitate growth, actualisation, and empowerment *with* others, taking a non-hierarchical approach in our appreciation of each other as unique beings, yet also understanding the inherently embedded nature of ourselves socially and relationally within systems of politics and oppression (Cooper, 2009; Winter & Charura, 2023a). It is with this lens that we approach the sections that follow, aiming to collaboratively explore how we can move anti-oppressive leadership forward as psychologists in practical, inclusive, and effective ways (Richards, 2018).

What Is Anti-Oppressive Leadership?

The term 'anti-oppressive' is defined by Galloway et al. (2020) as enacting practices that call out and engage in *critical dialogue* around racism, race, and oppression, in order to highlight the systemic barriers that maintain gaps for the minoritised. Strawbridge (1993) additionally acknowledges the inherent complexity within the term 'oppression', as it also encompasses *structural* differences in power, as well as the *personal* experiences of being targets of oppression in separate domains such as gender, sexual orientation, age, impairment, class, and race, and all the intersectional touchpoints between them. The use of the term 'anti-oppressive' can therefore become nebulous in nature, being regularly utilised but poorly understood, and without a 'clean definition' (Galloway et al., 2020, p. 490).

We therefore propose a plain English definition of anti-oppressive leadership as follows:

> "Anti-oppressive leadership is a dynamic, reflexive, and equitable approach to leadership. It is grounded in practices which *actively* and *critically* challenge social division, including racism, sexism, intersectional exclusion, or oppression of any kind. It aims to use power collectively and relationally *with* others to purposefully influence and facilitate tangible change. This can be structural or systemic, political, or social change. Anti-oppressive leadership means being aware of our power and using it to create space for integrating diverse knowledge, skills, and methods beyond traditional norms, with a firm commitment to social justice in action."

A Shared Philosophical and Theoretical Underpinning

Anti-oppressive leadership is underpinned by a shared radical humanist psychology represented by the collective works of Fanon (1990) and Cooper (1980), whose existential lens offers an explanation of how an individual's self-concept can be undermined by an adverse social, cultural, economic and political environment. This complex inter-relationship between political structure and ideology, culture, and mental health therefore demands that any attempt to ensure equality for those outside the mainstream should be accompanied by a radical change in cultural values (Hopton, 1997).

When radical humanist psychology is applied to anti-oppressive practice in this way, it can provide a theoretical framework for devising, implementing and justifying anti-oppressive strategies. This should include, for example, routine consultation with service users about service provision or evaluation, aiming to combat political activity and enhance feelings of self-worth and personal empowerment.

We also draw on theoretical understandings which share a commitment to social justice at their core (Winter & Charura, 2023a). As Oulanova, Hui and Moodley (2023) note, in psychology we need 'decolonising psychological theories and practice' which 'create a critical space' (p.13). This includes drawing on an understanding of psychological professions (and therefore of psychological leadership) as colonial and engaging with the important frameworks of Critical Race Theory (Delgado & Stefancic, 2023) and intersectionality (Crenshaw, 1989). These provide theoretical scaffolding for understanding the ways in which our intersectional identities and our social, cultural, historical positionings influence our interactions as anti-oppressive leaders. Further, understanding epistemic (in)justice helps us to understand the need to engage in open, egalitarian and collaborative meta-communication and dialogue (Winter & Charura, 2023b).

Why Systemic Disruption Is Necessary in Leadership

Historically, leadership has 'been a blank canvas on which we paint the fantasies of imperialism, white supremacy, capitalism and patriarchy' (Liu, 2020, p. 125). It is often romanticised through seemingly charismatic, transformational or ethical models of leadership which have been vulnerable to corruption, where even the most seemingly benevolent and inclusive leaders still enact racial, gendered or colonial oppression

(Liu, 2020). Systemic disruption is therefore urgently required to rock the foundational concepts of leadership, shifting them from the individual and their inherent or acquired traits towards anti-oppressive leadership practices which aspire to offer everyone an equal playing field.

Yet, even contemporary frameworks of 'inclusive' leadership are at risk of visibly othering competent individuals or enhancing *hypervisibility,* where an individual's differences are heavily scrutinised (Nishii et al. 2022). The language of 'diversity and inclusion', whilst well-intended, also implies an acceptance of people, skills, and qualities that differ from the white-dominant standards (Ahsan, 2022), where the leader holds the power to decide how much to diversify from the existing norms and who to include and share power with.

Therefore, there is an urgency to reflexively explore our systemic positionality and reflect on whether our attempts to 'give voice' (Braun & Clarke, 2022, p. 160) to marginalised individuals 'who speak quietly or not all' (Richards 2018, p.17), is enabling equality and equity or having the opposite effect. Anti-oppressive leadership, in contrast actively promotes *systems advocacy,* where leaders focus on partnering with communities or individuals to address specific systemic issues by setting goals and developing action plans to ensure they receive the necessary support to thrive (Lee & Humphrey, 2023).

Oppressive practices at a systemic level can also be seen to manifest through cultural ideologies and norms which affirm certain identities and marginalise others (Ezzani, 2020). Therefore, if we are to become truly anti-oppressive in our leadership practices, we must engage in a dynamically reflexive process aimed at changing complex patterns of social relationships that are often embedded in organisational structures, and embrace a stance as 'critical activists' breaking the cycle of systemic oppression and inequity (Ezzani, 2020, p. 230).

Having explored the concept of leadership in its historic guise, we propose that it should not be redeemed, but instead collaboratively re-imagined (Liu, 2020). As practitioner psychologists, we have an opportunity to theorise and practise anti-oppressively together based on our learnings. This requires acting collectively to decolonise our minds and relate differently to others by utilising a *power-with* approach to leadership (Proctor, 2021), and also to each other within our psychological professions (Liu, 2020).

Therefore, the section that follows explores the core principles for how we can *practically* model anti-oppressive leadership individually and collaboratively as practitioner psychologists.

Core Principles

We propose the following core principles or five Cs for anti-oppressive leadership:

1. Continuous self-awareness

As practitioner psychologists, we recognise the importance of self-awareness in therapy to ensure that we are conscious of our beliefs, values, intentions, and the assumptions, biases and prejudice we hold (Hedges, 2010). When our assumptions are unchallenged, they impact the way we understand the client, our choice of practice, and the therapeutic alliance (Brown, 2019). This is applicable to our leadership roles also, as our assumptions and biases will impact upon the way we understand colleagues (both our 'leaders' and our 'followers') and how we communicate with them. Self-awareness in the context of anti-oppressive practice is being critically conscious from a personal level to a systemic level, moving from locating the problems within an individual or group to critically examining the external inequalities and injustice (Brown, 2019). We propose that it is essential for anti-oppressive leaders to both maintain ongoing self-awareness and foster such practice within the team. Practically, this could be done by engaging in reflective spaces which promote reflexive self-awareness or in individual reflection. For example, by using Gibbs' (1988) reflective cycle.

2. Collective and relational reflective and reflexive practice

In therapeutic practice and research, reflexivity is a conscious and critical process of reflecting on our identities, positions, personal experiences, meanings, and patterns (Etherington, 2017). We propose that anti-oppressive leaders support the team to move beyond individual reflexive practice, engaging in collective and relational reflexivity. Cultivating collective reflexivity within the team helps leaders to demonstrate humility, openness, and respect (Leblanc et al., 2022), and to create a collective leadership space where all voices are welcome. Relational reflexivity also ensures that a mechanism of feedback and adjustment is practised, based on the needs of the members (Hedges, 2010). Facilitating relational reflective spaces for others could include, for example, the use of the University of Leeds' Structured Peer Group Supervision Model (Green, 2024).

3. Critical conversations

Critical conversations will always involve naming and discussing injustices, whether they directly impact our lives, or the people we serve. These conversations are often emotionally intense, with inherent risks involved to enable these much-needed dialogues (Arao & Clemens, 2013). Instead of aiming to create a safe space without risks, or a brave space that drains the members of marginalised groups, it would be more helpful and achievable to create an *accountable space* where all members are responsible for their participation and are committed to learning, self-reflecting, and giving space (Ahenkorah, 2020). We propose that anti-oppressive leadership goes beyond merely implementing this accountable space; it also involves supporting team members to facilitate these *critical conversations* to happen in accountable manner. For example, by providing reflective and reflexive anti-oppressive facilitator training, or by using supervision to support team members and diffuse any impacts of critical conversations.

4. Community involvement

Contemporary branches of psychology, such as community psychology, have provided us with new lenses and ways of thinking about service users and the therapeutic relationship; shifting from an individualistic and deficit-focused view to valuing the strengths, wisdom and *collaboration* that are located within the community (Nelson & Prilleltensky, 2010). Methods of engagement can include participatory action research, peer support groups, and creative expressive art projects, with the aim of joining forces, capitals and knowledge to target the root cause of social injustice (Lunghy et al., 2023). We propose that anti-oppressive leadership collectively utilises leaders' (and those individuals, teams, and service cultures they are responsible for) knowledge, power and resources to encourage community engagement; to model an anti-oppressive culture and ethos when working with communities, reminding team members of the purpose of the community project and returning power to the members of the community, while remaining vigilant of any risk of tokenism, co-opting and distraction.

5. Combatting systemic power, politics, policy and privilege

Whilst internal changes are crucial and should be prioritised, without external changes, individuals, communities and groups will continue to face the same structural power, oppressions and prejudice that brought them to the service in the first place. We believe anti-oppressive leadership is about recognising the team's power and responsibility to influence and act. We recommend leaders engage the team and service users in a collaborative exercise using tools such as the 'Five Ts' policy engagement principles by Pike (2019) i.e. targeting (to the right audience), translation (getting the message across), timing (at the right time), tools (using the most effective channels), and talk (building connections, networks and relationships), to plan realistic and attainable policy influence actions and goals. We also advocate for bringing in like-minded people from other disciplines, within and outside of the organisation, to address the gaps in knowledge, experience, and skills, as well as noticing the blind spots in the existing plan and practice. Reflective facilitators are trained to work with marginalisation, inter-group power dynamics and inter-professional rivalries, valuing open enquiry towards complexity, difference, and emotive responses. By using an external reflective facilitator, a safe, supportive, and blame-free environment can be provided where the facilitator encourages dialogue, whilst modelling qualities such as congruence, acceptance, and empathy that are not always inherent in team dynamics (Marshall et al., 2024). We would recommend inviting an external facilitator from outside of the organisation to enable these anti-oppressive conversations with the team or organisation as a whole.

Anti-Oppressive Leadership in Action

We understand that each leadership context presents its own set of challenges; therefore, we therefore offer a list of reflective questions to facilitate readers in formulating practical actions (not just words) based on the 5C principles for the self, team, organisation, or community in which they serve, acting as a strategic tool to instigate change at both the macro and micro level (Figure 22.1).

Opportunities and challenges

Finally, we consider together the opportunities and challenges practitioner psychologists have to develop and grow authentically as anti-oppressive leaders in our current systems and contexts. In this section, we take inspiration from Erikson's (1950) psychosocial stages of development, where, as individuals grow and develop, there are often

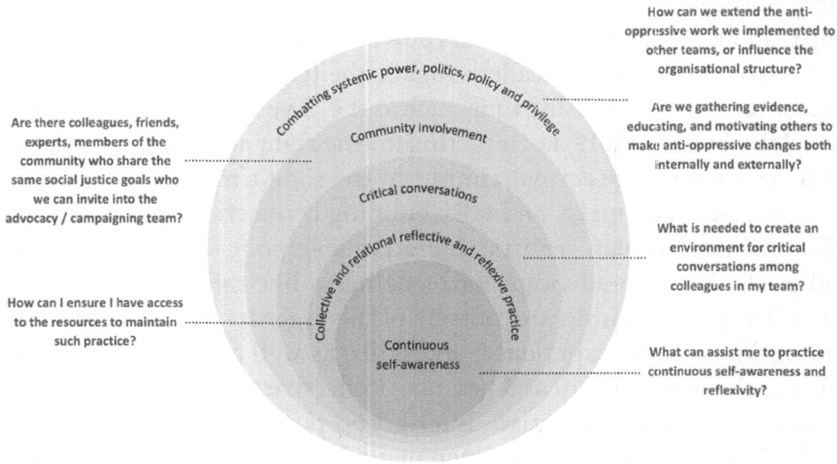

Figure 22.1 Reflective questions.

opposing psychological tendencies; if the virtue (or in this case the 'antidote') is adopted, it can help to resolve the current challenge or conflict (Orenstien & Lewis, 2022). We, therefore, consider what we see as the five main challenges and opportunities in anti-oppressive leadership as follows:

1. **Blind spots vs Self-awareness (antidote: reflection and reflexivity)**

Reflection and reflexivity can help us to become more self-aware, to evaluate and manage our own emotions and behaviours objectively so that they align with our social justice values and standards (Duval & Wicklund, 2008). By embracing these practices, not only do we become more privately self-aware, noticing our own blind spots curiously and reflexively, but we also become more consciously aware of how we are in public with others and how we can behave in ways that are anti-oppressive.

2. **Isolation vs Community (antidote: relationship and attachment)**

Michelle Obama stated that 'If we're going to out-innovate and out-educate the rest of the world, we've got to open the doors for everyone… We need all hands-on deck, and that means clearing hurdles for women and girls'. We embrace this anti-oppressive notion that we need *all* hands on deck, taking it one step further and asserting that anti-oppressive leadership is the responsibility of the *whole community*. It is in uniting with each other relationally, forming safe and secure attachments with others who have a similar anti-oppressive agenda (Bowlby, 1988), that we find our collective power *with* one another to combat oppression and social isolation (Proctor, 2021).

3. **Despair vs Action (antidote: hope and generativity)**

It is easy for us as psychological professionals to become despairing, feeling that change is impossible. Yet, the role of hope is an essential core of moral, social and political change (Stockdale, 2021). Hope can be seen as a desire or belief in change when faced with oppressive structures (Stockdale, 2021). It is therefore by embracing hope that we can harness generativity or positive action, both to care for ourselves and others as we create and accomplish tasks within our anti-oppressive agenda to care for and contribute positively to the next generations.

4. **Stagnation vs Creativity (antidote: innovation and change)**

Given our newfound hope for change, we may then feel stagnation in terms of what practical steps to take as anti-oppressive leaders. This is where leaning into collective creativity can be helpful. Creativity has the ability to bring communities together, facilitating collaboration and collective action to address social justice issues. By using creative spaces, workshops, and community-driven projects, creativity can empower individuals to become the agents of change and drive social innovation and transformation (The Creativity Conference, 2024).

5. **Oppression vs Identity (antidote: anti-oppressive practice)**

Identity is intricately bound to oppression, as identity is connected to what we look like, how we identify as an individual or group, and how we differentiate from one another (Dominelli & Campling, 2002). Therefore, our differences can become politicised, creating superior-inferior polarity, or borderlands policed by both sides of the binary divide (Dominelli & Campling, 2002). For us to move forward collectively with an anti-oppressive stance, we must therefore practically embrace the 5Cs in this chapter, using our reflective and reflexive stance to harness a collective, social justice identity for change.

We close this chapter reflecting on our hope that by embarking upon this collaborative journey together, exploring the meaning, necessity, challenges and opportunities for anti-oppressive leadership as practitioner psychologists, we may move forward with a shared vision and agenda for change. We hope that we have provided tangible steps towards anti-oppressive leadership practices that are accessible to all practitioner psychologists in the contexts we serve. We acknowledge, however, that the work here is not done, but hope that with collaboration, creativity, and community, we might move social justice and anti-oppressive leadership forward collectively into our lives, workplaces, and communities.

Ideas in Brief

- Anti-oppressive leadership is a dynamic, reflexive, and equitable approach that actively challenges all forms of social oppression. It emphasises the collective and relational use of power to drive purposeful and inclusive change.
- Anti-oppressive leadership involves critical reflection on one's own social identities and actively disrupts systemic inequalities and oppression.
- Anti-oppressive leadership 5 C's are continuous self-awareness, collective and relational reflective and reflexive practice, critical conversations, community involvement, and combating systemic power.
- Anti-oppressive leadership faces challenges such as blind spots, isolation, despair, stagnation, and persistent oppression. Strategies such as reflexivity, relational support, and collective innovation help to counter such challenges.

References

Ahenkorah, E. (2020, September 21). Safe and brave spaces don't work (and what you can do instead). *Medium*. https://medium.com/@elise.k.ahen/safe-and-brave-spaces-dont-work-and-what-you-can-do-instead-f265aa339aff

Ahsan, S. (2022, February 16). EDI: Endless distraction and inaction. *The Psychologist*. https://www.bps.org.uk/psychologist/edi-endless-distraction-and-inaction

Arao, B., & Clemens, K. (2013). From safe spaces to brave spaces: A new way to frame dialogue around diversity and social justice. In L. M. Landreman (Ed.), *The art of effective facilitation: Reflections from social justice educators* (pp. 135–150). Routledge.

Bowlby, J. (1988). *A secure base: Parent-child attachment and healthy human development*. Routledge.

Braun, V., & Clarke, V. (2022). *Thematic analysis: A practical guide.* Sage.

Brown, J. D. (2019). *Anti-oppressive counseling and psychotherapy: Action for personal and social change.* Routledge.

Cooper, D. (1980). *The language of madness.* Pelican.

Cooper, M. (2009). Welcoming the other: Actualising the humanistic ethic at the core of counselling psychology practice. *Counselling Psychology Review, 24*(3&4), 119–129. https://mick-cooper.squarespace.com/new-blog/2021/5/1/welcoming-the-other-actualising-the-humanistic-ethic-at-the-core-of-counselling-psychology-practice

Crenshaw, K. (1989). Demarginalizing the intersection of race and sex. *University of Chicago Legal Forum, 1*(8). http://chicagounbound.uchicago.edu/uclf/vol1989/iss1/8

Delgado, R., & Stefancic, J. (2023). *Critical race theory* (4th ed.). New York University Press.

Dominelli, L., & Campling, J. (2002). Oppression, social divisions and identity. In J. Campling (Eds.), *Anti-oppressive social work theory and practice.* Palgrave. https://doi.org/10.1007/978-1-4039-1400-2_3

Duval, S., & Wicklund, R. A. (2008). *A theory of objective self-awareness. Johnson research foundation colloquia social psychology. A series of monographs, treaties and texts, Vol. 17 of social psychology.* Academic Press.

Erikson, E. H. (1950). *Childhood and society.* Norton.

Etherington, K. (2017). Personal experience and critical reflexivity in counselling and psychotherapy research. *Counselling and Psychotherapy Research, 17*(2), 85–94. https://doi.org/10.1002/capr.12080

Ezzani, M. (2020). A principal's approach to leadership for social justice: Advancing reflective and anti-oppressive practices. *Journal of School Leadership, 31*(3), 227–247. https://doi.org/10.1177/1052684620908347

Fanon, F. (1990). *The wretched of the earth.* Penguin

Fassinger, R. E., & Shullman, S. L. (2017). Leadership and counseling psychology: What should we know? Where could we go? *The Counseling Psychologist, 45*(7), 927–964. https://doi.org/10r.g1/107.171/0770/1010101000010717744425

Galloway, M. K., Cllin, P., James, S., Vimegnon, H., & McCall, L. (2020). Culturally responsive, antiracist, or anti-oppressive? How language matters for school change efforts. *Equity and Excellence in Education, 52*(4), 485–501. https://doi-org.manchester.idm.oclc.org/10.1080/10665684.2019.1691959

Gibbs, G. (1988). *Learning by doing.* Further Education Unit [FEU].

Green, D. (2024, September 6). *Leeds model of structured peer group supervision.* https://mymedia.leeds.ac.uk/Mediasite/Showcase/default/Presentation/497b1e52ed0249cda505b175e8b1e3d71d

Health and Care Professions Council [HCPC]. (2023, July 20). *The standards of proficiency for practitioner psychologist*. https://www.hcpc-uk.org/standards/standards-of-proficiency/practitioner-psychologists/

Hedges, F. (2010). *Reflexivity in therapeutic practice*. Palgrave Macmillan.

Hopton, J. (1997). Anti-discriminatory practice and anti-oppressive practice: A radical humanist psychology perspective. *Critical Social Policy, 17*(52), 47–61. https://doi-org.manchester.idm.oclc.org/10.1177/026101839701705203

Leblanc, P.-M., Rousseau, V., & Harvey, J.-F. (2022). Leader humility and team innovation: The role of team reflexivity and team proactive personality. *Journal of Organizational Behavior, 43*(8), 1396–1409. https://doi.org/10.1002/job.2648

Lee, C. C., & Humphrey, M. (2023). Advocacy and working with individual clients beyond traditional therapy models. In L. A. Winter & D. Charura (Eds.), *The handbook of social justice in psychological therapies: Politics, power, change* (pp. 179–188). Sage.

Liu, H. (2020). *Redeeming leadership: An anti-racist feminist intervention*. Bristol University Press.

Lunghy, E., Zlotowitz, S., & Wallis, L. (2023). Critical community psychology & participatory action research. In L. A. Winter & D. Charura (Eds.), *The handbook of social justice in psychological therapies: Power, politics, change* (pp. 198–209). Sage.

Marshall, T., Keville, S., Cain, A., & Adler, J. R. (2022). Facilitating reflection: A review and synthesis of the factors enabling effective facilitation of reflective practice. *International and Multidisciplinary Perspectives, 23*(4), 483–496. https://doi.org/10.1080/14623943.2022.2064444

Marshall, C., Rehman, I., Winter, LA. & Wynn, G. (2024). Training Psychologist Therapists for Social Justice. In R. Tribe and D. Bhugra. (Eds.). Social Justice, Social Discrimination and Mental Health: Theory, Practice, and Professional Issues (pp. 215-228). Routledge

Nelson, G., & Prilleltensky, I. (2010). *Community psychology: In pursuit of liberation and well-being*. Palgrave Macmillan.

Nishii, L. H., & Leroy, H. (2022). A multi-level framework of inclusive leadership in organisations. *Group & Organization Management, 47*(4), 683–722. https://doi.org/10.1177/10596011221111505

Obama White House Archives. (2011, September 26). *Remarks by the First Lady at National Science Foundation family friendly policy rollout*. The White House. https://obamawhitehouse.archives.gov/the-press-office/2011/09/26/remarks-first-lady-national-science-foundation-family-friendly-policy-r

Oulanova, O., Hui, J., & Moodley, R. (2023). Engaging with minoritised and racialised communities 'inside the sentence'. In L. A. Winter & D. Charura

(Eds.), *The handbook of social justice in psychological therapies. Power, politics, change* (pp. 10–21). Sage.

Orenstein, G. A., & Lewis, L. (2022). *Erikson's stages of psychosocial development.* StatPearls Publishing. https://www.ncbi.nlm.nih.gov/books/NBK556096/

Pike, L. (2019, May 2). *The '5 Ts' of policy engagement: PolicyBristol's approach to supporting academics.* PolicyBristol Hub. https://policybristol.blogs.bris.ac.uk/2019/05/02/the-5-ts-of-policy-engagement-policybristols-approach-to-supporting-academics/

Proctor, G. (2021). *The dynamics of power in counselling and psychotherapy: Ethics, politics and practice* (2nd ed.). PCCS Books.

Richards, C. (2018). Leadership in counselling psychology: Sexuality and gender. *Counselling Psychology Review, 33*(2), 17–20. https://doi.org/10.53841/bpscpr.2018.33.2.17

Stockdale, K. (2021). *Hope under oppression.* Oxford University Press.

Strawbridge, S. (1993). *Towards anti-oppressive practice in counselling psychology.* British Psychological Society Special Group in Counselling Psychology 4th Annual Conference 1993, United Kingdom. https://study.sagepub.com/node/38391/student-resources/further-reading-and-case-studies/chapter-12-working-with-difference-a-1

The National Health Service Leadership Academy [NHS]. (2024, July 20). *Our leadership way.* https://www.leadershipacademy.nhs.uk/organisational-resources/our-leadership-way/

The Creativity Conference. (2024, August). *Creativity and social justice: How creatives can make a difference.* https://www.creativityconference.is/blog/creativity-and-social-justice-how-creatives-can-make-a-difference

Winter, L. A., & Charura, D. (2023a). *The handbook of social justice in psychological therapies. Power, politics, change.* Sage.

Winter, L. A., & Charura, D. (2023b). Core principles for social justice informed therapeutic work. In L. A. Winter & D. Charura (Eds.), *The handbook of social justice in psychological therapies. Power, politics, change* (pp. 63–76). Sage.

Identity and Leadership 23

Understanding the Meaning for Clinical Psychologists

Professor Jan Hughes and Professor Gary Latchford

Introduction

For many years, clinical psychology was described by clinical psychologists themselves as a young profession, but this is clearly no longer true, with the first clinical psychology course in the UK being founded almost 80 years ago. In the early years, clinical psychologists struggled to widen their scope of practice from assessment to delivering therapy. With growing confidence, later developments such as 'new ways of working' (Lavender & Hope, 2007) emphasised group work and leadership as a core part of the role of a clinical psychologist. Throughout those first decades, clinical psychologists situated themselves in relation to the longer-established and more powerful profession of psychiatry. Over time, however, they expanded their practice into different settings, working alongside multiple different professions and developing new roles. Fast forward to current practice, and clinical psychologists find themselves a relatively long-established profession embedded in many different NHS settings, at a time when there has been a massive and unprecedented expansion of the psychological professions. Quite naturally, the NHS expects clinical psychologists to step forward to help shape and lead NHS mental health services, as reflected in the NHS Long Term Plan (2019) and the Darzi report (2024), but are clinical psychologists embracing this aspect within their professional identity, and if so, how?

This chapter will focus on identity and leadership in three different areas: the professional, the conceptual, and the personal.

DOI: 10.4324/9781003492399-29

Leadership and the Professional Identity of Clinical Psychologists

The tension between the relative importance of therapy and research as key parts of the clinical psychologist's identity has been present since the earliest days of the profession. 'Scientist-practitioner' remains a common description. Though critical appraisal and evidence-based practice remain key, few engage in research after qualification. Most aspiring clinical psychologists are interested in delivering therapeutic interventions, and during their careers, they typically develop expertise in particular areas of practice or particular therapies. How do they respond to opportunities to develop leadership roles?

A qualitative study of university-based academics is potentially illuminating (Rehbock et al., 2022). Academics typically don't seek leadership roles; their identity is bound up with knowledge and skills. In this study, those who identified as a leader tended to rebrand this as a 'mentor' or 'manager', or someone effecting change in wider systems – a 'shaper'. Might clinical psychologists adapt the concept of leadership in similar ways, reluctant to discard the clinical identity that often motivated them to seek a career in the first place?

Leadership in the NHS encompasses mentorship and supervision, management and system change, and this feels consistent with improving clinical outcomes for those using services. There has certainly been an acknowledgement of other approaches of influence alongside one-to-one therapy; for example community psychology or campaigning for political change, the argument being that this has a greater impact on wellbeing than seeing individual service users, and reconciling this as an important aspect of professional identity.

A recent scoping review of qualitative studies found that professional identity in clinical psychology evolves over the course of a career, following relative growth and stability during training and the years following (Schubert et al., 2023). This is very individual, and there is a complex interplay for those with a dual identity – those with lived experience or those who identify with a minoritised group, for example. They found a need for personal and professional boundaries to be maintained, and also a challenge in rising to the expectations of the role. There is a sense of what one should be as a clinical psychologist – and in the UK this certainly is associated with leadership – but also a fear of not being competent. This fear often starts in training. Many clinical psychology trainees report feeling 'imposter syndrome' when they get on a course.

This might be reinforced by reflection, humility, and compassion being such key attributes of the profession. Another potential influence is that as understanding increases during training, trainees may become more aware of what they don't know – conscious incompetence – and this may remain with them on qualification. The hope is that practice increases competence and confidence in abilities, but this may be easier for skills used more often and more widely agreed on, such as clinical skills, than those that may be seen as more peripheral or harder to define, such as those relating to leadership.

One potential barrier to taking up leadership roles is the conflation of leader and manager. Taking management roles can be one way – though not the only way – of providing leadership in the NHS. Many are reluctant, seeing management as distancing themselves from the clinical work that often inspired their career choice in the first place. There is, however, pressure on clinical psychologists to adopt new roles in the changing landscape of promotion since the agenda for change. At one time, promotion could be sought in recognition of the development of high-level therapeutic skills, but this is now much less likely, higher banded roles being associated with increased levels of responsibility.

There is also an expectation that clinical psychologists will take a leadership perspective, whatever the band of the post they are in, moving away from a simple association between leadership and more senior posts. At a time of expansion of the psychological professions, the level and duration of the training of clinical psychologists means that they have something to offer, whatever the context of their post.

Two notes of caution. First, though national developments have long advocated for clinical psychologists to develop leadership roles in the NHS, and this is explicitly recognised in the new contracts for clinical psychology training in England, in practice this is not the day-to-day experience of many NHS psychologists. Many services have been slow to change, seeing only long waiting lists and the need for clinical psychologists to see service users, reluctant to support any activity that takes them away from this. Second, adopting a leadership position does not mean telling others what to do. One reason for the reluctance of clinical psychologists may be a fear that it will mean passing on advice to colleagues who may well be much more experienced than they are. In truth, there are many different ways to embody leadership, and they benefit hugely from the clinical skills of compassion, empathy and formulation that are already established as fundamental parts of the clinical psychology identity.

The Concept of Leadership

There is a conceptual dimension to taking on leadership roles. We all grow up with stereotypes of what a leader – and a good leader – looks like. Models of leadership have evolved over time, from 'great man' models that focus on the achievements of individuals from history, to situational, transactional, transformational, and more recently relational, inclusive, and dispersed models of leadership. Such models are covered in greater detail in the chapter by Tony Lavender in this volume, but for now we want to highlight that the trend has been to appreciate that leadership does not happen in a vacuum. Particular social situations facilitate particular styles of leadership, and successful leaders operate within an interpersonal context. Our understanding of the main tenets of leadership continues to evolve over time, but two popular current models seem particularly useful for those working in healthcare: the Compassionate Leadership Model (West, 2021) and the Inclusive Leadership Model (Hollander, 2012). Both seem to us to embody the clinical skills fundamental to the practice of clinical psychology.

The Compassionate Leadership Model focuses on the relationships between the leader and those they work with, and in turn, between everyone in an organisation. It puts compassion at the centre – a sensitivity to the suffering of the self and others and the desire to help. When embodied by the leader, the suggestion is that it influences the entire culture of the organisation. Through compassionate engagement with the people they work with, listening and understanding rather than judging, compassionate leaders make their staff feel valued and respected, and encourage them to treat others in similar ways. That's the theory at least. It does seem to work – resulting in staff with higher morale, fewer absences, and generally greater motivation, with clear implications for improved patient care (West, 2021). We acknowledge, though, that it can seem difficult to hold compassion as a central principle in times of financial challenge or organisational change.

It's easy to see the similarity between core therapeutic skills and the key elements named in the model – the five Cs of consciousness; curiosity; compassion; competence; and courage. Adopting a compassionate leadership style should therefore feel like a good fit for clinical psychologists. It is certainly far from the authoritarian leadership stereotype many still hold, though of course these may be based on personal experience of being led.

Inclusive Leadership is a related model – in fact, it's hard to imagine a successful compassionate leader who is not also inclusive. It refers to a leadership style that focuses on creating a diverse workforce who feel respected and fairly treated in a psychologically safe environment, something that the NHS has not always achieved (Kings Find, 2022). The notion of inclusion can sometimes be open to different interpretation, but Korkmaz et al. (2022) in a systematic review of inclusive leadership models, argue that the key components are fostering uniqueness and diversity of staff, strengthening feelings of belongingness, showing appreciation for staff, and supporting initiatives across the organisation, such as those to increase diversity. The elements considered to be crucial in inclusive leadership (the six Cs): commitment; courage; cognizance of bias; curiosity; cultural intelligence; collaboration also seem like a roll call of principles most clinical psychologists would be happy to align with.

The conceptual basis of these more recent developments in thinking about leadership is similar and seems a natural fit for clinical psychologists in terms of the values that underpin the profession. In order to fulfil their potential in leadership roles, clinical psychologists need to see leadership as a part of their professional identity, and promoting these more modern ideas of leadership is one way of doing this.

It's helpful too to highlight the principles underlying these new models. As described above, there is acknowledgement in the profession of the importance of influencing systems outside of the therapy room. One thing that may help clinical psychologists see leadership as a natural part of their identity is recognising the transferability of skills from the therapy room to leadership contexts. These core skills relate to the ability to sit and contain a situation, to be able to hear and listen to multiple perspectives and assess the issue in hand; to formulate using a number of different models; to use this formulation to inform the best course of action. As can be seen above, a compassionate and inclusive stance is common to both roles. Taking on a leadership role can be seen as extending these skills to gradually influence wider and wider systems.

Finally, another aspect that may potentially be a barrier for clinical psychologists is the potential for abuse of power. Power is certainly an aspect of any leadership role. Most are only too aware of individuals who seek leadership roles for the power it confers, or the boost to their ego they imagine it brings. Clinical psychologists may be reluctant to take leadership positions lest they be seen by others as having a similar motivation. Power or influence may also be used for the good of the service and those using it; however, it's notable that the recent leadership models described above have no role for the ego of the leader, but assume that they share a common set of values to support others, service users, and staff. This is arguably particularly so in public bodies or not-for-profit organisations such as the NHS. Such values are likely to echo the personal values of many clinical psychologists, and stepping up to a leadership role could be seen as the most effective way of enacting them.

We ought to acknowledge, however, that taking a leadership role may lead to situations where the individual values of the psychologist may sometimes conflict with decisions being made in the organisation. Some settings, such as forensics may produce particular conflicts between personal and institutional values, but this might be true in very many settings at different times. The truth is that though being exposed to these conflicts may be uncomfortable, it does offer an opportunity to try to do something about them not often afforded to the individual clinician. It can, at times, be trying but, as the American comedian and political commentator Jon Stewart once said, 'if you don't stick to your values when they are being tested, they're not values, they're hobbies' ("The Daily Show", January 22, 2009).

Leadership and the Personal Identity of Clinical Psychologists

This chapter tries to bring together the themes we have discussed and asks you to reflect on your position in relation to them. Here are some questions for you to consider as you carry on reading:

- Why did you want to become a clinical psychologist?
- What matters to you – what are your core values?
- Did you have a role model in mind when you started your path to training?
- What aspects of clinical psychology were embodied in your role model? A therapist? A leader?
- If you think of a leader in your professional life now, who comes to mind? Do you see them as a good leader or a bad leader?
- What sort of leader would you like to be?

In this final section, we will consider leadership in terms of personal identity. A major factor to take into account is our life-long journeys into the role and the things that have influenced us on this journey, for good or ill. This includes our social background, personal experiences, intersectionality regarding the ways we identify – often conceptualised using the Social Graces model (Burnham, 1992) – and the power and privilege we hold. We will all have been influenced by experiences before, during and after we undertook professional training. For some, how we identify in terms of lack of privilege may affect this journey. For example, having the experience of coming from a working-class background, and/or from a marginalised group may mean that we struggle more with our confidence in some settings, and have had few or no clear role models.

We earlier discussed the tendency of trainee clinical psychologists to experience imposter syndrome and speculated on how this might change after training. It certainly appears that self-efficacy in terms of leadership is slow to change. In a study of 68 newly qualified clinical psychologists using the Leader Efficacy Questionnaire (Hannah & Avolio, 2013), the leadership self-efficacy reported by participants was considerably lower than a normative sample of UK undergraduate students (61.04 vs 79.33) (McTiffin, 2022). This may reflect something of the difference in culture between the US and UK, but it is still a surprise to see such a difference between any professional group and undergraduate students. It would be interesting to see if leadership self-efficacy actually reduces after qualification for clinical psychologists as they become more aware of the complexities of the role. Leadership self-efficacy is certainly important – in this study it was found to be significantly related to motivation to lead (McTiffin, 2022).

How might our confidence in applying ourselves to leadership roles change? Clinical psychology training certainly impacts our sense of self. It leads to the development of meta-competencies in terms of managing and understanding clinical and professional relationships. We automatically develop formulations to help us understand situations on a large and small scale. Our growing self-awareness gains a new layer as we build a professional identity and discover an ability to extend our sphere of influence, but one inevitably influences the other, in both directions.

One of the most important factors in change is the development of relationships – change happens through and because of relationships. As described earlier, relationships are at the core of more recent models of leadership. This is mirrored by the many years of psychotherapy research highlighting the importance of the therapeutic alliance, the client's early rating of which is the most consistent predictor of later change (Baier, Kline, & Feeny, 2020). Similarly, the relationship between supervisor and supervisee (supervisor alliance) has emerged as one of the most important factors in supervision (Watkins, 2014). Recent literature focusing on leadership for clinical psychologists has also emphasised the importance of relationships (e.g. Evans, 2023; Cartmell, 2020; Messham, 2018; Corrigall; 2015).

However, even if persuaded it is a good thing to do, for clinical psychologists, leadership is perhaps the most exposing aspect of the role, one that for many might not have been considered when initially pursuing a career in the profession. Even if they feel more confident that they have something to offer in a leadership role, adapting to being 'seen' by peers, becoming more visible as a leader and therefore more likely to be judged by others may be a difficult step to take. It's unlikely everyone will agree with everything you do as a leader. Many will have been exposed to leadership that they saw as 'bad' in the past, but even being a 'good' leader will sometimes involve difficult choices – or easy choices with difficult consequences for some. There will sometimes be a need to take an 'expert' position and have a voice for the good of others, and this will not always be universally popular, particularly when advocating for change in long-established institutions or practices. This may come naturally to some, but for others, this may take some preparation. Such a position may seem at first to be at odds with the natural tendency of clinical psychologists to 'come alongside' others to collaborate. We don't think so. We suspect that the skills of clinical psychologists, in fact, make them particularly suitable for making difficult ethical decisions and attempting to carry others with them afterwards. Clinical psychologists may have a difficult relationship with power and be particularly mindful of the potential for power to be abused; in itself, this is a useful awareness, but not a reason to disengage.

Leadership roles will, then, sometimes involve having to make difficult decisions and sometimes involve a challenge to our values. In a study looking at dilemmas in decision-making in clinical psychology leaders, Messham (2018) found tension can arise when trying to act in a way that feels necessary but appears potentially incongruent with our values. Sometimes difficult choices will have to be made involving challenging conversations and the need to be clear and direct. Sometimes boundaries will need to be set, and people need to be pushed to act in ways that challenge a system. There can sometimes seem to be an incongruity between these processes and wanting to prioritise the relationship, linked to a human need to be liked at work. We have found it helpful to disentangle the need to be liked as a leader from the need to be respected. Gaining respect from followers (and having equal respect for them) is crucial – and in turn also makes it far more likely that you will be liked!

What Can Help?

What might the barriers be to clinical psychologists taking up leadership roles?

The first has certainly been an opportunity in the past, but this is clearly changing with increasing demand for clinical psychologists to do just that.

The second might be misunderstanding what leadership is and what clinical psychologists might have to offer. The DCP has been important in this. Leadership was one of the roles highlighted in new ways of working in 2007, and in 2010 the DCP produced a first leadership development framework for clinical psychology. The framework was aimed at clinical psychologists at all stages of their careers, arguing that 'our core psychological competencies and relationship expertise in engagement and collaboration can serve as valuable tools for effective leadership.' The framework also gave practical advice on developing leadership skills and proposed a leadership competency framework. More recently, the psychological professions network has produced a discussion paper on leadership and management in the psychological professions (2020), and there have also been calls for a revision to the original DCP competency framework (Rao & Mason, 2023).

The third might be the lack of self-efficacy described above. Training programmes have a role here and already focus on the skills and personal and professional development aspects of emerging leadership, supporting the trainees to incorporate leadership into their core identity as a clinical psychologist. Many programmes feature leadership placements in the third year, where trainees can see and join clinical psychologists taking leadership roles in different organisations.

The fourth might be a lack of training and support for clinical psychologists in leadership positions. This is changing. The NHS Leadership Academy offers leadership programmes to support leaders from a variety of NHS professions at different stages of their careers, which many clinical psychologists have attended. Meanwhile, the BPS/DCP published a report on supporting and developing leadership skills for psychologists working in health and social care in 2021 (BPS/DCP, 2021), and the DCP has put together the Clinical Psychologists as Leaders programme. This targets the development of leadership skills of clinical psychologists across the career span through leadership training and a mentoring programme, which addresses challenges some colleagues may face in taking up leadership roles, for example, those from the global majority. The mentoring programme has proved hugely popular, with 149 mentees and 54 mentors initially signing up for the scheme (Rao, Cate & Pote, 2023), which suggests that we are seeing a change in the way clinical psychologists view leadership.

Why Is All This Important?

This is a moment in history where the current relational concepts of leadership and the values of our profession are coalescing, alongside a recognition of the importance of our profession from policy drivers in the NHS. As a profession, we need to overcome our reticence to use our skills in a different forum and to embrace leadership roles when we have the opportunity. We have described the challenges this may bring. It may also bring significant rewards. Some of these will be around our personal identity – satisfaction with doing something well, pride in our efforts being recognised and respected, and maybe rewarded, though sometimes this will not happen – though this may sometimes feel like unwanted attention. Some of the rewards, however, will relate more to our professional identity – the opportunity to use our skills to effect the greatest change for the greatest number of people. Whether others see this or not, this is also perhaps the most important personal consequence. Effective leadership is about using influence as widely as we can to make a difference to as many as we can. This surely, at heart is our most important value.

Ideas in Brief

- The identity of CPs as leaders has evolved over the 80 years of the profession.
- Some of the current key leadership models align with CP values, e.g. compassionate and inclusive leadership
- Some of the tasks of leadership relate directly to the skills of a CP (e.g. assessing complexity, formulating, intervening) but with a wider sphere of influence
- Our identity as a leader is inextricably linked to our personal identity and the power and authority we feel.
- Understanding this can help us to use our influence as widely as we can to make a difference to as many as we can.

References

Baier, A. L., Kline, A. C., & Feeny, N. C. (2020). Therapeutic alliance as a mediator of change: A systematic review and evaluation of research. Clinical Psychology Review, 82, 101921. https://doi.org/10.1016/j.cpr.2020.101921

British Psychological Society/Division of Clinical Psychology. (2010). *Clinical psychology leadership development framework*. British Psychological Society/Division of Clinical Psychology.

British Psychological Society/Division of Clinical Psychology. (2021). *Leadership development and support for clinical psychologists working in health and social care*. British Psychological Society/Division of Clinical Psychology.

Burnham, J. (1992). Approach-method technique: Making distinction and creating connections. *Human Systems, 3*(1), 3–27.

Cartmell, H. (2020). *Exploring the relationship between authentic leadership, workplace wellbeing and attachment insecurity amongst clinical psychologists working in the NHS*. Unpublished D.Clin.Psychol thesis, University of Leeds.

Corrigall, F. A. (2015). *The experience of successful leaders: An IPA study on senior female clinical psychologists*. Unpublished D.Clin.Psychol thesis, University of Leeds.

Darzi, A. (2024). Independent investigation of the NHS in England. Available at https://www.gov.uk/government/publications/independent-investigation-of-the-nhs-in-england

Evans, Sophie Louise. (2023). *Exploring clinical psychologists' experiences of being leaders in CAMHS*. Unpublished D.Clin.Psychol thesis, University of Leeds.

Hannah, S. T., & Avolio, B. (2013). *Leader efficacy questionnaire*. Mind Garden.

Hollander, E. (2012). *Inclusive leadership: The essential leader-follower relationship*. Routledge. https://doi.org/10.4324/9780203809914

Korkmaz, A. V., van Engen, M. L., Knappert, L., & Schalk, R. (2022). About and beyond leading uniqueness and belongingness: A systematic review of inclusive leadership research. *Human Resource Management Review, 32*(4), 100894. https://doi.org/10.1016/j.hrmr.2022.100894

Lavender, T., & Hope, R. (2007). *New ways of working for applied psychologists in health and social care: The end of the beginning: Summary report*. British Psychological Society/Division of Clinical Psychology.

McTiffin, M. (2022). *How are leadership self-efficacy, leadership self identity, and leadership style related to motivation to lead in newly qualified clinical psychologists'*? Unpublished D.Clin.Psychol thesis, University of Leeds.

Messham, L. S. (2018). *Exploring clinical psychologists' experiences of leading within clinical teams in relation to their values*. Unpublished D.Clin.Psychol thesis, University of Leeds.

NHS England. (2019). *The NHS long term plan*. Available at https://www.longtermplan.nhs.uk/

Psychological Professions Network. (2020). Leadership and management in the psychological professions: Discussion paper. Available at https://www.ppn.nhs.uk/resources-url/publications/35-leadership-and-management-in-the-psychological-professions-discussion-paper/file

Rehbock, S. K., Hubner, S. V., Knipfer, K., & Peus, C. V. (2022). What kind of leader am I? An exploration of professionals' leader identity construal. *Applied Psychology, 72*(2), 559–587. https://doi.org/10.1111/apps.12389

Rao, A. S., Cate, T., & Pote, H. (2023). Supporting leadership development through mentoring. *Clinical Psychology Forum, 363*, 58–62. https://doi.org/10.53841/bpscpf.2023.1.363.58

Rao, A. S., & Mason, B. (2023). Examining leadership competencies. Are our leadership skills future ready? *Clinical Psychology Forum, 363*, 63–73. https://doi.org/10.53841/bpscpf.2023.1.363.63

Schubert, S., Buus, N., Monrouxe, L. V., & Hunt, C. (2023). The development of professional identity in clinical psychologists: A scoping review. *Medical Education, 57*(7), 612–626. https://doi.org/10.1111/medu.15082

The Kings Fund. (2022). What is compassionate leadership? Available at https://www.kingsfund.org.uk/insight-and-analysis/long-reads/what-is-compassionate-leadership

Watkins, C. E. (2014). The supervisory alliance: A half century of theory, practice, and research in critical perspective. *American Journal of Psychotherapy, 68*, 19–55. https://doi.org/10.1176/appi.psychotherapy.2014.68.1.19

West, M. (2021). *Compassionate leadership: Sustaining wisdom, humanity and presence in health and social care.* Swirling Leaf Press.

24 Leading Antiracism in Health and Care Systems

Dr Lorraine Gordon

At a time when the UK's National Health Service (NHS) is described as 'broken' by a Labour government, more than ever, health and care leaders need to build trust with their disenfranchised workforce and the communities they serve (Darzi, 2024). This chapter highlights health inequalities in mental healthcare with a focus on ethnicity and the impact on Black communities. It discusses the crucial role of leaders in creating a cultural shift towards antiracism (Jones, 2018) and suggests how organisations can add value through partnership working. The ideas discussed in this chapter may well apply to wider minoritised groups. This chapter considers national drivers highlighting the urgency for redress (NHS England, 2020), among political factors such as the Black Lives Matter movement (The Guardian, 2021). In a volatile, uncertain, complex and ambiguous socio-political and economic environment, it is near-impossible for health and care leaders to innovate and create beacons of antiracism without co-production with local communities.

Leaders Embodying and Imparting Values

Embodying an inspiring value-based vision, is a crucial aspect of leadership. Setting clear aims and ambitions that show the benefit to the end user and give employees a sense of purpose, is essential for any organisation or brand. When the National Health Service (NHS) was formed in 1948, it was the first time the UK had universal healthcare provision free at the point of use and delivered based on need rather than the

DOI: 10.4324/9781003492399-30

ability to pay (Darzi, 2024). As such, it was intended to be a great leveller (Gordon, 2020). The Windrush generation were people from Caribbean islands who were deemed British citizens prior to their journey to 'The Motherland', and were invited to the UK to help rebuild post-war Britain (Olusoga, 2019). They were an essential part of the NHS workforce from its inception and contributed to its early success. However, despite the principles on which the NHS was established, policies, practices, attitudes, and behaviours endemic in wider British society permeated its fabric and frustrated its ability to discharge its solemn duty (Institute of Health Equity, 2024). Inequality was present in the NHS both for the workforce it relied on to deliver care and treatment and the patients it was created to serve. Workers who had been qualified professionals in their country of origin faced hostility and discrimination and were given lower-status jobs (Vernon, 2023). All-the-while, members of the public, with nowhere else to turn when in need of statutory health provision, found themselves on the receiving end of, at best, a second-class service and, for many, overt racism (Institute of Health Equity, 2024). Trust in institutions funded by taxpayers that were unwilling and unable to meet their needs was understandably lacking (Gordon, 2021b).

Leadership Mandate to Tackle Health Inequalities

Alarmingly, health inequalities persist; this is exemplified by the design and delivery of care and treatment to racialised groups (Marmot, 2024). The Covid 19 pandemic brought to the fore the impact of decades of negligence, a consequence of inadequately addressing the diverse needs of the growing multicultural population (Olusoga, 2019). Racialised healthcare workers on the frontline and people from the global ethnic majority in the UK general public were disproportionately affected by Covid-19, with a higher morbidity and mortality rate (Gordon, 2020). With mental health being described as a 'Cinderella service' lacking parity of esteem with physical health provision (Eaton & Hunt, 2024), one might imagine the disparity for racialised groups would be felt even more acutely here. To reform the NHS so that it can deliver on its stated aims and principles, it is essential leaders focus on stakeholder analysis and engagement (Gordon, 2021c), to understand the population's strengths and needs using data and non-hierarchical relationships with Black-led organisations.

Health inequity is a wicked problem impacting, among others, mental health patients of African and Caribbean descent (Marmot, 2024).

Following the review of the Mental Health Act in 2018, where it was found that Black people are many times more likely to be detained than their white counterparts, NHS England (NHSE) outlined a national strategy to advance mental health equalities. Effective communication from leaders is critical to the process of change and the cultural shift that is required (NHSE, 2020). Publications like the one produced by NHSE set the strategic direction, which signals to managers and leaders the actions they must take and the key messages they need to deliver to ensure buy-in from the wider organisation and partners. It is imperative to critically review mental health service provision for people of African descent. Sadly, people from the global ethnic majority living in the UK, such as those with African, Caribbean, or Asian backgrounds, are disproportionately impacted by mental health problems, with poorer treatment outcomes than white British people (Institute of Health Equity, 2024). There is an opportunity for leaders within mental health organisations to challenge systems and processes that maintain inequity.

The Compelling Momentum of Social Action

In the year 2020, the resurgence of the Black Lives Matter movement was precipitated by the brutal, racist murder of George Floyd in the USA. The author was tasked with leading work on improvements for Black service users and carers in parts of South London, through the implementation of the Patient and Carer Race Equality Framework (PCREF), an approach to reimagine mental health services. The use of this framework provided rich insights into the power of partnership working with service users, carers and community members. The PCREF was mandated nationally to eradicate inequity in access, experience, and outcomes for racialised groups in England, in line with the Equality Act (2010).

The success of this approach is dependent on leaders involving key stakeholders. There is an opportunity to redesign mental health care with Black people through partnership working with key community groups and engagement with Black-led organisations. Olaseni Lewis was a 23-year-old Black man unlawfully killed whilst restrained by 11 police officers when he was an inpatient on a psychiatric ward in a South London hospital in 2010. Olaseni's untimely, tragic and wholly preventable death (Justice for Seni, 2020), highlighted the urgent problem of racial inequity in service provision (Gordon, 2021b). Leaders must build trust in relationships with Black communities through openness and transparency, admitting to past and ongoing failures to enable meaningful partnership working. This allows organisations to redesign mental health services and prevent the disproportionate use of restraint, seclusion, and detention for Black inpatients in mental health services. Co-production involves partnership working to develop and provide meaningful interventions whilst valuing the contribution each party adds. Zeilig et al. (2020), demonstrated the successful use of co-production with mental health patients. Yet, the evidence of leaders pursuing antiracism through co-production between mental health service providers and Black communities in South London remains insufficient.

Addressing Culture-Bound Needs

'Ubuntu', an African philosophy, is a concept that at once humanises self and the other, and can be interpreted as, 'I am because we are' (Nobles, 2015). Taking an African-centred approach, one places value on collectivism and the spiritual connection between humans and all that is within the universe. Great African thinkers hold that our interrelatedness is prized far above material wealth (Wissing et al., 2020). A study of African psychology elucidates an African-centred worldview from which to understand well-being, as opposed to a Eurocentric outlook. Meaning can be derived from adversity, leading to growth and a breakthrough in self-awareness (James-Myers, 1993).

This chapter is primarily concerned with adults of working age. However, taking a whole lifespan approach, perinatal women, like elderly Black people, present with numerous culture-bound needs (Gordon, 2021a). In the USA, Black women have been shown to have undiagnosed mental health problems, whilst at the same time, having trouble accessing mental health services. Woods-Giscombe et al. (2016), studied the spiritual needs of participants in their research and showed that cultural awareness within mental health services was vital to reduce inequity in service accessibility. Similarly, Black women who had experienced post-natal depression were shown to benefit from their religious faith and involvement at church (Keefea et al., 2016). In their study, the cohort under investigation were relieved of stress and had improvements in their family relationships because of their spiritual practices (Keefea et al., 2016). Elsewhere, it is argued that inclusive, supportive places of worship themselves can positively impact emotional well-being (Newbold, 2016). For Black people who migrated to Canada, it was established that accessing a place of worship was helpful both for spiritual and mental well-being (Newbold, 2016).

For older adults, the use of mental health services diminishes (Turner et al., 2019). This was shown to have a detrimental effect on those Black communities in the USA, in terms of their quality of life. Turner et al. (2019), argue that embracing a faith-facilitated engagement with mental health providers is enabling for service users. A potential barrier to engagement, however, was the medical model's lack of sensitivity to terms commonly used among those communities. Older Black people in their cohort tended to use more colloquial terms that services failed to pick up on (Akinyemi et al., 2018). Such research indicates that leaders need to attend to diversity in help-seeking behaviours. Appreciation of the role faith plays and knowledge of language that is meaningful to communities is important.

Efforts to aid the well-being of Black people must follow the wisdom of African ancestors (Nobles, 2015). Leaders in mental health services are encouraged to learn from an approach that aligns human consciousness with the Divine. Black people may have a deeper knowledge of themselves as spiritual, rather than solely being viewed by others through a Eurocentric lens, a lens which is limited by preoccupation with their physical characteristics. Returning to the notion that interrelatedness is pivotal to the well-being of Black people, using a co-production approach offers a method of engaging local Black communities in the prevention of severe mental illness, thus reducing inpatient admissions and the likelihood that they will be disproportionately detained, restrained, and secluded. Indeed, such an approach could provide a means of healing Black communities from racialised trauma. Antiracism is an active process that health and care leaders must embrace to disrupt the systemic and structural oppression of Black people through engagement with local communities in a culturally congruent manner.

Reducing inequity in mental health service provision for Black inpatients involves partnership working with stakeholders, where the solution to the problem depends on the perspective of the viewer. There are multiple solutions to a problem from the standpoint of various stakeholders. This diversity of opinion and insight is crucial for leaders to draw on to reimagine mental health services, so that services meet the needs of racialised groups. Therefore, an important recommendation of this chapter is for leaders to address culture-bound needs by engaging Black service users, carers and local Black communities to gain an understanding of the problems around inequity, particularly in terms of the disproportionate use of detention, restraint and seclusion against Black people, from their vantage point.

Strategic Leadership

Historically, strategic leaders concerned themselves with forecasting. However, in contemporary strategy, there is recognition that it is not possible to predict the future; rather, to imagine possible futures whilst firmly in the present. Leaders need to reach beyond existing demands and focus on Black service users as a new market for the delivery of mental health services in innovative ways. Blue ocean strategy involves persistently striving for value innovation (Kim & Marborgne, 2015), in an agile, iterative way, as successful companies like Apple or IBM have demonstrated.

Scaling up a business offer to reach a new market, in this case, differentiating to meet the needs of Black communities, necessitates leaders propelling an organisation in a new direction of growth (Kim & Marborgne, 2015). However, there is a risk that business model expansion leads to increasing complexity within an organisation. Anticipating the risk makes it possible to generate solutions, such as enhancing communication, to keep colleagues and others engaged with the strategy. To achieve the objectives inherent within the strategy, an organisation's systems and processes must be aligned.

Whilst plans may be robust, it is not possible to predict every event. Stakeholders' competing interests could obstruct attempts to agree and implement an innovative strategy designed to meet the needs of Black people. There may be key people within or outside of an organisation whose interests lead them to reject the ideas of differentiation or diversification. There may well be stakeholders who benefit from the status quo where the needs of racialised communities remain unmet. Therefore, leaders introducing change into systems may present a challenge, which for some, will be akin to a grieving process (Burns, 2020). Hence, negotiation and an agile process of refinement are crucial elements that may result in an emergent strategy.

Systematic monitoring of performance alerts managers to any deviation from the strategy and the risk of a deficit in delivery on embedding antiracism. To that end, monitoring the implementation of a strategy to reduce health inequalities through controls such as key performance indicators is an important motivating factor for the workforce. This is in addition to inspiring, emerging transformational narratives, enabling leaders to engage hearts and minds. A well-structured mission statement enables communication up and down reporting lines and mobilises people in one direction. Often, the pervasive position or 'reality', with regard to inclusion, is that some people have a privileged vantage point with opportunities afforded to them. This is not dissimilar to the white privilege (Gordon, 2021d) service users with white skin are afforded. However, Black service users find themselves disadvantaged, and starting from a position akin to being 'buried in the ground' in comparison to their white counterparts, they cannot engage on an equal footing in a meaningful way when the system and structures are rigged against them. The notion of equality, where individuals are given the same opportunities, neglects to accommodate the disadvantage inherent in systems and processes that use a given norm from which to treat everyone else in the same colour-blind way. 'Equity', however, is where everyone has the resources they need to participate in a meaningful way; no one is at a disadvantage (Gordon, 2021b). This is an enabling, inclusive environment where no one group is privileged over the other and every perspective has value. Furthermore, the barriers to inclusion and participation are removed for everyone, and all can experience a sense of liberation and an opportunity to actively participate in each activity.

Executive leadership teams where organisations receive public funds to provide mental health services must adopt a position of cultural humility (Mosher et al. 2017), so they can listen to and learn from the contribution of Black service users, carers and local communities. Lacking diversity in the boardroom, as found in the leadership of many publicly funded mental health providers, prevents creative thinking and reduces the relevance and effectiveness of the service, harming its reputation.

There is an opportunity for health and care leaders to build trust with their global majority workforce and the diverse communities they serve (Darzi, 2024). There are a myriad of options available for leaders providing mental health services that would add value for Black communities and move towards antiracism. Many of the considerations for leaders stated below may well apply to wider minoritised groups:

- Tailor business models towards reaching a new market where the needs of the growing multicultural population are addressed (Kim & Marborgne, 2015)

- Engage in partnership working with faith groups and other Black-led organisations supporting Black communities to promote well-being within those groups.
- Create an enabling, inclusive environment where no one group is privileged over the others and previously under-represented perspectives are valued.
- Remove barriers for Black people so they experience a sense of liberation and have opportunities to actively participate
- The executive leadership teams in mental health systems should adopt a position of cultural humility, listening to and learning from the contribution of Black service users, carers and local communities

Ideas in Brief

There is inequity by ethnicity in the provision of mental health services

The inequity disproportionately impacts Black people amounting to race discrimination which is illegal and morally unacceptable

Leaders have an imperative to create a cultural shift towards antiracism

Leadership in antiracism involves attention to structural inequalities, embodying an inspiring value-based partnership vision, cultural humility and respect for diverse cultural and faith-based practices

References

Akinyemi, E., Watins, D.C., Kavanagh, J., Johnson-Lawrence, V., Lynn, S., & Kales, H. C. (2018). A qualitative comparison of DSM depression criteria to language used by older church-going African-Americans. *Aging and Mental Health, 22*(9), 1149–1155. https://doi.org/10.1080/13607863.2017.1337717

Burns, L. (2020). *Elisabeth Kubler-Ross: The rise and fall of the five stages of grief.* Available at: https://www.bbc.co.uk/news/stories-53267505

Darzi, A. (2024). Independent Investigation of the National Health Service in England. [Online] Available at: https://www.gov.uk/government/publications/indepedent-investigation-of-the-NHS-in-england [Accessed 1 12 2024]

Eaton, E., & Hunt, A. (2024). Does willingness to pay differ for mental and physical health? *Value in Health, 27*(10), 1417–1425. [Online] Available at: https://www.sciencedirect.com/science/article/pii/S1098301524027487

Equality Act. (2010). Available at: https://www.legislation.gov.uk/ukpga/2010/15/part/7/crossheading/special-provision-for-political-parties

Gordon, L. (2020). Everyone should feel uncomfortable about the number of BAME staff dying from Covid. Health Service Journal, May. [Online] Available at: https://www.hsj.co.uk/workforce/everyone-should-feel-uncomfortable-about-the-number-of-bame-staff-dying-from-covid/7027696.article#commentsJump [Accessed 1 12 2024]

Gordon, L. (2021a). *Is co-production a useful way to engage communities of African descent in African-centred wellness to prevent severe mental health problems?* Pearson College Study.

Gordon, L. (2021b). *The Maudsley: A platform empowering black and mixed black communities to prevent severe mental illness*. Pearson College Study.

Gordon, L. (2021c). *Purposeful leadership and management: Black lives matter.* Pearson College Study.

Gordon, L. (2021d). *Business case: Using technology to prevent severe mental illness in black communities*. Kent University Study.

Institute of Health Equity. (2024). *Structural racism, ethnicity and health inequalties in London*. [Online] Available at: https://www.instituteofhealthequity.org/resources-reports/structural-racism-ethnicity-and-health-inequalities

James-Myers, L. (1993). *Understanding an afrocentric world view: Introduction to Optimal Psychology.* Kendall/Hunt Publishing.

Jones, C. P. (2018). Toward the science and practice of anti-racism: Launching a national campaign against racism. *Ethnicity & Disease, 28*(1), 231–234. https://doi.org/10.18865/ed.28.S1.231

Justice for Seni. (2020). *The Olaseni Lewis campaign for justice and change.* Available at: https://www.justiceforseni.com/#:~:text=Justice%20for%20Seni%20%E2%80%93%20The%20Olaseni%20Lewis%20Campaign,voluntary%20patient%20at%20the%20Bethlem%20Royal%20Hospital%2C%20Croydon

Keefea, R. H., Brownstein-Evans, C., & Polmanteer, a. R. R. (2016). "I find peace there": How faith, church, and spirituality help mothers of colour cope with postpartum depression. *Mental Health, Religion and Culture, 19*(7), 722–733.

Kim, W. C., & Marborgne, R. (2015). *Blue ocean strategy: How to create uncontested market space and make the competition irrelevant*. Harvard Business School publishing.

Marmot, M. & Allen, J. (2024). A programme for greater health equity for the next UK Government. The Lancet, 403(10445), pp. 2675-2677.

Mosher, D. K., Hook, J. N., Captari, L. E., Davis, D. E., DeBlaere, C., & Owen, J. (2017). Cultural humility: A therapeutic framework for engaging diverse clients. *Practice Innovations, 2*(4), 221–233. https://doi.org/10.1037/pri0000055

Newbold, B. A. a. B. K. (2016). Religion/spirituality, therapeutic landscape and immigrant mental well-being amongst African immigrants to Canada *Mental Health, Religion and Culture, 19*(7), 674–685.

NHS England. (2020). *Advancing mental health equalities strategy.* NHS England. [Online] Available at: https://www.england.nhs.uk/wp-content/uploads/2020/10/00159-advancing-mental-health-equalities-strategy.pdf

Nobles, W. W. (2015). From black psychology to Sakhu Djaer: Implications for the further development of a pan African black psychology. *Journal of Black Psychology,* 41 , 1–16.

Olusoga, D. (2019). *Windrush: Archived documents show the long betrayal.* Observer special report: Windrush scandal. [Online] Available at: https://www.theguardian.com/uk-news/2019/jun/16/windrush-scandal-the-long-betrayal-archived-documents-david-olusoga

The Guardian. (2021). *Protesters in London mark anniversary of George Floyd death.* [Online] Available at: https://www.theguardian.com/world/2021/may/22/anti-racism-protesters-gather-in-london

Turner, N., Hastings, J. F., & Neighbors, H. W. (2019). Mental health care treatment seeking among African Americans and Caribbean blacks: What is the role of religiosity/spirituality? *Aging and Mental Health, 23*(7), 905–911.

Vernon, P. (2023). What does Windrush 75 mean for the NHS? *Race and Health Observatory.* [Online] Available at: https://www.nhsrho.org/news/what-does-windrush-75-mean-for-the-nhs/

Wissing, M. P., Wilson Fadiji, A., Schutte, L., Chigeza, S., Schutte, W. D., & Temane, Q. M. (2020). Motivations for relationships as sources of meaning: Ghanaian and South African experiences. *Frontiers in Psychology, 11.* Article 2019. https://doi.org/10.3389/fpsyg.2020.02019

Woods-Giscombe, C., Robinson, M. N., Carthon, D., Devane-Johnson, S., & Corbie-Smith, G. (2016). Superwoman schema, stigma, spirituality, and culturally sensitive providers: Factors influencing African American women's use of mental health services. *Research, Education and Policy, 9*(1), 1124–1144.

Zeilig, H., Gee, B., Teague, B., Wilson, J., & Hackman, C. (2020). Foregrounding the perspectives of mental health service users during the covid-19 pandemic. *Mental Health and Social Inclusion, 24*(3), 131–133.

PART SIX

THE TAO OF LEADERHOOD IN PRECARIOUS TIMES

TOWARDS FUTURE HORIZONS

25 A Relational Model of Leadership and Its Risks

Dr Anton Obholzer

It seems odd that a book on rethinking leadership in the present day, as applied in the Clinical, Counselling and Health Psychology field, should include a chapter on the risk to those who hold or aspire to hold a leadership role. Given the book's focus on managing complexity and leading change to enable thriving workplaces, it is essential to include a section on the risks inherent in the task of leadership.

There are various sources of pressure and anxieties that leaders face and manage. Leadership often involves multiple tasks such as making decisions, containing and managing uncertainty and work-related anxieties; venturing into uncharted territories; and being accountable for initiating actions and outcomes that have an impact on the people and organisations being led. There are risks inherent in taking up such tasks. Leaders also have personal anxieties arising from their inner and outer world realities. Working in a pressured complex environment makes leaders vulnerable to isolation, untested assumptions, disconnect with the system realities, and ruptures in engagement.

One of the key tasks of leadership is to have an inward and outward focus and remain engaged with the primary task as embedded in their organisational role. The task may shift over time and is often faced with various pressures, such as resources and competing expectations from the service members and stakeholders. The risk of being derailed from performing the task cannot be underestimated. The focus can be diverted by external demands activating internal anxieties such as being admired, loved, feared, hated, and dismissed, requiring an ongoing balancing act to get back to the task in role.

DOI: 10.4324/9781003492399-32

Nowadays, both locally and globally, the pressure is not only on leadership, however that is defined, but increasingly on so-called efficiency and financial probity. As a result, the essential Human Relations component of the work is under constant threat of being replaced by electronic and mechanical means, including the use of AI. Human contact is cut short or replaced by medication or by using other techniques and technologies. The strain of survival anxiety and competition amongst individuals and organisations is on the increase as relentless financial pressures often give rise to survival strategies and rapid solution-seeking actions such as restructuring, financial re-modelling, and redundancy cycles. The chapter focuses on the impact of these various external and internal pressures on leaders' ways of thinking and relating to their environment.

Humility, Inquiring Mind and Risk Awareness in Leadership

One of the impacts is the adoption of a form of leadership that is insensitive and destructive to human individuality, creativity, and health, both in its physical and mental expression. The resultant leadership, whether in the inner world of the leader's orbit or at any of the other levels of the leadership pyramid—whether in one's inner world, in the world of personal relationships, with partners or children, or in one's professional identity—where 'certainty of role and perspective' becomes a form of intellectual imprisonment. In a wider sense, in the role of leaders, one might find oneself as the rigid representative of a particular sectarian professional approach, be it psychoanalytical, behavioural, or in the mode of any of the other 'professional religions'. These cripple the capacity for appropriate professional flexibility and a wider perception of events. The debate is thus blunted and leads to dull conformity, which can, it is true, be quite welcomed at times by leadership.

As a result, the leader is at risk of 'turning a blind eye' either in their inner or personal family role or else in work settings—resulting in disengagement with others holding different perspectives. It is as if there is only one approved way of seeing things. Everything else is seen as irrelevant, whereas in fact, it might very well be a positive contribution to the debate and resultant decision. The risk for those lower down the pecking order is to conform, thus depriving the system of growth or innovation. The leadership might welcome the pseudo-calmness, but the risk is that any questioning is seen as sabotage, and eventually the entire management leadership system collapses. Without an awareness of these processes, it becomes more likely that the new regime will repeat the mistakes of the past.

Humility, risk awareness and attention to one's responses to anxieties are the cornerstones of success and need to be monitored regularly from an independent consultancy resource. Even then, it must be acknowledged that leadership in the mental health and social systems is among the most demanding roles in the NHS and society. Attention to the impact of pressures on one's state of mind and behaviour is important to mitigate such risks for meaningful, fulfilling and effective leadership. The interplay of the group and internal processes such as risk perceptions, self-doubt, fear of failure, resistance to new ideas and conflicts, and disavowal of rivalry and competition are some of the important considerations.

The leader's state of mind needs to be seen as the weather vane of the conscious and unconscious 'psychic winds' that frequent the institution.

The examples of the leader succumbing to one of the risks of expecting conformity of diagnosis are as follows.

A female member of staff engaged in a sexual act with an inmate in a prison. The usual approach would be to see the event as the result of the psychopathology of the staff member and that the incident needs to be dealt with through disciplinary action. That might very well be necessary, but it completely misses the point for the leadership to view the incident solely as an individual matter rather than also as a symptom of a subterranean unconscious dynamic in the organisation. The underlying dynamic is one of sexuality and its manifestations in the organisation and the acting out of perversion by all concerned, staff and prisoners. If this perspective is not understood and addressed, it will remain under the carpet and be a constant blight and handicap, sabotaging the reparative and positive ambitions and attempts of the staff and organisation.

Another example would be of a leader becoming personally and institutionally authoritative-authoritarian, supposedly in the service of growth and role development. The question needs to be asked: what is the reason for this emotional shift? The answer lies in the fact that the existing leadership approach has failed and has then been tilted into a management direction in an attempt to address the problem of staff resistance. If not addressed, it does act as a brake on the observation, thought and intervention and leads to the altered state of mind of the leader's frustration and his plans failing. If noted by the leader and his entourage, this needs to be seen as an institutional warning sign rather than as a matter of individual diagnosis.

Any leadership dynamic, whether individual or organisation, must therefore always make room for other ways of seeing and diagnosing the way ahead, apart from the agreed ones. The core question asked in all cases is: *what else might be going on that we have missed, and that needs addressing to remove the inevitable roadblock?*

The risks and pressures in leadership roles are inevitable and cannot be overlooked. Leaders need to stay alert and manage such risks and pressures thoughtfully. Tensions in taking up the task of management and the authority to hold others accountable are inescapable. They can put the relational dimension under strain, raising conflict with the containing function of the leadership role. The hardest challenge for a leader is figuring out and doing the right thing regardless of the personal or professional negative impact on them.

Risk aversion is not the solution—instead, thoughtful engagement is. This requires investment in thinking/consultative spaces for ongoing learning and setting up support systems for self and others to foster work-life balance and thriving workplaces.

Ideas in Brief

Following are the key points from my experience of leadership.

- Risk and emotional labour are inherent in the task of leadership.
- Attention to institutional, work-based, and personal anxieties arising from one's inner and outer world realities is an important leadership task.
- Internal and external pressures, alongside covert and overt organisational dynamics, can derail leaders from their primary task and role-taking.
- Watch out for the pull to turn a blind eye and seek rapid understanding and solutions. Consider what else might be going on that has been missed, and needs addressing.
- Inquiry into the leader's state of mind can provide useful insights into the conscious and unconscious organisational dynamics impacting the task and workplace well-being.
- Leaders need to stay alert to the importance of managing one's personal and organisational life.
- Not everyone sees the world in the same way—beware of one's assumptions and prejudices.

- Engage with other perspectives to unstick blockages and foster creativity and innovation.
- Humility, an inquiring mind, risk awareness, thoughtful undertaking of authority, attention to internal and external sources of anxiety, and awareness of personal and collective biases are important cornerstones of success. They need to be observed and monitored regularly. An independent consultancy resource and the cultivation of reflective spaces can help.
- Invest in sources of support and reflection to foresee and manage pressures and risks impacting the uptake of effective leadership and to enhance fulfilment at work.

References

Beggan, J. K., Allison, S. T., & Goethals, G. R. (2023). *The hazards of great leadership: How and why leaders harm those they lead*. Lexington Books.

Heifetz, R. A., & Linsky, M. (2002). *Leadership on the line: Staying alive through the dangers of leading*. Harvard Business School Press.

Obholzer, A. (2022). *Workplace intelligence: Unconscious forces and how to manage them*. Routledge.

Simpson, P., French, R., & Harvey, C. (2002). Leadership and negative capability. *Human Relations, 55*(10), 1209–1226. https://doi.org/10.1177/001872670205501002

26 Centring Leadership around the Communities We Serve

Truth, Hearing and Ceding Power

Joanne Hemmingfield

Beyond Myself to All of Us

Work involves looking beyond ourselves: Psychological professionals serve everyone in the whole of the community.

The whole community is everyone of all ages, from the very oldest to the very youngest. All should be included, from the most outspoken to those who have been oppressed so much that, to them, communication seems pointless. "Everyone" includes those with the greatest sense of entitlement to those who feel like they don't count. The whole community comprises those whose mother tongue is the same as mine and those with whom we don't share a spoken language. All are served, irrespective of possession of a smartphone, having an internet connection at home, or being able to fill in an "easy online form".

However, services may not have a fuller representation of the community. Similarly, psychological services do not represent the whole community. Inevitably, care for young people will be provided by someone who is older, and care for our elders is likely to be given by someone who has not matured to that extent. How can the connection be maintained with post-pandemic youth culture and with our elders and beyond? Co-production with these communities, using the tools of cultural humility, can help us.

In the UK, working for the National Health Service (NHS) confers privilege. Many NHS psychological services are dominated by white,

DOI: 10.4324/9781003492399-33

able-bodied women. They almost inevitably communicate verbally rather than non-verbally and are confident and articulate, often with a middle-class accent. Communication is littered with acronyms, technical terms, and jargon. Visible differences in skin tone are occasionally seen, and visible disability is even less frequent. There is pressure to keep invisible differences hidden. It is all about what we see on the surface.

Appearances are overly valued in our increasingly materialistic world. The "beauty" industry and plastic surgery are massive industries. It is in these industries' interests for us to equate success and happiness with spending money on "improving" our appearance. To understand the experiences of our clients, we must be people who go beyond the surface, beyond skin-deep, to see more of the whole person, their history, what matters most to them, and not just what is wrong but what is strong. To build services that work for the whole community, with a focus on those underserved, we have to humbly and seriously embark on a journey of understanding.

It is concerning that in the UK, where I live, the individual and independence have become idealised. Have we thrown out the baby with the bathwater, dismissing the importance of connection, a sense of identity from where we have come from and who we are?

Connection and relationships are forfeited at our peril. It is in conversations together that we can keep one another safe from poor choices and extreme behaviour. Within relationships, we can encourage one another to be brave and take risks. In trusting, safe, open systems, there is the potential for health and well-being. We can co-create our understanding of what is holding us back and co-create the solutions. The cultural and intergenerational fractures run deep, but we can nurture seeds of love and respect to start to re-establish and restore wholeness.

Fresh Green Shoots in the Face of Impossibility: Beyond Cultural Competence to the Hopefulness of Cultural Humility

With such a challenge ahead, no one person can have the understanding to shape services appropriate to the whole community. What are leaders to do? Tervalon and Murray-Garcia (1998) have shared with us helpful wisdom about how to learn more about one another with their model of Cultural Humility. Firstly, they invite us to view culture beyond social identities, which are little more than judging by appearances.

Most people belong to many different groups and communities, and their actual sense of who they are as a person may or may not relate to obvious things we might notice "at first sight". We are more than the amount of melanin in our skin, our hairstyle, our clothes, and whether our name is familiar or not to your ear. Humans are complicated and dynamic, as are the groups to which they belong to.

The culturally humble learn to engage with their shifting privilege from situation to situation, being aware of dominant voices and those less heard. Working together, we can share the tasks of identifying problems and co-creating solutions with the widest community possible. Aspiring towards coproduction whilst embracing cultural humility is the way forward.

Coproduction and the Ladder of Participation

Differences in power can be understood through the ladder of participation (Arnstein, 1969) (Figure 26.1). The ladder of participation is a helpful tool to understand how we might make decisions together.

Arnstein's Ladder of Participation

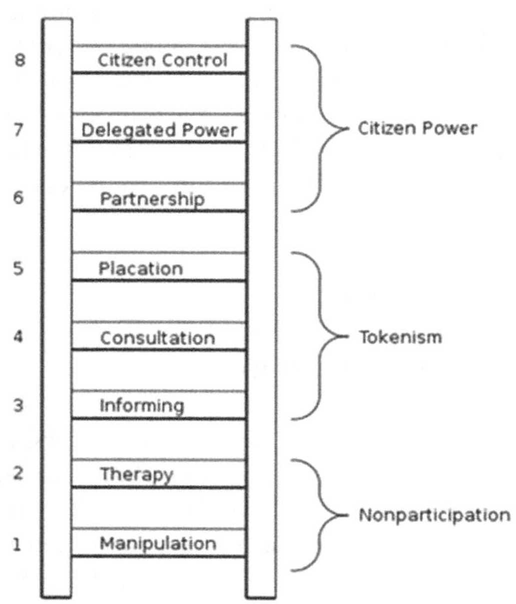

Figure 26.1 Ladder of participation (Arnstein, 1969).

Coproduction is, in essence, groups of people working equally together. Usually, one of the groups is more powerful than the other, e.g. people who work for a service provider. The second group is less powerful, for example, people who use the services of the service provider.

In cultural humility, the conversation began around ethnicity, whereas my experience of coproduction has primarily been with people who have been described as having mental health issues. These groups are not separate and distinct but instead are made up of people with different patterns of strengths, vulnerabilities, and allegiances. To generalise, however, in both cultural humility and coproduction, there are differences in power between two parties. In coproduction, there may be more of a focus on a task or a purpose, e.g. service redesign. The question asked is to what extent each group contributes to deciding why we are working together, any discussions that take place, and any decisions that are made; that is, the purpose, the process, and the impact? Alternatively, how might we judge an afternoon's workshop or an entire project?

It is essential that the least powerful group assess the level of participation. When the most powerful of the groups "mark their own homework", being sensitive to the efforts they themselves will have made, they are usually overly generous to themselves. It is when the least powerful group has the opportunity to evaluate coproduction anonymously that the most telling and relevant scores and feedback emerge.

Coproduction is an opportunity to interrogate the reasons why things are the way they are, to examine assumptions, and to consider flexible ways of working based on person-centred or community-centred approaches. Like in cultural humility, it is about taking the perspective of curiosity that "I don't know everything." It is about groups that have a different culture; in my case, this has often been people like me who have used mental health services. Being part of this group and having worked alongside people with lived experience of using mental health services, I hope that I can not just listen but also hear and understand what matters most.

When working with the Division of Clinical Psychology in the British Psychological Society in the UK, for 15 years I had the privileged position of seeing what was important to (some) psychologists. Often, people who use the services of psychologists and those providing services wanted the same thing; often, but not always. Now, working for a Health and Social Care NHS Trust in the UK, I can gain insight into some of the opportunities and barriers to the change that people who use services want.

The task can start to feel impossibly large. How do we even keep in mind the widest community? The challenge is enormous – partly because this challenge has been neglected. We can, however, start where we are. It is within diverse views and life experiences that we can co-create understanding and solutions. All parties need to be welcomed at the decision-making table. Those who have been marginalised and historically excluded will initially question if they are indeed welcome. Is the process tokenistic or meaningful?

Professional people are expected to be able to work in any place. NHS Trusts have their own premises, may hire out conference venues and hotel rooms for larger meetings. People who use our services tell us that they feel very uncomfortable in these venues. We must go to community venues – we must go to them. Meeting in a location that someone else is familiar with is essential. What is important to me will not be important to you. What I take for granted may be an issue for someone else. As we respect others' preferences, we let go of our own power. Might I feel uncomfortable to start with in an unfamiliar place? Possibly. Might it mean travelling to a part of the city that I am unfamiliar with? Yes. May I wonder about how to get there – sure. Is it worth it – absolutely! What is more, when meeting in community venues, my experience is that something almost magical starts to happen – the welcome and feeling of mutual respect and appreciation start to rebuild trust.

Addressing Power Imbalances by Centralising the Marginalised

An important role of leadership is to seek out the experiences of the marginalised and centralise them.

Case Study 1: In the Division of Clinical Psychology, Expert by Experience (people who have used services) annual events, there was a progression of centralising the marginalised over time. The initial launch event in London was well received. Feedback included that the people with lived experience speaking from the front and in the audience were adults who had had mental health challenges. The clinical psychologists who worked with children and those who worked with older people wanted to know how their clients were to be represented. This was a fair question that we committed to addressing. To centralise these groups who had been marginalised, we worked alongside these two groups of psychologists to connect with their clients. Between us, we designed the next event focused on a lifespan approach. We started the two-day event with older people sharing a human rights approach to living well with dementia. As the event progressed down the lifespan, someone of working age performed a one-man show about how alienating, dehumanising, and disempowering.

The feedback from this event was very positive, but we were asked, what about the experiences people described as having intellectual disabilities? So at the next event, we centralised this group but held on to a lifespan approach.

Case Study two: In Sheffield Health and Social Care NHS Foundation Trust, we have run workshops for people who have Complex Emotional Needs, individuals who may have been diagnosed with a personality disorder. The term "personality disorder" is widely rejected by people with lived experience as an attack on their identity. In a society that is often unhelpfully cold, clinical, and even brutal in the way we approach one another, the sensitivity that some of the people in the group experience could represent something that we all could learn from.

We wanted everyone to be clear about what sort of help is available, who offers what and what is important to service users, including that respectful words are used to describe their experiences. Our hope is that this will result in some useful, easy-to-understand information from the perspective of those who have used our services.

During a workshop, in the break, those of us facilitating were approached by one of the groups who said that she had her hand up for some time but had not been noticed. Those who were more confident were holding the floor. We had allowed the conversation amongst the group to become more of a series of monologues. The facilitators were a little nervous about not "closing down" the more confident. Over the remainder of that session and subsequent sessions, we used a range of techniques to rebalance the group and centralise those who had felt marginalised by their level of confidence at that time in that setting.

Making informed choices for ourselves is key. As we make our own decisions and consider the impact of these, we can rebuild our own autonomy and pave the way for recovery.

All groups have the power to help and heal or to harm. It is beholden on all of us to lead the groups that we are part of in a way that is inclusive. There must be a place for anyone and everyone who wants to be a part of that group, whether that be our family, a friendship group, work colleagues, scouts or a faith group. All communities should have safe spaces to discuss and debate their values. Everyone should be able to have a voice and be heard.

Service providers, for example, UK NHS Trusts, come from a history of hierarchy and top-down decision-making. Much of the language sounds similar to military language. The "command and control" model that is useful in emergencies and surgery is not as useful in mental health. There are mental health "officers." Decisions made by NHS England are described as coming from "on high," almost as if they came from an angelic host. Decision-making is traditionally top-down. Senior leaders do not always explain the thinking or reasoning behind decisions. There is sometimes a sense of a patriarchal approach. Sometimes, things seem to be as they are "because I say so."

Have those who have opened the doors got the skills to hear?

Steven Covey (1989) talks about listening to hear. Counsellors are skilled in active listening and can support colleagues in developing this skill. To hear, we must put to one side any thought of what we might want to say next and just connect with another perspective in a non-judgemental and curious way. Are psychologists prepared to do this outside the therapy room, or are they tempted to think that leadership is a separate and distinct task? One of the most important contributions psychologists could make might be to train colleagues in communication skills, particularly listening.

What if what people are saying to us is hard to hear? My role is coproduction in an acute mental health organisation. People who deliver the service are collaborating with people who use the services. At the beginning of the relationship, experts by experience, people who have been service users, will challenge the process. They say, "What is the point of working with you on this? This organisation has been asking these same questions for decades and nothing changes." This question is confronting and can be hard to hear for some colleagues. It can be taken personally. The manager might think, "I'm a good person, I'm well intentioned, I work hard, I do a good job, my colleagues are all busy working hard – how can this person imply that we are stuck in something that is not ideal?" Our job is to demonstrate that we can hear confronting views. We can learn to look like we are listening, but what does it take to really hear? What does it take to change the system based on what we have heard?

How do leaders help us reach beyond being personally offended by challenging views and connect with the voice of difference? It is essential that we are able to hear challenges from our citizens, and how to do this from the widest community, not just those who feel most comfortable speaking up. There is a strong history of healthcare workers whistle-blowing and raising issues. The "Hello, my name is" campaign was initiated by a nurse who found herself receiving healthcare from people who did not even bother to introduce themselves. The name badges that many of us wear now were designed to remind us to connect as fellow humans and retain the warmth of a personal introduction.

The issues at Mid-Staffordshire Hospital, which led to the Francis Report, were initially raised by a nurse (Francis, 2013). When we look at the Thirwell Inquiry report (2025), when a nurse continued to murder babies – even the medics were not listened to by the managers. These cases illustrate just how hard it can be for systems to hear and respond appropriately, to lay to one side personal reputations and maintain the image of the organisation.

There are senior managers making decisions who may have very little understanding of clinical issues. Even the most sensitive clinicians, although attuned to the issues are often so used to speaking in NHS-speak that they may be unable to communicate in a helpful way with members of the public.

How do we, when we speak with the public, resist the temptation to teach them our language of service structure, pathways, diagnoses, treatments, interventions, medications, etc.? How can we find a way to have a conversation in laypeople's terms? Are we prepared to carefully unlearn speaking in therapy-speak, using terms like "thoughts" instead of "cognitions"? Can we describe to anyone, a 14-year-old or to our grandma, what the issues are?

Why Is It So Easy to Miss the Truth?

Neglecting different perspectives occurs when we rush for efficiency, driven by willful blindness (Heffernan, 2012). In reality, even working with colleagues can be challenging. The NHS is siloed in parts, and the competitive business model of the 1980s has obscured our shared purpose. A key aspect of the NHS Five Year Forward View (2014) was the emphasis that we're responsible not just for those who meet service criteria but for the health of the entire community. We must ensure access to services for all, not just those with privileged connections. How often have we heard of colleagues using their power to help those they know navigate services? What about those without such connections? This cannot continue, especially when systems are strained and too focused on therapy. New, innovative approaches that empower people and share knowledge should be celebrated. Cultural humility and co-production can help redefine problems and co-create solutions.

Sometimes, when some people's voices are not heard, disaster can continue unchecked. Margaret Heffernan (2012), describes a process of "Willful Blindness." In a small town in Northwest America, a gas meter reader noticed that as they went from one person's house to another, an alarming number of people had a particular form of cancer. The main source of income in the area was mining a chemical, vermiculite. This vermiculite, a particularly toxic form of asbestos, was everywhere in the town, including the children's school playground. The facts were overwhelming, but it took a long time for the community to be prepared to see what was staring them in the face.

Some realities are so hard that they are practically impossible to face. We cannot allow this to be the case in psychological services and wider health and social care. The systems are often interconnected and play a part in quality of life. As leaders, we need to be able to connect with the widest community of citizens and journey together on a shared path of transformation across systems.

As well as supporting colleagues in developing these approaches, it is important to keep checking the order that one's own house is in. For instance, let's not be complacent about the therapy offer. Although those most skilled in this usually find it is still hard to build therapeutic relationships of trust and honesty, it is easy to lean into our existing assumptions when we judge another. Therapy can be extremely helpful and is often described as lifesaving. Once trained, what happens in the room, though, is too often shrouded in mystery. We put a high level of trust in what happens behind closed doors, rightly protecting the client's confidentiality; however, is this at the risk of ensuring the integrity of the experience? Are there things that might happen in the therapy room that the therapist should have taken to supervision but was too afraid to do so? It's so important to retain a healthy level of scepticism about the helpfulness of all approaches to mental distress and to support all our service users in being able to ask questions about their care.

A Golden Age of Psychology?

Psychological professionals in health care settings are often placed in positions of authority. They are looked up to by the public. Increasingly, citizens are looking to them even more than to medics or priests of the past. People tend to think that if you have wisdom in one area, you have wisdom in all areas. This is a dangerous temptation. We should be careful to temper what we say depending on the level of expertise that we have and always be prepared to say when we don't know. This is the essence of helpful humility in leadership.

Simply Human or Super-Human – What Sort of Leaders Do We Want?

A strong leader is often framed as someone who is prepared to make tough decisions. There are times of crisis when difficult decisions may need to be made quickly. However, this cannot be the only approach. It is possible to be aware of our vulnerabilities, know that "we do not know" and continually be prepared to grow and change. Great leaders are not right all the time. The ancient Greeks told tragic stories of the fall of great kings. Shakespeare took up this theme in his tragedies. These leaders were blind to their fatal flaws and were tempted by pride or "hubris". People who are put on pedestals often come crashing down – we are not meant to be idolised. We are all human. I vote for leadership that is simply human. It is understanding our humanity and how little we might know that brings us to learning from one another and rejecting the false sense of being superhuman. Be courageous and humble as you walk your journey of leadership – I, for one, wish you well.

Ideas in Brief

- Leaders should collaborate with communities using co-production and cultural humility.
- Embrace humanity and avoid "superhuman" expectations.
- Acknowledge and take responsibility for mistakes.
- Drive genuine learning and change, not tokenism.

References

Arnstein, S. R. (1969). A ladder of citizen participation. *Journal of the American Institute of Planners, 35*(4), 216–224. https://doi.org/10.1080/01944366908977225

Covey, S. R. (1989). *The seven habits of highly effective people: Restoring the character ethic*. Simon & Schuster.

Francis, R. (2013). *Report of the Mid Staffordshire NHS Foundation Trust public inquiry: Executive summary*. The Stationery Office. Retrieved on April 20,

2025, from https://www.gov.uk/government/publications/report-of-the-mid-staffordshire-nhs-foundation-trust-public-inquiry

Granger, K. (n.d.). *Hello my name is... A campaign for more compassionate care.* Retrieved on April 20, 2025, from https://www.hellomynameis.org.uk/

Heffernan, M. (2012). *Wilful blindness: Why we ignore the obvious—at our peril.* Simon & Schuster.

NHS England. (2014). *Five year forward view.* Retrieved on April 20, 2025, from https://www.england.nhs.uk/publication/nhs-five-year-forward-view/

Tervalon, M., & Murray-García, J. (1998). Cultural humility versus cultural competence: A critical distinction in defining physician training outcomes in multicultural education. *Journal of Health Care for the Poor and Underserved,* 9(2), 117–125. https://doi.org/10.1353/hpu.2010.0233

Thirwell Inquiry. (2025). *[Title pending].* [Details to be confirmed upon publication].

27

Leadership for an Anxious Future

Leading in a Technological Age

Stephen Murgatroyd

Introduction

In this chapter, the nature of change leadership, especially as it relates to technology driven innovation and change, will be explored and some features of evidence-informed post-pandemic change leadership in health systems will be examined. The key assumption is that change and uncertainty about "what's next" are constant and that leadership needs to be focused on both courage and anticipation. The guiding epigram for what follows is: "all problems are treasures from which we can improve."

The reason technology is a focus of this chapter is twofold. The first is that many health policy makers and systems funders see various technologies – AI-enabled therapies, robotic surgery, artificial intelligence used for diagnostics and treatment, 3-D printing of needed medical equipment, gene editing, new drug discovery systems using quantum computing, complex social media and their potential for reputation damage – as critical features of the futures landscape for health systems and patient care. In part, they are seen to offer greater efficiency and effectiveness, as technology is beginning to show superior performance to humans for specific tasks (Mollick, 2024), but also funders see technology as a strategy to contain cost growth.

The second is a simple observation: most technology change and transformation projects in health and other organisations fail. Studies by Deist et al. (2022), Krantz & Trainor (2019) and many others suggest that between 65% and 80% of all such change efforts in organisations

DOI: 10.4324/9781003492399-34

fail to deliver the expected results and sustained value over time. A key issue in the analysis of these failures is the importance of the culture of the organisation and the failure of leadership to engage at both the conscious and unconscious levels with the concerns and anxieties colleagues have about change in general, and technological change in particular (Mills & Murgatroyd, 1991). Peter Drucker is reported to have said "culture eats strategy for breakfast and transformation for lunch" (Guley & Reznik, 2019).

The speed of technological change is accelerating, as anyone following developments in AI and related technologies will attest. Given the speed at which the "next big thing" could arrive, understanding leadership as anticipation involving constant change management is an essential skill set for the contemporary leader.

The Shape of the Future

The discipline of anticipatory studies has been developing for some time, triggered by early science fiction writers such as H G Wells[1] and then by the emergence of trend analysis, scenario planning and the use of other futures tools to anticipate projected, possible, probable, preferred and cancelled futures (Miller, 2015; Poli, 2010; Urry, 2016; Couture & Murgatroyd, 2024). Rather than trying to predict the future, practitioners of future thinking seek to understand patterns, trends and developments that will lead to a range of possible, probable and preferred futures. They practise anticipation rather than prediction.

Leaders vary in the degree to which they use anticipation as part of their strategic work. Couture & Murgatroyd (2024), for example, suggest that there are several different anticipatory archetypes seen amongst leaders, only some of which truly leverage an evidence-informed understanding of possibilities to shape a preferred future. A great many leaders are simply reactive – "responding to the next thing while nudging the organisation forward" – something Rodgers describes as "muddling through" (Rodgers, 2021). Anticipatory leaders actively analyse and think about the future (Murgatroyd & Simpson, 2011).They plan and act by thinking back from the future: they imagine what 2030 or 2035 will need to look like if their organisation is to be successful, and then work back from that analysis to better understand what actions they should take in the present to make that future possible. Strategic planning becomes more about working from the future than from the present and projecting forward (Murgatroyd, 2015).

Emerging Technologies

In terms of health and care systems, we can already see technological developments beginning to emerge that will shape the future of care. Three, in particular, are worth noting here: (a) an expansion of AI as a diagnostic tool for psychological, medical and genetic conditions, including "real-time" diagnostics during certain procedures – e.g. MRI, colonoscopy, ECG; (b) the expanded use of integrated analytics for an individual patient or category of patients in which all available data from all sources are used to create a comprehensive picture of the person, their medical history, social and lifestyle behaviours and test data enabling much more personalised medicine; and (c) the growth of wearable and domestic robotics to better support wellbeing, healthcare and psychological wellbeing.

Such emerging systems will access and synthesise more medical knowledge and information than ever before. In the 1950s, medical knowledge was doubling every fifty years (Oss, 2023). According to IBM's analysis, by 2020, it was doubling every 73 days. Now, in 2024, in the age of AI, it is doubling every 11–12 hours.[2] It is impossible for humans to be "on top" of the knowledge available in a specific field of expertise, but it is not a challenge for the emerging AI systems. More of a challenge are issues of privacy, security, and data-integrity.

Just because something is possible does not mean it will happen or that implementation is "inevitable." What gets in the way, apart from underinvestment in technology infrastructure and the professional development needed to maximise the potential of any technology, is organisational culture and mindsets. Changing established work practices and mindsets is challenging. Doing so may involve union negotiations or re-education. It always involves courageous leadership. Indeed, the analysis of the failures of attempts at health system change and transformation suggests that the failure to address these issues is the principal reason most major technology-related transformations fail (Bayat et al., 2023; Masoud, 2022).

Leadership, Anxiety, Change

Let us unpack the cultural challenges leaders face and use some archetypes to help understand how culture becomes an issue of interpersonal dynamics. Benjamin Bratton is a Professor of Visual Arts and Director of the Centre for Design and Geopolitics at the University of California (San

Diego), where he has been exploring the complex relationships between technology, politics, and design, offering critical insights into the future of cities and urban life in an increasingly computational world. He has also explored the boundaries between people and the technologies they use (Bratton, 2016, 2021). Couture and Murgatroyd (2024) have leveraged some of his thinking and analysis and that of his colleagues (Bratton et al., 2021) to build a framework for understanding how individuals and groups react to threat, challenge, or change. This work builds on earlier work (Mills & Murgatroyd, 1991; Murgatroyd, 1988) which used models from Minuchin's systems approach to family therapy (Minuchin, 1974) and applied them to organisational change and development.

The "Bratton model," as it is referred to and which is summarised here, uses two dimensions:

- **The vertical: What We Pay Attention to**: This is the "sensing" dimension. It refers to the issues, developments, and activities to which we pay attention to. What do we attend to, whom do we attend to, and why? Some pay close attention to issues and concerns related to technology deployment and investigate possibilities and challenges. They feel a need to be informed. Others live their lives paying little or no attention to what is happening around them and are especially disdainful of the idea that "technology is the answer" since they do not know the question being asked.
- **The horizontal dimension: Connectedness and Engagement**: Some live their lives as if they were "masters of their universe" and see the world through the lens of "self." Yet others see the world through the lens of connections between people, land, and social action. In psychology, this is referred to as the relationship domain: it refers to whether one is motivated by self-interests (a sense of a separate atomistic self, personal accountability, and responsibility) or by a focus on the interconnectedness to others, both living and non-living (ecology, altruism, and transcendence).

When we combine these two dimensions, we create four personas that can be found in any higher education institution, shown in Figure 27.1.

Table 27.1 elaborates on how each persona identified here might respond to challenges, change, and transformation.

Organisations such as health teams have individuals in each of these four cells. What is more, on some issues, they will operate from one cell (e.g. highly focused collaborators on research), but on other issues, they will "switch" cells (e.g. the expert loner when it comes to their specialism

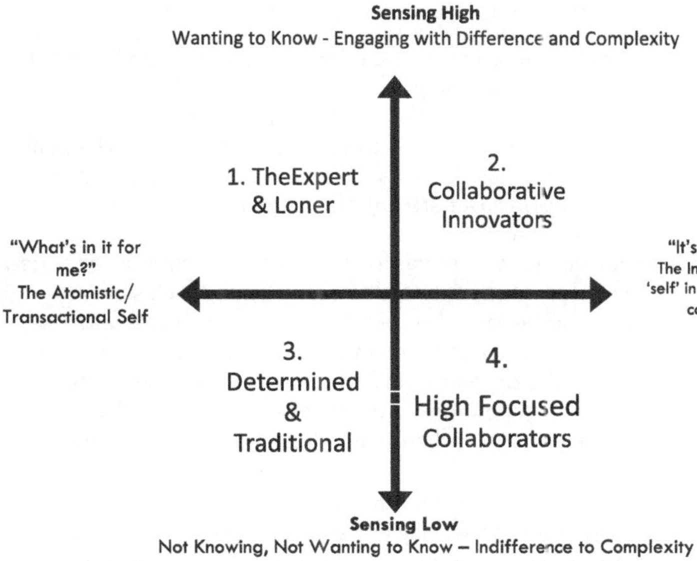

Figure 27.1 Couture and Murgatroyd (2024). Four personas.

in patient care). To make matters more complex, some are more easily influenced by the peer network than others, and some are deliberately cantankerous and contrarian based on a grudge about something that has happened to them. Human systems such as health teams are complex ego-systems which are difficult to navigate and often very difficult to change. This is one of the key reasons so many change and transformation projects struggle: failing to change the interpersonal dynamics, professional boundaries, and mindsets that determine patterns of work interactions (Skerritt et al., 2024). Though challenging work, it is key to the work of change leadership.

A shared understanding of why change is needed and what new roles each is expected to play is key to successful change. Change is more likely to be successful when it is supported by expert analysis and evidence of effective deployment in other organisations, especially other health teams. Though some see the deployment of a specific technology as the "change that is needed," most see change as an imposed burden. Any technology deployment needs to increase impacts on outcomes while at the same time reducing the burden of work for healthcare workers. Many technology deployments have almost no impact on patient outcomes and increase the work of employees – another key reason for failure.

Table 27.1 The four personas response to change and transformation

1. The Expert and Loner	Seeks to leverage their position in the institution but often look for more complex challenges and relationships while remaining self-interested. They look for status and recognition while continuing to act as an individual rather than as part of a collective. They provide advice and support but are not "team" players or natural collaborators.
2. Collaborative Innovators	These individuals are natural collaborators, curious, engaged and strongly committed to diversity and inclusion. They go beyond the idea of engaged clinicians and administrators and are activists and advocates for changes across the organisation and in the business processes. They are champions of innovative approaches. They share, engage and network. They are early adopters and problem-solvers.
3. Determined and Traditional	The institution is a safe base from which to enable their work, especially if they have job security. They are seeking to improve their patient's success and wellbeing: their clinical work and their patients are their focus. They want to get to care and practice in the way they have always done and get good feedback for doing so. The operate in very traditional (and often very good) ways, but they are not engaged in conversations about "new practices" and shun "innovation," "collaboration" or significant change involving technology. "I know what works!" They do what they have always done and often get good results.
4. Highly Focused Collaborators	This is the cell in which health professional's partner with others to engage in social action and collective activities, for example in relation to social issues, climate change or health. As "engaged educators and clinicians," they want their health system to have impact through social action and work with community partners (often leading such organisations) with the intention of achieving specific social change. They are always "up for" something new…and love to try new things in their teaching and in their assessments and, while they have reservations about technologies like AI, they will experiment under certain conditions.

Leadership, in the face of such challenges, depends on building what Africans refer to as a culture of Ubuntu – the idea that each of us is enabled by the presence of all – "I am because *we* are." Cultivating engagement, empowered teams capable of facing up to challenges and responding in agile and collective ways is at the heart of the work of leadership.

Making Change Possible

Post-pandemic, the nature of organisations has been changing, especially in health systems and organisations. There is now a deeper understanding of the value of compassionate leadership and a new understanding of the place of self-compassion, mutual care and social support in the workplace. There is also a new appreciation of agile responses at a local level to local conditions and circumstances and a recognition of the need to embrace local, national and international interdependencies. Colleagues now expect to feel respected, understood and cared for by their organisation. Given the global shortage of healthcare professionals, colleagues have choices.

These emerging developments place new demands on leaders, reinforced by the growing presence of new generations of workers who bring different values and mindsets. While always focused on performance and patient outcomes, leaders need now to always focus on their colleagues as persons with feelings, anxieties, and vulnerabilities – their whole selves, not just their thinking and action processes. What followers have come to expect is a leader who supports them through engagement, coaching, and mentoring rather than through command and control. Leaders need to grow and support their teams in a shift from an ego-driven organisation to a more agile ecosystem always ready to adapt to the "next big thing."

Enabling Possibilities

Building an Agile Organisation

Individuals and teams, leaders need to reimagine their organisation so that it is better able to be agile (Boustani et al., 2020), anti-fragile (Taleb, 2012) and resilient (Belasen, 2021). As technological-driven change dominates the coming decade in health systems, being able to respond nimbly, effectively and creatively will become a defining feature of leader behaviour.

There are many accounts of what it takes to build agile health and psychological service organisations. These five key actions are seen as key to developing the kind of innovation-enabling organisation that health systems now need:

1. Foster a culture of continuous learning, development and risk-taking (Cutrer et al., 2020).
2. Develop cross-functional teams and flatten hierarchies, and enable collaboration across health specialists (Çetin et al., 2023).
3. Adopt agile project-management practices for all core activities (Misra et al., 2024).
4. Implement data-enabled and evidence-informed decision making (Painuly & Sharma, 2023).
5. Prioritise environmental and resource sustainability in all that the organisation does (Thomas & Suresh, 2023).

Enabling the team and organisation to develop and sustain a strong sense of interconnectedness, commitment, and focus, as well as a feeling of "owning their future," is key to this work. It also helps to have fun and demonstrate the satisfaction that comes from achieving goals and making a difference to patients' lives. Building engaged teams that focus on success and have energy for the work is both demanding and satisfying work.

Leadership Development and Growth

To facilitate an agile organisation and to support the shift in mindset and culture needed to sustain an agile organisation, leaders need to grow and change too. They need to develop the knowledge and skills needed to help team members cope with uncertainty and anxiety; keep a focus on maintaining a high performing organisation while helping their teams adopt and adapt to future possibilities; they need to develop the skills of courage (Murgatroyd, 2023) and resilience (Aris & Murgatroyd, 2017) and keep focused on the purpose of the organisation (Rodgers, 2021).

Leaders will find themselves engaged in coaching team members for success in the emerging agile, technology-enabled organisation they are part of. Developing the skills of coaching and performance management for agility will be a key leadership development task.

Coaching Team Members for Success

Those who lead through coaching will find that their technical skills and experience can only be useful when they are matched by the effective and meaningful deployment of non-technical skills, as a series of studies by a team in Wisconsin has demonstrated (Greenberg et al., 2017). Key amongst these non-technical skills are empathy, warmth, genuineness, compassion, and active and engaged listening.

There is a range of coaching models that are used in healthcare organisations. Among the most popular is the GROW model (Whitmore, 2002, 2010; Spence & Grant, 2007), which involves these four steps:

Step 1: Agree the GOAL for this session.

Ask: What do we need to achieve together in this session?
Ask: How would you like to feel afterwards?

Step 2: Understand the current REALITY the coachee faces in relation to their work in the team.

Ask: How have things gone since we last connected?
Ask: What have you learned about the work we are doing and the situation you are in? What is working, not working, and what is new?

Step 3: Explore OPTIONS for learning, growth, and improvement in your professional skills.

Ask: What skills and understanding do we need to work on together for the next steps in the work we are committed to?
Ask: What else do we need to address and work on for you to feel good about your work?

Step 4: Identify the WAY forward for this work.

Ask: What do you need to research, review, or better understand?
Ask: What skills do you want to work on between now and our next coaching session?

Ask: What supports do you need to find, build, create, or engage to help you improve your work?
Ask: Can you connect with peers who can support you on this journey?

This kind of narrative and engagement can make a significant difference to performance, outcomes and the sense of well-being colleagues feel in the face of change and uncertainty. Indeed, there is a growing literature showing the efficacy of leadership as coaching in practice, especially in health systems (Boet et al., 2023; Haynal & Chioléro, 2022). Various refinements of the GROW model have been explored, and some valuable insights about the language of coaching have emerged (Fleishhacker & Graf, 2024; Hauser, 2017).

Some colleagues may need more than coaching. They need mentoring to bring out their full potential and to enable them to become more engaged, effective, and involved in what they do. Coaching is focused on "the work"; mentoring is focused on personal growth and development – on becoming (Bennis, 2009). Leaders develop not just capabilities through coaching, but capacities and imagination through mentoring (Aris et al., 2024; Murgatroyd, 2024a, 2024b).

Conclusion: The Future Isn't What It Used to Be

As the opening of this chapter made clear, this is an anxious time of rapid change, and many colleagues find both the nature and speed of change challenging. The future is increasingly non-linear, brittle, and challenging – creating pressure on leaders to perform. One key to being able to do so is ensuring that leaders are healthy and taking care of their physical and mental health. Leaders need to develop personal mastery (Murgatroyd & Simpson, 2011) and find a work-life balance that maintains their energy, commitment, and passion for leading an agile team (Hooda et al., 2023). Failing to do so could lead to burnout, project failure, and low morale.

Leaders also need to build a community of trust and compassion, focused on both caring for each other and self-care. Change requires stamina and support, care and concern, compassion and focus. All of these are outcomes of mutual trust within a team (West, 2021).

The future may involve complex interactions between people, technology, and systems. What is needed, more than anything, is a sense of adventure and possibility linked to purpose, courage, and skill (Rodgers, 2021). After all, no one said leadership cannot be fun.

Reflective Questions

This chapter explores the expectations and challenges leaders will face in developing an agile culture, able to adapt to technology-enabled change. They may also have to shift the culture and mindsets of colleagues, who may be resistant to the new world of working with a co-intelligent AI partner. Here are some questions to reflect on:

1. What are the cultures and mindsets within your team at this time, and how might these need to change to enable the team to be more agile and receptive to technology?
2. When you look at the Bratton persona (see pages 385 to 387), who on your team fits where and what are the implications of this for your work as a leader?
3. What is most likely to get in the way of technology-enabled change within your team, and how might you overcome these challenges?
4. From a personal point of view, what knowledge, skills and capabilities do you need to develop to lead an agile, responsive and innovative organisation that embraces technology as a key feature of its future?

Ideas in Brief

- In a rapidly evolving, tech-enabled world, leaders must balance strategic foresight with psychological safety, building cultures of trust, energy, and support.
- **Foster agility through mindset shifts.** Embrace innovation by addressing cultural resistance, supporting learning, and guiding teams through mindset changes necessary for AI-integrated, agile working.
- Sustainable leadership in anxious times demands personal mastery, compassion, and a clear sense of purpose to prevent burnout and build adaptive capacity.
- **Embrace technology as a partner.** Lead the integration of emerging technologies with curiosity, skill, and humanity – seeing digital change not as a threat but as a catalyst for transformation and connection.

Notes

1 H G Wells suggested the need for universities to teach futures studies in 1901 – see https://www.wnrf.org/cms/hgwells.shtml
2 See https://www.linkedin.com/pulse/human-knowledge-doubling-every-12-hours-amitabh-ray/

References

Aris, S., Rao, A., Roycroft, P., & Clutterbuck, D. (Eds.). (2024). *Mentoring in health, social care and beyond: Handbook for practice, training and research*. Pavilion.

Aris, S., & Murgatroyd, S. (2017). *Beyond resilience – From mastery to mystery. A workbook for personal mastery and transformational change*. Lulu Press.

Bayat, M., Kashkadan, T., Khodadost, M., Shokri, A., Fattah, H., Seporro, F. G., Younesi, F., & Khalilneszhad, R. (2023). Factors Associated with failure of health system reform: A systematic review and meta-synthesis. *Journal of Preventive Medicine and Public Health, 56*(2), 128–144. https://doi.org/10.3961/jpmph.22.394

Belasen, A. (2021). *Resilience in healthcare leadership: Practical strategies and self-assessment tools for identifying strengths and weaknesses*. Routledge.

Bennis, W. (2009). *On becoming a leader*. Basic Books.

Boet, S., Etherington, C., Dion, P.-M., Desjardins, C., Kaur, M., Ly, V., et al. (2023). Impact of coaching on physician wellness: A systematic review. *PLoS ONE, 18*(2), e0281406.

Bratton, B. H. (2016). *The stack: On software and sovereignty*. MIT Press.

Bratton, B. H. (2021). *The revenge of the real: Politics for a post-pandemic world*. Verso.

Bratton, B., Boyadjiev, N., & Axel, N. (2021). *The new normal*. Park Books.

Boustani, M., Azar, J., & Solid, C. A. (2020). *Agile implementation: A model for implementing evidence-based healthcare solutions into real-world practice to achieve sustainable change*. Morgan James.

Çetin, S., Ergün, E., & Tekingündüz, S. (2023). The effect of agile leadership characteristics of academic staff on organizational agility: A study in higher education. International *Journal of Leadership in Education, 26*(2), 367–384

Couture, J-C., & Murgatroyd, S. (2024). *Educational futures for school leadership: Evidence-informed strategies for managing change*. Routledge.

Cutrer, W. B., Pusic, M. V, Gruppen, L. D., Hammoud, M. M., & Santen, S. A. (2020). *The master adaptive learner*. Elsevier.

Desist, M., Reusch, A., & Barwinski, R. (2022). Digital mess up – Why digital organizational initiatives fail. *Academy of Management Proceedings*, 1 July 6th. https://doi.org/10.5465/AMBPP.2022.16646abstract

Fleischhacker, M., & Graf, E-M. (2024). A closer look into the 'black box' of coaching – Linguistic research into the local effectiveness of coaching with the help of conversation analysis. *Coaching: An International Journal of Theory, Research and Practice, 17*(1), 119–141. https://doi.org/10.1080/17521882.2024.2312295

Greenberg, C. C., Ghousseini, H. N., Pavuluri Quamme, S. R., et al. (2017). Wisconsin surgical coaching program. A statewide surgical coaching program provides opportunity for continuous professional development. *Annals of Surg*ery, *267*(5), 868–873. https://doi.org/10.1097/SLA.0000000000002341

Guley, G., & Reznik, T. (2019). Culture eats strategy for breakfast and transformation for lunch. *Jabian Journal*, Fall. https://journal.jabian.com/wp-content/uploads/2019/10/701_JJ_Fall_19_Culture_Eats_Strategy.pdf

Hauser, L. (2017). The science behind powerful questioning – A systemic questioning framework for coach educators and practitioners. *Philosophy of Coaching – An International Journal, 2*(2), 51–68. http://dx.doi.org/10.22316/poc/02.2.04

Haynal, V., & Chiolëro, R. (2022). *Coaching physicians and health care professionals – Supporting workplace wellbeing and high-quality care.* Routledge.

Hooda, D. S., Singh, J., & Patil, A. A. (2023). An analysis of work-life balance in the healthcare industry. *Pacific Business Review International*, June 12, 2023. Available at https://www.researchgate.net/publication/381118501_An_Analysis_of_Work-Life_Balance_in_the_Healthcare_Industry#fullTextFileContent

Krantz, J., & Trainor, K. (2019). The myth of rationality – Why change efforts so often fail. Chapter in J. Krantz & K. Trainor (Eds.), *The unconscious at work*. Routledge. Available at: https://www.taylorfrancis.com/chapters/edit/10.4324/9781351104166-22/myth-rationality-james-krantz-kay-trainor

Masoud, R. (2022). Digital transformation in healthcare. *International Journal of Scientific and Research Publications, 12*(7), 379–382. https://doi.org/10.29322/ijsrp.12.07.2022.p12744

Miller, R. (2015). *Making experimentalist leadership practical: The theory and practice of futures literacy* [mimeo]. Centre for Strategic Education.

Mills, A., & Murgatroyd, S. (1991). *Organizational rules – A framework for understanding organizational action*. The Open University Press.

Minuchin, S. (1974). *Families and family therapy*. Harvard University Press.

Misra, S., Jadeja, R., & Mittal, M. (2024). *Practical approaches to agile project management*. IGI Global.

Mollick, E. (2024). *Co-intelligence – Living and working with AI.* Portfolio.

Murgatroyd, S. (1988). Consulting as counselling – The theory and practice of structural consulting. In M. L. Gray (Ed.), *Consulting and education.* Cassell.

Murgatroyd, S. (2015). *How to rethink the future – Making use of strategic foresight.* Lulu Press.

Murgatroyd, S. (2023). *Becoming courageous: The skills of courage.* Lulu Press.

Murgatroyd, S. (2024a). Mentoring leaders for courage. In S. Aris, A. Rao, P. Roycroft, & D. Clutterbuck (Eds.), *Mentoring handbook – Approaches for health and social care.* Pavilion.

Murgatroyd, S. (2024b). Changing minds through futures focused mentoring. In S. Aris, A. Rao, P. Roycroft, & D. Clutterbuck (Eds.), *Mentoring handbook – Approaches for health and social care.* Pavilion.

Murgatroyd, S., & Simpson, D. G. (2011). *Renaissance leadership – Rethinking and leading the future.* Lulu Press.

Oss, M. (2023). *Leading in a time of knowledge doubling.* Open Minds, August 21st. Available at https://openminds.com/market-intelligence/executive-briefings/leading-in-a-time-of-knowledge-doubling/

Painuly, S., Sharma, S., & Matta, P. (2023). Artificial intelligence in e-healthcare supply chain management system: Challenges and future trends. *International Conference on Sustainable Computing and Data Communication Systems (ICSCDS)*, 569–574. Available at: https://api.semanticscholar.org/CorpusID:258335433

Poli, R. (2010). The many aspects of anticipation. *Foresight, 12*, 7–17.

Rodgers, C. (2021). *The wiggly world of organization – Muddling through with purpose, courage and skill.* Routledge.

Skerritt, D., Parsons, J., Stewart, M. L., Schrimper, M., & Rainone, N. (2024). Going all in: Why employee "will" can make or break transformations. *McKinsey Quarterly.* Available at https://www.mckinsey.com/capabilities/transformation/our-insights/going-all-in-why-employee-will-can-make-or-break-transformations

Spence, G., & Grant, A. M. (2007). Professional and peer life coaching and the enhancement of goal striving and well-being: An exploratory study. *The Journal of Positive Psychology, 2*(3), 185–194. https://doi.org/10.1080/17439760701228896

Taleb, N. N. (2012). *Anti-fragile – Things that gain from disorder.* Random House.

Thomas, A., & Suresh. M. (2023). Readiness for agile-sustainability in healthcare organizations. *International Journal of Quality and Service Sciences, 15*(2), 15th May. https://doi.org/10.1108/ijqss-06-2022-0056

Urry, J. (2016). *What is the future?* Polity.

West, M. A. (2021). *Compassionate leadership: Sustaining wisdom, humanity and presence in health and social care.* Swirling Leaf Press.

Whitmore, J. (2002). *Coaching for performance: Growing people, performance and purpose.* Nicholas Brealey

Whitmore, J. (2010). *Coaching for performance – Principles and practice of coaching and leadership.* Nicholas Brealey.

28

Why We Need a Paradigm Shift

Thoughts from Young Leaders

Dr Olga Luzón, Dr Hannah Shaw, Dr Sarina Afzali, Charlotte Baribeau, Dr Arshia Choudhury, Dr Maryam Haghiran, and Dr Saim Kirhan

Emerging Landscape of Clinical Psychology[1]

Over the past two decades, the role of clinical psychologists within the National Health Service (NHS) has significantly broadened, evolving beyond the traditional domain of expert therapists to encompass consultancy, strategic leadership, and service development (Hunt et al., 2024). This shift shows growing recognition that psychologists are well positioned to lead services and influence organisational culture.

Since the British Psychological Society published the Clinical Psychology Leadership Development Framework (BPS, 2010), which emphasised the importance of leadership across the career lifespan and levels of practice, clinical psychology has embedded leadership at all stages of the career trajectory (BPS, 2017). The UK doctoral training programmes consider leadership a core competency (BPS, 2025). The Health and Care Professions Council (HCPC) stresses that psychologists should be competent in working with teams and organisations at a macro level to create environments that promote mental well-being (HCPC, 2023). The Fit for the Future: 10 year Health Plan (NHS, 2025) identifies clinical psychologists as key leaders in delivering integrated care and system-wide transformation. Clinical psychologists are, therefore, expected to leverage their expertise to address complex

DOI: 10.4324/9781003492399-35

psychosocial and health-related challenges that impact individuals, families, and communities.

Simultaneously, over the last decade, there has been an increased recognition that mental health is profoundly influenced by wider determinants, including socio-economic factors such as housing, employment, education, access to healthcare, and systemic inequalities like racism, discrimination, and social exclusion. These factors are known to significantly contribute to disparities in mental health outcomes across populations (WHO, 2014). Addressing health inequalities through developing inclusive services represents a significant challenge for a profession that has been historically criticised for lacking diversity and reinforcing Eurocentric and colonial perspectives, which pathologise non-Western cultural expressions of distress (Harper & Speed, 2012). Mills (2014), among other authors, argue that mainstream psychology has often failed to consider the social, historical, and political contexts contributing to mental health issues, instead promoting individualistic and depoliticised models of distress.

Recent events such as Black Lives Matter, the disproportionate impact of COVID-19 on non-white populations, and the Windrush scandal have further highlighted the pressing need to address health inequalities and the pervasive systemic racism within societal institutions, including mental health services (Dawes et al., 2022; Thomeer et al., 2023; Reicher, 2024). Such events have prompted the re-evaluation of the profession's standards, recognising the limitations of current systems and the role psychologists must play as leaders in addressing broader societal injustices that directly or indirectly affect population mental health. The BPS has increasingly prioritised anti-racism, diversity, and inclusivity in training, practice, policy, and research (BPS, 2021). It recognises that the profession must better reflect the diversity of the population it serves by supporting mentoring and access schemes, advancing anti-racism and decolonisation initiatives, and fostering inclusive practices. Similarly, the HCPC has updated its Standards of Proficiency (2023) to ensure that psychologists are equipped to address complex psychosocial challenges faced by marginalised communities and emphasises that psychologists must "promote and protect the service user's interests at all times" and "actively challenge barriers to inclusion" (HCPC, standard 2.2).

While this discourse has been largely embraced, it has also faced criticism. Some members of the profession have expressed concerns about the growing emphasis on social justice, framing it as an encroachment of political ideology into clinical practice. The BPS's monthly publication, *The Psychologist*, has been accused of promoting a 'left-wing agenda' by focusing disproportionately on issues of racism, decolonisation, and diversity, and overlooking other facets of psychology (Dennis Relojo-Howell, 2020). Critics argue that ideological biases could negatively impact clinical practice (Silander et al., 2020), and that therapists should remain politically neutral to avoid alienating clients with differing ideological views (Mather, 2020). However, others suggest that maintaining impartiality perpetuates systemic issues that marginalise certain groups, both within therapy settings and in wider society (Patel, 2003). Many believe that the inclusive and culturally sensitive approaches recommended by current BPS and HCPC guidelines, whilst valuable, fall short of addressing the problem. They propose that existing leadership structures often uphold, willingly or not, a *status quo* of failing to challenge entrenched power dynamics or adequately confront the complexities of racism and xenophobia, both within the profession and society at large (Wood & Patel, 2019). Instead, they call for a shift towards a social justice and human rights approach to effectively address the root causes of poor mental health and inequalities that affect both service users and practitioners (Fernando, 2017; Luzon et al., 2023; Patel, 2020).

Global Mental Health and Social Justice

We argue that clinical psychologists, as leaders, must take a more proactive stance in advocating for systemic change. To address global challenges and the needs of increasingly diverse communities, the profession must move beyond mere inclusion and diversity efforts. It should engage in profound systemic reform and challenge entrenched power structures that perpetuate inequality and injustice (Patel, 2019; Fernando, 2017). It has been argued that the role of clinical psychologists in leadership positions is not merely to treat distress but to advocate for a more just and equitable society (Patel, 2003). Ultimately, clinical psychology must recognise that neutrality in the face of systemic inequality is not an option; otherwise, it may invertedly contribute to such inequalities (Wood & Patel, 2019).

The ongoing global refugee crisis and the far-right riots in some parts of the UK in 2024 are pertinent examples of the urgent need for psychology to raise its profile and adopt a more proactive, visible, and human-rights approach to care. The United Nations High Commissioner for Refugees reports unprecedented numbers of forcibly displaced people worldwide driven by ongoing conflicts, political instability, and the climate crisis, and numbers will continue to grow (UNHCR, 2022). Mental health services must be prepared to address the unique needs of these populations, who are at heightened risk of developing mental health issues, such as post-traumatic stress disorder, anxiety, and depression, due to the compounding effects of pre-migration trauma, the migration journey itself, and post-migration adversities such as discrimination, socio-economic disadvantage, and systemic barriers to accessing care (Silove et al., 2017; Priebe et al., 2016). Effective support requires culturally appropriate (Bhui, 2022), community-based mental health interventions with interpreters and cultural mediators (Tunariu & Tribe, 2017; Venables et al., 2021). It also demands committed leadership to integrate these practices and adopt a human-rights-based framework that centres social justice in psychological practice (Patel, 2020).

Clinical psychologists possess advanced formulation skills that enable them to analyse and influence individual and systemic levels within organisations, which is crucial for driving structural change. The HCPC Standards of Proficiency for Practitioner Psychologists (2023) emphasise that a critical role of psychologists is to apply these skills to enhance multidisciplinary teams' psychological understanding of the experiences and presentations of those they work with. This dual perspective – being embedded within the system while also stepping back to observe its (power) dynamics – positions psychologists uniquely to address and challenge problematic organisations. However, disrupting the *status quo* in clinical psychology can be particularly challenging due to the deep-rooted traditions and established practices that have long governed the profession, the NHS, and wider society. For this, it is necessary to acknowledge the influence of whiteness and other dominant cultural norms and institutional practices that maintain the *status quo*, which primarily benefit those in positions of power and limit opportunities for diverse perspectives and transformative change. Psychologists must remain vigilant, hold themselves accountable to professional standards, and actively advocate for positive change, even when this change goes against historically held assumptions, rather than succumbing to inertia or reluctance.

A Diverse Leadership Reflective of Communities

To achieve transformative change, leadership in clinical psychology must also address barriers, discrimination, and inequalities within the profession itself, including the lack of diversity among practitioners (Ahsan, 2020) and the scarcity of female leaders (Hoyt & Simon, 2024).

Clinical psychology as a profession continues to be dominated by white, middle-class, female psychologists and is not representative of the communities it serves (York, 2019). Reports from the NHS Confederation (2022) show that individuals from racialised communities encounter significant barriers to accessing and advancing to senior positions in clinical psychology, demonstrating a pervasive "glass-ceiling" effect and systemic racism.

Furthermore, whilst women comprise about 80% of qualified educational and clinical psychologists in the UK, they remain underrepresented in senior leadership roles and earn less than their male counterparts, who are more likely to hold higher-paying roles despite being fewer in numbers (ONS, 2019; Palmer et al., 2020). From an intersectionality perspective, women of colour face further prejudice and discrimination in reaching and navigating leadership roles, and experience unique and often insurmountable barriers (Hancock, 2007). Diverse leadership can offer a wider range of perspectives and foster a culture of inclusivity better equipped to serve diverse communities (McIntosh et al., 2019). The profession must promote leadership pathways for psychologists from minoritised backgrounds to ensure that leadership is representative (Tribe & Bell, 2018; Patel, 2019). Initiatives such as the NHS and BPS aspiring clinical psychologist access and mentoring schemes (George et al., 2024) are effective strategies for addressing barriers for underrepresented groups (Oldridge, 2019), but it is imperative to consider the lifespan of career progression as well. Allyship plays a crucial role, for established leaders, peers, and colleagues, by actively supporting women and other underrepresented groups and bolstering their legitimacy in leadership roles.

Nonetheless, representative leadership and giving people a "seat at the table" are not enough in isolation. Building psychologically safe organisational cultures, where people feel able to speak up, requires a multi-faceted approach (Hunt et al., 2021). Leaders need to facilitate continuous and active feedback loops where everyone is involved in decision-making and able to raise concerns or challenge existing structures. Instead of isolated Equality, Diversity, and Inclusion (EDI) initiatives, there is a need for brave and compassionate leaders who actively embrace their own and others' discomfort and defences (Ahsan, 2020).

The Power Threat Meaning Framework (Johnstone et al., 2018) could serve as a useful meta-framework to make sense of the multiple ways human distress is influenced by sociocultural context and negative operations of power in society. There needs to be protected time embedded in job plans to address anti-racist practices and policies, where teams are encouraged to develop a critical stance towards Western psychological models and ways of practising. Effective and culturally sensitive supervision is essential in this process (Vekaria, 2023), supporting psychologists to build confidence in their expertise and develop critical thinking and cultural awareness (HCPC, 2023). Eliciting individual and shared values and strengths within a system may also help teams to develop a sense of belonging and shared direction. Teams and professionals are unable to do this if they feel burnt out, silenced, and hopeless. Leaders need to promote staff wellbeing and challenge the perceived stigma associated with asking for help in clinical psychology (Tay et al., 2018). Whilst fostering diverse and supportive leadership is crucial, it is also important to recognise that generational shifts in how leadership is perceived present new challenges and opportunities. These shifts offer a chance to cultivate a workplace culture that embraces innovation and is equipped to respond to global mental health needs.

Generational Differences in Leadership Approaches and Challenges for Young Leaders

Significant generational changes in values, life experiences, technological abilities, cultural trends, and historical events have emerged between Baby Boomers, Generation X, Millennials, Generation Z, and, soon to join the profession, Generation Alpha.[2] These changes profoundly influence how leadership is conceptualised across these groups. To effectively influence organisational culture and drive change, leaders must steer organisations beyond traditional hierarchical structures based on power differences and status. Instead, they should embrace agile organisational models that value autonomy, participative processes, and shared decision-making. Such models promote higher visibility for everyone in the organisation, maximise technological advances, and enhance connectivity amongst the workforce. Younger generations highly value leaders who mentor, empower, and promote transparency and social responsibility. The absence of such qualities is often viewed as archaic and outdated, hindering progress and perpetuating imbalances and inequalities (Alam, 2023; Valenti, 2019).

Newly qualified clinical psychologists in the UK NHS typically start at the *Band 7* level according to the Agenda for Change system (Department of Health, 2004). This level demands advanced expertise, significant managerial responsibilities, and specialist knowledge within a multidisciplinary team. However, the transition from doctoral training to this role often creates a discrepancy between the expectations placed on new practitioners and their actual managerial experience, leading to tension between their confidence and their perceived role within the team.

Despite their position of relative power and the extensive training they have undergone, newly qualified psychologists may struggle to leverage their skills effectively. Imposter syndrome and self-doubts (Chrousos et al., 2020; Maftei et al., 2021) can undermine their confidence, making them hesitant to share innovative perspectives that could lead to positive change. This challenge is compounded by the hierarchical structures and unspoken norms within the profession, which can lead to young leaders being dismissed or marginalised, particularly when they propose changes that challenge established practices (Burnes, 2004). Such resistance can further isolate young leaders and discourage them from advocating for change, thereby perpetuating the *status quo*. Social factors like race, gender, and socioeconomic status can further complicate their leadership journey, often leading to additional experiences of discrimination and exclusion (Martinot, 2010). The interplay of these social dynamics with professional stressors and internalised expectations can contribute to burnout, even early on in their professional careers (Nadal, 2017).

To address these challenges and support emerging leaders, it is crucial to provide adequate support, including allyship, mentorship, and opportunities to meaningfully effect change early on in their careers (Lawrence et al., 2022). Leadership and management training and placement experiences that focus on and value leadership activities may also build the confidence and expertise of junior staff (Hassett et al., 2021). Meaningful responsibilities and opportunities to take on tasks such as developing advocacy groups, guidelines, working on community centred partnerships, engagement with public health initiatives and leading action research are all actionable strategies that would support the development of relevant competencies. Other strategies could include fostering networks and peer support, having role models who look like "us," and senior leaders who demonstrate inclusive practices and promote an active, non-defensive dialogue about systemic issues. Such measures can help mitigate feelings of powerlessness and empower young leaders, ultimately fostering a more supportive environment for innovation and progress within the profession. The efficacy of these strategies should be the focus of ongoing review, making systems accountable through transparent governance structures open to scrutiny and feedback.

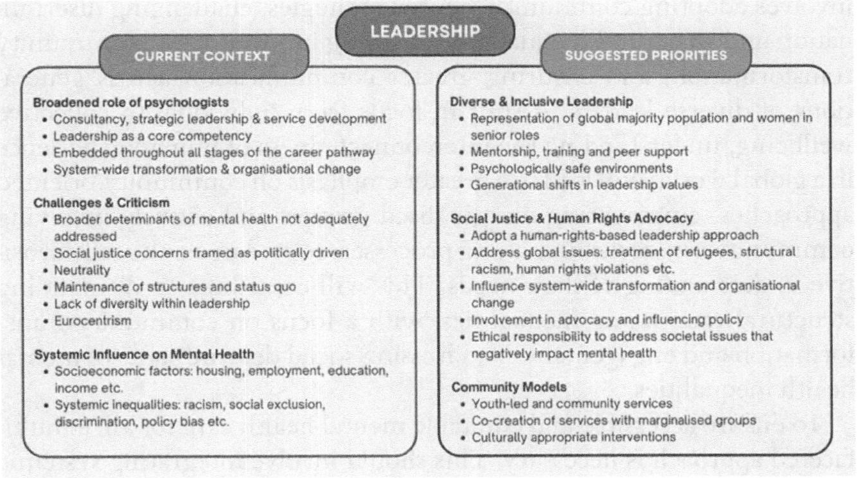

Figure 28.1 Key themes in the current leadership landscape requiring prioritisation.

There are excellent examples of innovative services where young leaders are pioneering new models of community-based interventions to better serve marginalised groups. Arts Against Knives (AAK) and MAC-UK are prime examples of organisations founded and led by young leaders who co-create services with and within the communities they serve. AAK tackles youth violence by engaging young people in creative projects that offer safe spaces for skill-building and personal growth. MAC-UK reimagines mental health support by getting out of the clinic and meeting young people where they are. By working in partnership, these organisations foster long-term engagement and ensure that services and interventions are culturally relevant and accessible to groups who are often excluded from mainstream support. These organisations demonstrate how young leaders can disrupt traditional approaches and implement community-based models addressing social inequalities and mental health needs, showcasing collaborative, non-hierarchical, and creative leadership. Figure 28.1 presents a summary of key themes relevant to the current leadership landscape within clinical psychology and highlights three critical areas that the authors propose should be prioritised moving forward.

Closing Remarks

The field of clinical psychology is undergoing a necessary transformation towards a more comprehensive and inclusive approach. This change involves adopting community-focused strategies, challenging discrimination and structural inequalities, fostering innovation for community transformation, and ensuring greater communication across generations of diverse leaders. A shift in focus from individual to collective wellbeing, understanding the interconnectedness of human experience in a global world, will lead to a greater emphasis on community-oriented approaches, empowering marginalised groups, and actively involving communities in decision-making processes, rooted in a culturally sensitive understanding of their needs. This will contribute to dismantling structural racism and inequalities, with a focus on community transformation and engagement in addressing social determinants of mental health inequalities.

To ensure accessible and equitable mental health care for all, a multifaceted approach is necessary. This should involve integrating systemic thinking, community partnership, workforce support and development, and critical advocacy for policy reforms that reflect the needs of patients and professionals. Leaders in clinical psychology must engage with policymakers to influence real change and ensure that the healthcare system is responsive to diverse populations and evolving needs. At times, the involvement of mental health professionals in issues that are perceived as political may create discomfort or resistance within established leadership. However, remaining neutral perpetuates inequalities and directly impacts communities, teams, and individuals' mental health. It is the individual responsibility of all leaders to use their privileged position to advocate for an expanded understanding of the profession's role in societal issues, emphasising ethical responsibility to address the broader determinants of mental wellbeing (Rahim & Cooke, 2019). A human-rights-partnership based approach that advocates for social justice and incorporates professional obligations into everyday clinical practice, service design, research, and policy is required to bridge the gap between traditional clinical practice and the evolving needs of communities (Patel, 2020).

Ideas in Brief

- Mental health disparities are increasingly recognised as stemming from systemic inequalities, socio-economic factors, and racism. The profession needs to engage in profound systemic reform and challenge entrenched power structures that perpetuate inequality and injustice.

- Clinical psychologists are uniquely positioned to advocate for systemic reform, challenge inequitable power dynamics, and address broader social justice issues. Neutrality in the face of systemic inequalities is increasingly viewed as complicity, urging psychologists to adopt proactive, transformative leadership approaches that reflect and empower diverse communities.
- Culturally sensitive decolonised approaches and leadership that actively advocate for positive change, even when this change goes against historically held assumptions, are to be promoted.
- The profession must address its lack of diversity, particularly in leadership roles, and implement inclusive practices that empower underrepresented groups and foster more representative and transformative leadership.
- Aspiring leaders value collaborative and community-led approaches over traditional hierarchies. Young leaders need to be supported to create opportunities for innovation to drive systemic change.

Notes

1 The authors of this chapter span across the clinical psychology career span from training to qualified levels. Our intention is not to speak for all 'young leaders' but rather to give voice to those who share our concerns, hopes, and reflections on aspects of leadership that matter to us. Whilst the focus of this chapter is on clinical psychology, and its practice within the UK National Health Service, we believe the dilemmas, reflections, and suggestions will also be relevant to other branches of psychology and contexts.

2 Baby Boomers (1946–1964), Generation X (1965–1980), Millennials (1981–1996), Generation Z (1997–2012), Generation Alpha (2013–2025)

References

Ahsan, S. (2020). Holding up the mirror: Deconstructing whiteness in clinical psychology. *Journal of Critical Psychology, Counselling and Psychotherapy, 20*(3), 45–55. https://egalitarianpublishing.com/JCPCP/2020/jcpcp2003_Ahsan.html

Alam, A. (2023). *Navigating generational waves: Leadership's response to Gen Z work values and its effect on organizational evolution*. https://doi.org/10.13140/RG.2.2.11531.67363

Bhui, K. (2022). A Refugee rose of competencies and capabilities for mental healthcare of refugees. *British Journal of Psychiatry Open, 8*(2), e45. https://doi.org/10.1192/bjo.2022.11

British Psychological Society. (2017). *Practice Guidelines (3rd ed.)*. https://www.bps.org.uk/guideline/bps-practice-guidelines-2017https://www.bps.org.uk/guideline/bps-practice-guidelines-2017

British Psychological Society. (2025). *Standards for the accreditation of doctoral programmes in clinical psychology*.

British Psychological Society. (2021). *Racial and social equalities in action: What can possibly go right?* Report.

Burnes, B. (2004). Kurt Lewin and the planned approach to change: A re‐appraisal. *Journal of Management Studies, 41*(6), 977–1002. https://doi.org/10.1111/j.1467-6486.2004.00463.x

Chrousos, G. P., Mentis, A. A., & Dardiotis, E. (2020). Focusing on the neuro-psycho-biological and evolutionary underpinnings of the imposter syndrome. *Frontiers in Psychology, 11*, 1553. https://doi.org/10.3389/fpsyg.2020.01553

Dawes, D., Amador, C., & Dunlap, N. (2022). The political determinants of health: A global panacea for health inequities. *Oxford Research Encyclopedia of Global Public Health*. https://doi.org/10.1093/acrefore/9780190632366.013.466

Department of Health. (2004). *Agenda for change: Modernising the NHS pay system*. https://www.nhsemployers.org/system/files/2021-06/tcs-handbook-version-2004.pdf

Fernando, S. (2017). *Institutional racism in psychiatry and clinical psychology*. Springer eBooks. https://link.springer.com/content/pdf/10.1007/978-3-319-62728-1.pdf

George, A. M., Millar, J. F. A., & Faheem, A. (2024). Measuring impact: A prospective evaluation of a mentoring scheme for aspiring clinical psychologists from black, Asian and Minority Ethnic backgrounds. *Mentoring & Tutoring Partnership in Learning, 32*(3), 344–360. https://doi.org/10.1080/13611267.2024.2342829

Hancock, A. M. (2007). When multiplication doesn't equal quick addition: Examining intersectionality as a research paradigm. *Perspectives on Politics, 5*(1), 63–79. https://doi.org/10.1017/S1537592707070065

Harper, D., & Speed, E. (2012). Uncovering recovery: The resistible rise of recovery and resilience. *Studies in Social Justice, 6*(1), 9–26. https://doi.org/10.26522/ssj.v6i1.1066

Hassett, C. L., Gresswell, D. M., & Wilde, S. V. (2021). Motivation to lead in trainee clinical psychologists: Service evaluation of a UK doctorate programme. *The Journal of Mental Health Training, Education and Practice, 16*(6), 442–453.

Health and Care Professions Council. (2023). *Standards of proficiency: Practitioner psychologists*. https://www.hcpc-uk.org/globalassets/resources/standards/standards-of-proficiency---practitioner-psychologists.pdf

Hoyt, C. L., & Simon, S. (2024). Social psychological approaches to women and leadership theory. In S. R. Madsen (Eds.), *Handbook of research on gender and leadership* (pp. 65–83). Edward Elgar Publishing. https://doi.org/10.4337/9781035306893.00015

Hunt, D. F., Bailey, J., Lennox, B. R., Crofts, M., & Vincent, C. (2021). Enhancing psychological safety in mental health services. *International Journal of Mental Health Systems, 15*, 1–18. https://doi.org/10.1186/s13033-021-00439-1

Hunt, M. G., Schmitz, T. M., Vail, W., & Opperman, K. (2024). Training, skills, and leadership experience: The need to expand clinical psychology training as illustrated by psychology leadership stories. *Psychological Services*. https://doi.org/10.1037/ser0000846

Johnstone, L., & Boyle, M. (2018). The power threat meaning framework: Towards the identification of patterns in emotional distress, unusual experiences and troubled or troubling behaviour, as an alternative to functional psychiatric diagnosis. *Counselling Psychology Review, 33*(1), 57–59. https://doi.org/10.53841/bpscpr.2018.33.1.57

Lawrence, J. A., Davis, B. A., Corbette, T., Hill, E. V., Williams, D. R., & Reede, J. Y. (2022). Racial/ethnic differences in burnout: A systematic review. *Journal of Racial and Ethnic Health Disparities*, 1–13. https://doi.org/10.1007/s40615-020-00950-0

Luzon, O., Afzali, S., Baribeau, C., Bhatoa, R. S., Choudhury, A., Dale, A., Haghiran, M., Kirhan, S., Powell, B., Shaw, H., Surendran, P., & Wong, C. L. M. (2023). Agents of change: A vision for psychology through the lens of tomorrow's leaders. *Clinical Psychology Forum, 363*, 74–85. https://doi.org/10.53841/bpscpf.2023.1.363.74

Maftei, A., Dumitriu, A., & Holman, A. C. (2021). "They will discover I'm a fraud!" The imposter syndrome among psychology students. *Studia Psychologica, 63*(4), 337–351. https://doi.org/10.31577/sp.2021.04.831

Martinot, S. (2010). *The machinery of whiteness: Studies in the structure of racialization*. Temple University Press.

Mather, R. D. (2020, July 16). Conservative psychologist wanted. *Psychology Today*. https://www.psychologytoday.com/au/blog/the-conservative-social-psychologist/202007/conservative-psychologist-wanted

McIntosh, M., Nicholas, H., & Huq, A. H. (Ed.). (2019). *Leadership and diversity in psychology: Moving beyond the limits*. Routledge. https://doi.org/10.4324/9780429432606

Mills, C. (2014). *Decolonizing global mental health: The psychiatrization of the majority world*. Routledge.

Nadal, K. L. (2017). "Let's get in formation": On becoming a psychologist–activist in the 21st century. *American Psychologist, 72*(9), 935. https://www.researchgate.net/profile/Kevin-Nadal/publication/322111787_Let's_get_in_formation_On_becoming_a_psychologist-activist_in_the_21st_century/links/606fafb5a6fdcc5f779085ca/Lets-Get-In-Formation-On-Becoming-a-Psychologist-Activist-in-the-21st-Century.pdf

NHS England. (2025). *Fit for the Future: 10 year Health Plan for England*. https://www.longtermplan.nhs.uk/

https://www.longtermplan.nhs.uk/

NHS England. (2019). *The NHS long term plan*. www.longtermplan.nhs.uk/publication/nhs-long-term-plan

NHS Confederation. (2022, June 17). *Shattered hopes: Black and minority ethnic leaders' experiences of breaking the glass ceiling in the NHS*. https://www.nhsconfed.org/publications/shattered-hopes-NHS-BME-leaders-glass-ceiling

Office for National Statistics. (2019). *Employment and labour market*. https://www.ons.gov.uk/employmentandlabourmarket/

Oldridge, K. (2019). A grounded theory study exploring the contribution of coaching to rebalancing organisational power for female leaders. *Coaching Psychologist, 15*(1). https://psycnet.apa.org/record/2019-33760-001

Palmer, W., Schlepper, L., Hemmings, N., & Crellin, N. (2020). *The right track: Participation and progression in psychology career paths*. Nuffield Trust. https://www.nuffieldtrust.org.uk/sites/default/files/2021-07/nuffield-trust-the-right-track-pipeline-of-psychologists-web2.pdf

Patel, N. (2003). Clinical psychology: Reinforcing inequalities or facilitating empowerment?. *The International Journal of Human Rights, 7*(1), 16–39. https://doi.org/10.1080/714003792

Patel, N. (2019). Human rights-based approach to applied psychology. *European Psychologist, 24*(2). https://doi.org/10.1027/1016-9040/a000371

Patel, N. (2020). Critical human rights-based approach to applied psychology: Context and power. In P. Hagenaars, M. Plavšić, N. Sveaass, U. Wagner, & T. Wainwright (Eds.), *Human rights education for psychologists* (pp. 61–76). Routledge. https://www.taylorfrancis.com/chapters/edit/10.4324/9780429274312-6/critical-human-rights-based-approach-applied-psychology-nimisha-patel

Priebe, S., Giacco, D., & El-Nagib, R. (2016). *Public health aspects of mental health among migrants and refugees: A review of the evidence on mental health care for refugees, asylum seekers and irregular migrants in the WHO European Region*. World Health Organization: Regional Office for Europe. https://iris.who.int/handle/10665/326308

Rahim, M., & Cooke, A. (2019). Should clinical psychologists be political? In W. Curvis (Eds.), *Professional issues in clinical psychology* (pp. 81–91). Routledge. https://www.taylorfrancis.com/chapters/edit/10.4324/9781351056267-10/clinical-psychologists-political-masuma-rahim-anne-cooke

Reicher, D. (2024, August 7). Hush now, don't explain: A perverse commentary on the 2024 riots. *The Psychologist*. https://www.bps.org.uk/psychologist/hush-now-dont-explain-perverse-commentary-2024-riots

Relojo-Howell, D. (2020, March 3). The Psychologist in a time of polarisation. *The Psychologist*. https://www.bps.org.uk/psychologist/psychologist-time-polarisation

Silander, N. C., Geczy, B., Jr., Marks, O., & Mather, R. D. (2020). Implications of ideological bias in social psychology on clinical practice. *Clinical Psychology: Science and Practice, 27*(2). https://doi.org/10.1111/cpsp.12312

Silove, D., Ventevogel, P., & Rees, S. (2017). The contemporary refugee crisis: An overview of mental health challenges. *World Psychiatry, 16*(2), 130–139.

Tay, S., Alcock, K., & Scior, K. (2018). Mental health problems among clinical psychologists: Stigma and its impact on disclosure and help seeking. *Journal of Clinical Psychology, 74*(9), 1545–1555. https://discovery.ucl.ac.uk/id/eprint/10042161/1/Scior_Full%20Manuscript%20Jan%202018.pdf

Thomeer, M. B., Moody, M. D., & Yahirun, J. (2023). Racial and ethnic disparities in mental health and mental health care during the COVID-19 pandemic. *Journal of Racial and Ethnic Health Disparities, 10*(2), 961–976. https://doi.org/10.1007/s40615-022-01284-9

Tribe, R., & Bell, D. (2018). Social justice, diversity and leadership. *The European Journal of Counselling Psychology, 7*(1), 111–125. https://doi.org/10.5964/ejcop.v6i1.145

Tunariu, A., & Tribe, R. (2017). Working with interpreters. In L. A. Winter & T. Hanley (Eds.), *The SAGE handbook of counselling and psychotherapy* (pp. 536–541). SAGE.

United Nations High Commissioner for Refugees. (2023, June 14). *Global trends: Forced displacement in 2022*. UNHCR. https://www.unhcr.org/sites/default/files/2023-06/global-trends-report-2022.pdf

Valenti, A. (2019). Leadership preferences of the millennial generation. *Journal of Business Diversity, 19*(1), 75–84.

Vekaria, B., Thomas, T., Phiri, P., & Ononaiye, M. (2023). Exploring the supervisory relationship in the context of culturally responsive supervision:

A supervisee's perspective. *The Cognitive Behaviour Therapist, 16*, e22. https://doi.org/10.1017/S1754470X23000168

Venables, E., Whitehouse, K., Spissu, C., Pizzi, L., Al Rousan, A., & Di Carlo, S. (2021). Roles and responsibilities of cultural mediators. *Forced Migration Review, 66*, 27–28. https://www.proquest.com/scholarly-journals/roles-responsibilities-cultural-mediators/docview/2547073293/se-2

Wood, N., & Patel, N. (2019). Editorial: Being nice is not enough. *Clinical Psychology Forum, 323*. https://doi.org/10.53841/bpscpf.2019.1.323.1

World Health Organization and Calouste Gulbenkian Foundation. (2014). *Social determinants of mental health*. World Health Organization. https://www.who.int/publications/i/item/9789241506809

York, K. (2019, December 2). BAME representation and psychology. *The Psychologist*. https://www.bps.org.uk/psychologist/bame-representation-and-psychology

PART SEVEN

EPILOGUE

29 The Leadership Odyssey

Key Insights and Reflecting Forward

As we bring this exploration of leadership to a close, one thing becomes abundantly clear: leadership is not a static discipline but an evolving practice, shaped by context, complexity, and human connection. In turbulent times, our instinct is often to tighten control. Yet the real challenge and opportunity lie in loosening our grip: choosing presence over prescription, curiosity over certainty, and connection over command.

This book has explored a dynamic, interconnected world where constant evolution requires leaders to engage and adapt actively. From navigating a VUCA–BANI world to fostering systemic transformation, promoting wellbeing and psychological safety, cultivating inclusive transformation, and nurturing resilience and innovation amid uncertainty, this journey underscores that leadership is both an art and a science, grounded in clear purpose, relational intelligence, emotional maturity, adaptability, and systems thinking.

I am deeply grateful to the contributors whose diverse and incisive perspectives have shaped this dialogue on rethinking leadership. Their reflections, research, and lived experience have expanded traditional paradigms and illuminated new possibilities for psychology's role in leadership. This collective work exemplifies the power of collaboration and shared inquiry in advancing our understanding of leadership.

A deep dive into the chapters and their interconnected threads reveals a rich tapestry of ideas and practices. Each chapter offers a distinct lens, yet together they illuminate a broader vision of leadership—psychologically attuned, politically informed, adaptive, relational, ecologically and systemically grounded, inclusive, and rooted in learning. This final

DOI: 10.4324/9781003492399-37

chapter synthesises and amplifies recurring themes, insights, practices and challenges explored throughout the book. It draws on the collective wisdom of contributors, distilling their learning into a reflective overview of leadership today, and what it is becoming. Some chapters are named to illustrate key ideas, but all contributions have shaped this synthesis. Where not cited directly, their influence is nonetheless embedded in the insights and patterns reflected here.

This is not a conclusion, but an invitation for readers to pause, recalibrate, and reflect on how these themes resonate with their leadership journey and what else may be emerging for them.

From Defensive to Generative Leadership

At the core of this journey is the recognition that modern leadership is less about controlling complexity or merely exercising authority, and more about effectively navigating the intricacies of human systems and change. As waves of disruption sweep through organisations and societies, some leaders construct barriers, seeking to shield themselves and their teams from the turbulence. Others, however, choose to harness these very winds, transforming them into sources of energy, movement, and innovation.

Leadership models and approaches reflect a central theme across chapters, demonstrating how their dynamic use can support practice and ongoing generative learning in the role. As highlighted in the section on *Rising with the Tide* and *Phoenix Leadership*, effective leadership today is not about resisting change or attempting to insulate ourselves from unpredictability. Rather, it involves engaging with uncertainty and the evolving socio-technological world (Chapter 27) as a catalyst for growth, resilience, and transformation, while staying connected to the strategic core task.

Defensive leadership—often rooted in fear, perceived threat, overload, or vulnerability—tends to manifest in rigid hierarchies and an overreliance on control. When stakes are high or contexts feel chaotic, leaders may contract around tight control, a need for certainty, and an overemphasis on individual responsibility, rather than fostering shared accountability. This impulse is understandable: it seeks to reduce anxiety, impose order, and preserve authority. Yet, such approaches can stifle creativity, breed mistrust, and lead to stagnation (Raelin, 2011; Obholzer & Roberts, 1994).

Leaders who neglect both the rationale for change and its emotional dimensions risk fostering toxic cultures where compliance hinders creativity and critical thinking. This dynamic often emerges when efforts to restore control, though well-intentioned, are driven by anxiety, shame, or a need to reassert authority. For example, when institutional responses to discrimination rely solely on top-down directives to signal commitment to equality, they may deepen mistrust rather than resolve it. In contrast, when leaders acknowledge the emotional undercurrents and engage in sustained, inclusive dialogue, such as forums on equity, cultures can begin to shift: from silence to shared responsibility, from defensiveness to collective learning.

Generative leaders engage with disruption. Rooted in emotional maturity, agility and systemic awareness, they invite shared sense-making and collective resilience. They do not suppress anxiety; they contain it thoughtfully, creating psychological safety while enabling experimentation and growth. Rather than leading over others, they lead with others, guided by inquiry across key domains of relevance (Table 29.1).

While adaptive leadership enables systems to steady themselves amid disruption, generative leadership goes further, transforming uncertainty into an opportunity to co-create new futures. This contrasts with the common reflex to act quickly and restore control, even when deeper inquiry is needed (Heifetz, 1994). In crises, leaders may seek immediate answers, which can heighten anxiety and hinder learning. Uncontained anxiety fuels defensive patterns within individuals and relational systems

Table 29.1 Reflective enquiry prompts for generative leadership

Domains	Guiding Questions
Sense-making and Learning	What is emerging here What are we being asked to learn?
Mission and Alignment	How does this challenge affect our core purpose?
Contextual Awareness	What psycho-social-economic parameters require attention? Who are the stakeholders? Where is alignment needed?
Leadership and Power Dynamics	What is leadership's key task, and how can it be shared? What ethical issues are at stake?
Systems and Change	What transformational and transactional frameworks support navigating change?
Resilience and Support	What keeps the workforce focused and resourced in uncertainty?

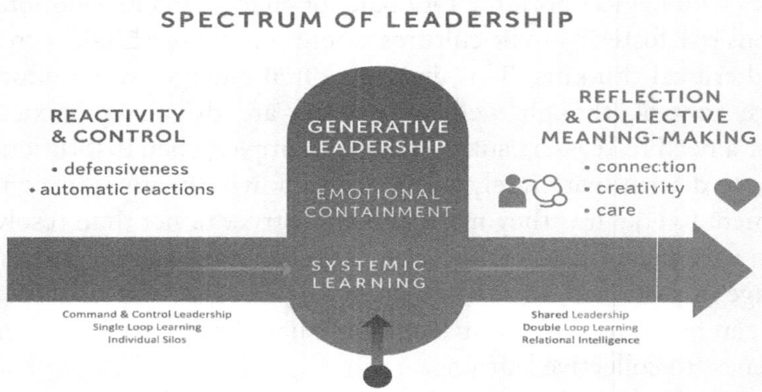

Figure 29.1 From reactivity and control to reflection and collective sense-making.

(Hirschhorn, 1990). Generative leaders recognise these dynamics and create holding environments—spaces for reflection, experimentation, and accountability to shared purpose. For instance, periods of major restructuring, such as when posts are downgraded or disbanded, often create a tense and uncertain emotional climate. Rather than defaulting to control or avoidance, leadership can engage with collective anxiety: naming it, seeking support through professional networks for them and their teams. This approach helps staff consider possibilities beyond their existing roles, exploring broader horizons, mobility, and innovative possibilities, rather than a collapse into fear, blame, or individualised shame.

This shift can be understood as a spectrum, from reactivity and control towards reflection and collective meaning-making that informs action (Figure 29.1). Generative leadership sits at the intersection of emotional containment and systemic learning to shape strategy and action. The aim isn't to remain in a generative stance at all times, but to return to it when it matters. All leaders are susceptible to defensiveness; the real work lies in recognising when we're being reactive and cultivating practices that reorient us towards the purpose, connection, creativity, and care.

Emotional Intelligence and Relational Depth in Leadership

Emotional maturity and relational intelligence are foundational to effective leadership, enabling a balance between strategic demands and the psychological conditions necessary for meaningful, sustainable work. A recurring theme throughout the book, particularly in Chapters 17, 18, 20, 21, and 26, is relational resilience: the capacity to remain grounded under pressure through deep self-awareness, emotional regulation, and the ability to foster environments where others feel safe, valued, and empowered to step into leadership themselves. Emotionally resilient leaders name, contain, and work with emotions in real time—shifting team dynamics from reactive patterns to responsive dialogue, from defensiveness to open inquiry. This is not a soft skill but a *system skill*, essential for adaptive learning, creative engagement, and psychological safety (Goleman, 2000; Edmondson, 2018).

A psychologically informed approach builds on these foundations. Leaders grounded in psychological insight and personal mastery understand that transformation rarely stems from structural fixes or top-down directives alone. True change involves supporting individuals and teams through distress, resistance, and uncertainty. By addressing the emotional tensions that often fuel organisational conflict and offering support for anxiety, such leaders help systems remain responsive, adaptive, and resilient (Scharmer, 2009; Garvey & Cooper, 2018).

Psychologically astute leaders create space for growth by recognising hidden dynamics—such as competition, envy, and unspoken loyalties—that obstruct collaboration and development. Think of such leaders as emotional thermostats: attuned to the emotional climate, they regulate their responses and recalibrate the environment to maintain a productive emotional temperature. Rather than relying on directive authority, they attend to the conscious and unconscious emotional levels with a "balance of mind" and a reality-rooted judgement to consider potential options to move forward (Hinshelwood, 2025). Through this, they enable others to stay engaged in the work, even when discomfort arises (Heifetz, Grashow, & Linsky, 2009). This is evident in organisations where, even under pressure, leaders engage their teams in shared planning and decision-making rather than acting alone.

In today's landscape of remote, hybrid work and an AI world, relational skills are not just valuable—they are essential. Drawing on both literature and lived experience, contributors to this book consistently underscore that effective leaders stay emotionally present in the face of conflict, ambiguity, and uncertainty. This presence enables teams to hold complexity rather than rushing to premature closure—a dynamic long recognised in psychoanalytic theory (Bion, 1961; Winnicott, 1960).

Such leadership demands emotional labour—absorbing organisational "toxins" while maintaining boundaries, perspective, and the capacity to stay grounded and respond constructively (Kets de Vries,

2006). It also requires *negative capability*: the ability to hold uncertainty and complexity without rushing to resolution (Wilkinson, 2006; Simpson, French, & Harvey, 2002). As some of the contributors highlight, this work is frequently invisible and ultimately unsustainable without structured support. Leaders, too, need containers—spaces such as supervision, coaching, mentoring, and peer consultation that allow for emotional processing, meaning-making, and restoration (Hawkins & Smith, 2013; Stokes, 2015; Aris et al., 2024).

A critical thread in this book is workforce wellbeing. Sustainable leadership requires enabling others to thrive and sustaining oneself. Part Five challenges the false divide between leadership and self-care. Burnout, over-functioning (taking on excessive responsibility to compensate for system gaps), and disconnection are signs of systemic strain, not personal failure. Wellbeing underpins a thriving work culture and demands a whole-systems approach grounded in shared responsibility and structural support. Emotional intelligence and relational depth are vital capacities that enable leaders to embrace ambiguity, foster inclusion, and honour courage alongside care. These qualities drive more humane, resilient, and flourishing futures.

From Direction to Co-Creation— Leading with Purpose in Collective Contexts

The key task of leadership is to hold purpose and direction while creating the conditions for collective growth through containment rooted in the reality of the situation (Hinshelwood & Mendes, 2025). Yet many risk taking it as a solitary endeavour, carrying the burden alone rather than engaging others in shared responsibility. This isolation can disconnect leadership from the very systems it aims to serve, limiting its potential and leaving vital relational dynamics untapped. Authentic leadership is not about hoarding power or seeking personal recognition but about sharing power and fostering collective ownership of the leadership process. Leadership, in this sense, is relational, distributed, and inclusive of followership. It involves enabling others to step into leadership roles and creating structures that support collective action, collaboration, and shared meaning-making. Leaders who embrace this mindset foster cultures of inclusion, trust, and mutual accountability—where diverse perspectives are not only valued but actively leveraged for collective growth (Raelin, 2011; Bourke & Dillon, 2018). In doing so, they strengthen the resilience and effectiveness of the systems they lead. For example, during periods of financial strain or uncertainty, leaders may feel pressure to act alone. Yet those who open the process—inviting staff into strategic conversations—can strengthen both trust and adaptability. Such approaches have been observed to surface new insights and foster shared ownership, contributing to more grounded and resilient organisational responses.

Themes of strategic leadership, shared power, and navigating emotional and systemic complexity are woven throughout the book, from the dedicated focus on strategic leadership (Chapter 7), eco-leadership (Chapter 2), and systems psychodynamic thinking (Chapter 4), to anti-oppressive, inclusive leadership practices in Chapters 22 and 28. The importance of emotional safety and relational trust, introduced earlier and developed in Chapters 19 to 21, has emerged as foundational to shared leadership. These chapters illuminate the conditions in which it can thrive: containment, empathy, and mutual support (Edmondson, 2019; Hawkins & Smith, 2013). This book calls for leadership rooted in purpose and shared humanity, where accountability meets emotional depth, and power is held with others, not over them. In a rapidly changing world, such co-creative leadership may be our most enduring and essential resource.

Nevertheless, working collectively is emotionally complex. Psychologically informed leadership not only fosters collective action but also acknowledges the emotional barriers that arise when groups attempt to work together under stress (Gersick, 1988; Kets de Vries, 2006; French & Vince, 2019). During times of uncertainty, defensive behaviours—such as denial or avoidance—can surface, often as unconscious attempts to shield individuals and groups from emotional discomfort. These barriers can hinder collaboration and stall progress, particularly in environments that demand emotional risk, care, or responsibility (Menzies Lyth, 1960).

Lawrence, Bain, and Gould's (1996) notions of "me-ness"—a defensive withdrawal into individuality to avoid the vulnerability and tension of group life, and "we-ness"—a fusion with the group that suppresses individuality, difference, or dissent—are helpful here. Both dynamics signal a loss of task focus and a drift into reactive or defensive modes. Leaders attuned to these unconscious processes play a critical role in providing containment (Obholzer & Roberts, 1994), helping teams process anxiety and return to the primary task with clarity, trust, and collaborative intent. Through such holding, they create psychologically safe environments where emotional experiences can be named, thought about, and worked through—ultimately supporting growth, resilience, and system-wide learning.

Like tuning an ensemble, the leader listens for discord and adjusts the relational rhythm, supporting both the strength of individual voices and the coherence of the whole.

A useful way to understand this leadership work is through the lens of "Me–We–World" (Figure 29.2).

- **Me**: attending to the inner landscape—self-awareness, emotional regulation, values, tasks, roles, alignment.
- **We**: navigating group dynamics, holding space for emotional risk, and cultivating trust and inclusion.
- **World**: holding a wider systemic view—organisational, ecological, political, societal—linking work to a broader purpose and environmental influences.

Focusing solely on "me" risks ego or isolation; only on "we" invites conformity; only on "world" risks burnout or fragmentation. Sustainable leadership weaves all three. This emotionally complex work requires not just intelligence but emotional elasticity—the capacity to hold discomfort, navigate tension, and transform fragmentation into generative friction.

Such labour is often invisible and unsustainable without support. Even emotionally attuned leaders can burn out. Sustaining collective leadership requires that this work be made visible and properly

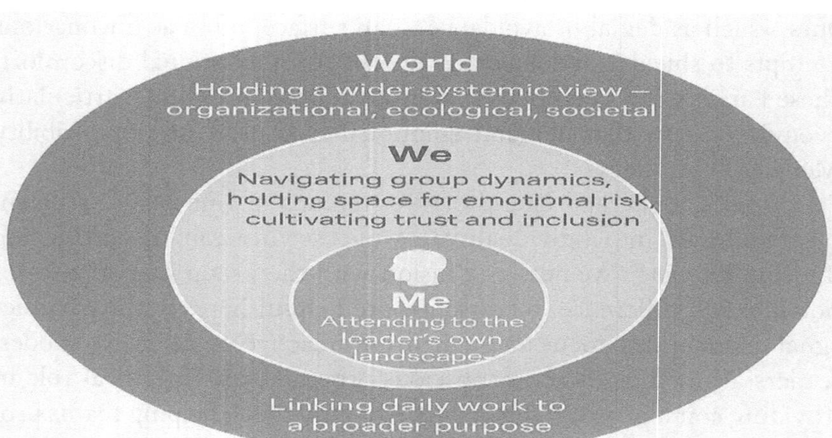

Figure 29.2 Leadership lens at Me–We–World.

resourced. Emotional literacy alone isn't enough—collective leadership depends on collective care. Workplace wellbeing, including that of those who lead, isn't peripheral; it fundamentally shapes culture, ethics, and sustainability.

The Courage to Lead with Humanity

As highlighted across this book, the call is to lead with courage—the courage to challenge the status quo, to engage in difficult conversations, and to advocate for change that benefits not just the individual but the collective. This thread runs through contributions on anti-oppressive leadership, trauma-informed practice, and compassionate care. It requires not only professional expertise but also a commitment to our shared humanity, ensuring that leadership is never reduced to personal gain or recognition, in contrast to many examples seen in organisational life.

True leadership, as explored in chapters on political acumen, systems thinking, and humility, involves fostering cultures of learning and inclusion, adapting one's approach to context, people, and the core task at hand (Raelin, 2016; Schein, 2010). Whether navigating organisational conflict (Chapter 13) or shaping equitable community-centred systems (Chapters 26 and 28), leading with humanity and humility requires strength and care.

Psychologists are uniquely positioned to lead in this way at all stages of their careers. By integrating psychological insight with leadership practice—and by embodying humility, self-care, and emotional acuity—they model what it means to lead with both backbone and heart. In times of difficulty, when decisions carry emotional weight, we must resist dehumanising others or labelling individuals as "troublesome." Spaces for reflection and dialogue are vital for ethical, inclusive decision-making grounded in integrity and care (Brown, 2018; Goleman, 1998). When organisations become fixated on outcomes, ethical considerations can come under intense pressure, risking marginalisation or compromise. In such moments, psychologically informed thinking is essential to help leaders remain attuned to the human and systemic costs of their decisions.

This is the challenge for psychologists and leaders alike: to reject the myth of the lone, heroic leader; to move beyond individual self-interest; and to support others in stepping into leadership. In this way, leadership becomes a shared endeavour, one rooted in empathy, humanness, trust, and commitment to building healthier organisations, communities, and societies.

Inclusion, Equity, and Diversity: Practice Amid Tension

Building on the ethical and psychological foundations explored earlier, this section turns explicitly to the theme of leadership in the face of structural injustice and marginalisation.

Inclusion, equity, and diversity are not the soft side of leadership; they are its ethical foundation. Not a checklist. Not a one-off training. But a sustained act of responsibility. To lead in today's complex systems is to confront how power operates, often invisibly, within our structures, cultures, and everyday decisions.

The realities are stark. Bullying, racism, microaggressions, and exclusionary norms persist across sectors. Whistleblowers who raise concerns often do so at great personal cost. People from racialised, disabled, LGBTQ+, and other minoritised backgrounds face systemic barriers to voice, advancement, and psychological safety. These are not isolated incidents or individual failings—they are embedded, structural patterns. Leadership plays a critical role in either perpetuating or dismantling them.

Situating this work within the historical context and evolution of psychology as a profession reveals its dual potential: to reinforce the status quo or to act as a transformative force in society. Psychology's engagement with social change—from early clinical roots to its current applications in public health, education, and policy—highlights both its influence and its responsibility. In cross-cultural and global leadership contexts, this responsibility is magnified, demanding cultural humility, awareness of colonial legacies, and sensitivity to how psychological constructs travel across cultural boundaries.

This challenge is taken up across the book, particularly in the section Breaking the Mould: Race, Culture, and Identity—Can Leadership Truly Transform Without Confronting Power Dynamics? (Chapters 22–24), which argues that leadership cannot evolve without a direct reckoning with race, identity, and systemic inequality. It interrogates power and empowerment, implicit bias—both conscious and unconscious—exclusionary norms, and the emotional labour required to resist dominant expectations. Leaders are called to use their influence to challenge inequity, redistribute power, and create inclusive leadership spaces. This means moving beyond traditional paradigms of control towards leadership that disrupts hierarchy and centres equity, mutual agency, and social responsibility.

This kind of leadership is transformative. It breaks with the status quo, resists exclusion, and fosters cultures where people can show up fully, especially those historically pushed to the margins. It requires the courage to challenge dominant narratives, centre lived experience, and lead with authenticity, even amid discomfort or resistance.

The work is difficult. Efforts towards inclusion often provoke defensiveness, discomfort, and pushback. Leaders may be accused of creating division when they name inequity or disrupt norms through initiatives such as widening access to marginalised groups. Yet these tensions are not barriers to leadership—they *are* the work of leadership, not only for those in formal Equality Diversity Inclusive specialist roles, but for all. As Kline (2020) reminds us, meaningful progress on racism and bullying demands both moral courage and systemic intervention. Failing to engage in this work doesn't just weaken leadership; it undermines the quality and equity of services delivered to diverse communities.

Leadership here demands cultural humility, critical self-reflection, and moral stamina. It means fostering environments where people can speak openly without fear—where, for example, a junior clinician raising concerns about discriminatory practice is met with listening, reflection, and reparative action, not silence or sanction. Such responses show accountable leadership. Because microaggressions often go unseen by those in dominant roles, change starts with awareness—and must be followed by accountability (Sue, 2010).

This requires reckoning with our complicity. A defensive or distant response risks scapegoating the complainant and blocking systemic reflection. Leaders, especially psychologists, must examine how their identities and privileges shape the systems they influence. As Turner and Sherwood (2021) note, progress lies not in isolated "bias training" but in embedding anti-oppressive practice into governance, resource allocation, and leadership development.

True leadership recognises that inclusion is not about perfection; it's about persistence. It means acknowledging when harm has occurred, responding with integrity, and transforming systems to reduce their recurrence. These moments, when difficult truths surface, are the crucibles in which accountable leadership is forged.

Inclusion is not an add-on to humane leadership—it is its most rigorous test.

Developing Leadership: A Path to Impact

This final theme synthesises insights from across the book to reflect on leadership as a dynamic developmental journey towards meaningful impact. Throughout this leadership odyssey, several interwoven themes have emerged—each highlighting the evolving nature of leadership in a complex and uncertain world.

At its core, leadership today is not about control, certainty, or rigid authority. It is about the capacity to navigate complexity dynamically with emotional intelligence and relational depth—seeing disruption not as a threat, but as a catalyst for growth and transformation. Generative leadership leans into uncertainty, asks powerful questions, and cultivates environments that support adaptability, collaboration, and shared meaning. This approach requires emotional maturity: deep self-awareness, the ability to regulate anxiety, and a commitment to fostering psychological safety. When coupled with clear purpose and direction, this stance creates space for reflection, connection, and resilience, buffering against burnout and enabling teams to thrive.

Leadership, as explored in this book, is fundamentally an ecological process: interconnected, collective, distinct from, yet enriched by, management acumen (Chapters 2 and 3). While leadership centres on vision, purpose, and people, leaders must also attend to strategic delivery and the operational dimensions of management. It flourishes when power is shared, voices are included, and trust is actively built. Psychologically informed leadership recognises the ethical dilemmas, dialectical tensions, and emotional undercurrents within organisations, offering direction and thoughtful containment amidst uncertainty. It involves holding space for discomfort without rushing to resolution, maintaining transparency, and enabling groups to stay engaged in the work. In today's complex landscape, leaders across politics, public services, and the private sector face intense financial pressures, competition for resources, environmental challenges, and demanding output expectations, to name a few (Chapter 1). Those drawing on psychological system-based insight do not bypass these realities but engage with them reflectively, navigating competing demands while attending to emotional climates, enabling meaning-making, and modelling ethical, values-driven decision-making under pressure, all while recognising the personal impact of such work.

Leadership today transcends disciplines. The approaches explored in this book apply across sectors: academia, healthcare, government, finance, and non-profits, because all human systems demand thoughtful, adaptive, and emotionally attuned leadership. Organisations are, after all, living human systems—rich with complexity, vulnerability, and potential. To evolve leadership for our time, interdisciplinary dialogue and cross-sector learning are essential. They open space for grappling with key tensions such as: What does it take to lead wisely, fostering purpose-driven systems in a world where ethical integrity may conflict with measurable outcomes, and care for people may clash with performance pressure? Can we remain in dialogue, value-led, task-focused, and human-centred while navigating these paradoxes?

Leadership development is not a solitary pursuit, nor can it be reduced to traits or technical training. It grows through role-taking, embracing ongoing responsibility, and sustaining relational connection with others. For this growth to flourish, organisations must create enabling conditions—authorising leadership across levels and embedding values of collaboration, compassion, and equity into their systems. This includes supporting both horizontal development (gaining new skills and knowledge) and vertical development (deepening leaders' capacity to think, relate, and act in more complex, adaptive ways) (Petrie, 2014; Sounding Board Inc., 2023). Psychologically informed leadership is supported not only by insight but by environments that nourish responsibility, reflection, and connection amidst complexity and paradox.

Psychologists already lead in meaningful ways—for example, shaping policy and advancing public and organisational wellbeing. Their understanding of human behaviour, emotional dynamics, and group processes equips them to navigate the tensions inherent in leadership roles. In public discourse, they bring nuance to complex issues such as trauma, identity, and power, while promoting equity through dialogue and systemic change. Through coaching and consultation, they build others' leadership capacities. At a systems level, they support organisations in moving from siloed hierarchies to more collective, resilient cultures. There is further potential to extend their influence by drawing on diverse branches of applied psychology and learning from adjacent disciplines.

Leading in complexity, however, requires more than insight. It calls for psychological, systemic, critical, political, intercultural and economic acumen—blending value creation with self-awareness, the capacity to hold paradox, stay relational under pressure, and navigate discomfort and unconscious group dynamics. As leadership often evokes anxiety and projection (Menzies Lyth, 1960; Obholzer & Roberts, 1994), psychologists must also invest in their own growth through supervision, peer support, and reflective practice. The insights explored in this book invite psychologists to step forward with greater clarity and confidence, while resourcing themselves for the emotional and systemic demands of leadership. In doing so, they can help shape healthier, more equitable systems where leadership is rooted in care, connection, and collective flourishing.

As we look ahead, several vital questions require attention:

- What will it take to shift from individual heroism to shared leadership, especially when the pull for self-recognition overshadows the need to uplift others?
- How can we support leaders to stay present with complexity, rather than defaulting to quick fixes or rigid certainty in high-pressure environments?
- What might leadership become when power and voice are more equitably distributed—when we lead within systems, not silos?

Additionally:

- How do leaders sustain themselves emotionally and ethically over the long haul, especially when change is slow, contested, or invisible?
- How do we remain accountable to those most impacted by our decisions, especially when their voices have long been marginalised?

Finally, reflecting on our practise:

- In what ways are we, consciously or unconsciously, reproducing the very dynamics we seek to change?
- What enables open, reflective debate on the ethical and paradoxical dilemmas of leadership, and how might such dialogue be cultivated, sustained, and protected within systems under pressure amid rising global conflicts?
- What does it mean to leave a leadership legacy defined not just by influence, but by stewardship and regeneration?

These questions call for deep reflection and systemic inquiry into power, politics, ethics, economics, sustainability, and the cultural dynamics that shape leadership. They demand both personal accountability and collective responsibility to sustain open, values-led dialogue in complex systems. But beyond introspection, they also require external action: from employers, institutions, policymakers, and professional bodies to lead with integrity and invest in the conditions that nurture future leadership. These actors may hold formal authority, but they are also part of the wider leadership system, subject to the same tensions, responsibilities, and opportunities for transformation. A collective, open dialogue—grounded in a systemic lens, mutual accountability, and critical ecological thinking—can support the reflective practices leadership now requires.

Leadership is not a title but a practice—one to be reimagined, shared, sustained, and renewed. This book offers no fixed blueprint, but a companion for the journey: a journey shaped by courage and inquiry. The authors have brought bold, diverse perspectives, debating conventional models and offering rich ways to understand and enact leadership. They position psychology not only as a lens but as a force for transformation.

As John Dewey reminds us, "We do not learn from experience…we learn from reflecting on experience." Leadership evolves through reflection, courage, and generative action. Through this process, we become the leaders our times demand—alive to complexity, rooted in humanity, and open to possibility.

References

Aris, S., Rao, A., Roycroft, P., & Clutterbuck, D. (Eds.). (2024). *Mentoring in health, social care and beyond: A handbook for practice, training and research.* Pavilion Publishing and Media Ltd.

Bion, W. R. (1961). *Experiences in groups.* Tavistock Publications.

Bourke, J., & Dillon, B. (2018). The diversity and inclusion revolution: Eight powerful truths. *Deloitte Insights.* https://www2.deloitte.com/insights/us/en/deloitte-review/issue-22/diversity-and-inclusion-at-work-eight-powerful-truths.html

Brown, B. (2018). *Dare to lead: Brave work. Tough conversations. Whole hearts.* Random House.

Dewey, J. (1933). *How we think: A restatement of the relation of reflective thinking to the educative process.* D.C. Heath and Company.

Edmondson, A. C. (2018). *The fearless organization: Creating psychological safety in the workplace for learning, innovation, and growth.* Wiley.

Edmondson, A. C. (2019). *Teaming: How organizations learn, innovate, and compete in the knowledge economy* (2nd ed.). Wiley.

French, R., & Vince, R. (2019). *Group relations, management and organisation.* Oxford University Press.

Garvey Berger, J., & Cooper, R. (2018). *Unlocking leadership mindtraps: How to thrive in complexity.* Stanford Business Books.

Gersick, C. J. G. (1988). Time and transition in work teams: Toward a new model of group development. *Academy of Management Journal, 31*(1), 9–41. https://doi.org/10.2307/256496

Goleman, D. (1998). *Working with emotional intelligence.* Bantam Books.

Goleman, D. (2000). Leadership that gets results. *Harvard Business Review, 78*(2), 78–90.

Hawkins, P., & Smith, N. (2013). *Coaching, mentoring and organisational consultancy: Supervision and development* (2nd ed.). McGraw-Hill Education.

Heifetz, R. A. (1994). *Leadership without easy answers.* Harvard University Press.

Heifetz, R., Grashow, A., & Linsky, M. (2009). *The practice of adaptive leadership: Tools and tactics for changing your organization and the world.* Harvard Business Press.

Hinshelwood, R. D. (2023). Unconscious anxieties in organizations. In B. Huppertz (Ed.), The psychology of organizations and workplace issues: Resolving everyday conflicts (pp. 73–82). Lexington Books.

Hinshelwood, R. D., & Mendes, T. (Eds.). (2025). *Containment, organisations and the working task.* Routledge.

Hirschhorn, L. (1990). The workplace within: Psychodynamics of organizational life. MIT Press.

Kets de Vries, M. F. R. (2006). *The leader on the couch: A clinical approach to changing people and organizations.* Jossey-Bass.

Kline, N. (2020). *The courage to lead: A mindfulness approach to confronting racism and bullying in organisations.* Routledge.

Kline, R. (2020). *Healing the wounds: The promise of mindfulness in organizational life.* Routledge.

Lawrence, W. G., Bain, A., & Gould, L. (1996). The fifth basic assumption: A leadership study. *Group Analysis, 29*(1), 77–90. https://doi.org/10.1177/053331649602900105

Menzies Lyth, I. (1960). A case study in the functioning of social systems as a defence against anxiety: A report on a study of the nursing service of a general hospital. *Human Relations, 13*(2), 95–121. https://doi.org/10.1177/001872676001300204

Obholzer, A., & Roberts, V. Z. (1994). *The unconscious at work: Individual and organisational stress in the human services.* Routledge.

Petrie, N. (2014). *Future trends in leadership development.* Center for Creative Leadership. https://www.ccl.org/articles/white-papers/future-trends-in-leadership-development/

Raelin, J. A. (2011). From leadership-as-practice to leaderful practice. *Leadership, 7*(2), 195–211. https://doi.org/10.1177/1742715010394804

Raelin, J. A. (2016). *Leadership-as-practice: Theory and application.* Routledge.

Scharmer, O. C. (2009). *Theory U: Leading from the future as it emerges*. Berrett-Koehler Publishers.

Schein, E. H. (2010). *Organizational culture and leadership* (4th ed.). Jossey-Bass.

Simpson, P., French, R., & Harvey, C. (2002). Leadership and negative capability. *Human Relations, 55*(10), 1209–1226. https://doi.org/10.1177/0018726702055010002

Sounding Board Inc. (2023). *The new leadership paradigm: Unlocking the potential of vertical development*. https://www.soundingboardinc.com/resources/whitepapers/the-new-leadership-paradigm

Stokes, P. (2015). *Peer supervision in organisations: A guide for practitioners*. Palgrave Macmillan.

Sue, D. W. (2010). *Microaggressions in everyday life: Race, gender, and sexual orientation*. Wiley.

Turner, A., & Sherwood, J. (2021). Embedding anti-oppressive leadership: A systemic approach to governance and development. *Journal of Organizational Change Management, 34*(4), 755–772. https://doi.org/10.1108/JOCM-11-2020-0347.

Wilkinson, H. (2006). *Uncomfortable learning: The role of negative capability in leadership*. [Report]. The King's Fund.

Winnicott, D. W. (1960). The theory of the parent-infant relationship. *International Journal of Psycho-Analysis, 41*, 585–595.

Glossary of Terms

Adaptive Leadership

A developmental and relational approach to leadership focused on navigating complex, uncertain, and systemic challenges. Adaptive leaders engage people in identifying underlying issues, shifting mindsets, and experimenting with new ways of working to foster resilience and long-term transformation. It emphasises learning, emotional intelligence, and mobilising collective energy rather than technical fixes.

See also: Change Leadership, Change Management

Advocacy and Policy Influence

Strategic actions aimed at shaping public policies, institutional practices, and systemic priorities through evidence, persuasion, and collaboration. In leadership contexts, this involves amplifying voices, influencing for impact and influence, challenging inequities, and working within or alongside decision-making structures and stakeholders to promote change aligned with strategy and ethical, psychological, and social values.

See also: Policy Development, Systems Leadership.

Agile Organizations

Purpose-driven, adaptive systems designed to navigate complexity and evolving contexts through decentralised decision-making, cross-disciplinary stakeholders' collaboration, and iterative learning. Rooted in agile principles, they foster responsiveness, innovation, and psychological safety, enabling leadership that is inclusive, systems-aware, and resilient in the face of change.

See also: Adaptive Leadership, Complexity Theory, Psychological Safety.

Anti-Oppressive Practice

A framework and set of actions aimed at actively challenging power imbalances, systemic oppression, and discrimination within organisations and society.

See also: Anti-Racism, Social Justice.

Antiracism

A proactive and sustained commitment to identifying, challenging, and dismantling racism in all its forms: individual, institutional, and structural. Antiracist leadership involves not only recognising the impact of racial inequity but actively transforming policies, practices, and power dynamics to create inclusive, equitable environments. It requires critical self-reflection, cultural humility, and collective responsibility.

See also: Racism, Structural Racism, Cultural Humility.

Anxiety

A psychological and physiological state marked by heightened alertness, worry, or fear in response to perceived threat or uncertainty. While often associated with clinical conditions, anxiety also functions as a signal emotion in leadership and organisational life, surfacing around threat, change, ambiguity, or relational tension. Understanding and working with anxiety is central to emotionally intelligent, psychologically attuned leadership.

See also: Emotional Intelligence, Psychological Safety, Stress.

Authenticity

The alignment between one's values, emotions, and actions, expressed with honesty and integrity in relationship to others. In leadership, authenticity involves showing up with self-awareness, transparency, and congruence—balancing inner alignment with relational sensitivity and systemic responsibility. It fosters trust, psychological safety, and deeper connections in complex and diverse contexts.

See also: Emotional Intelligence, Relational Leadership, Psychological Safety.

Authoritarian Leadership

A directive, top-down leadership style characterised by centralised control, limited input from others, and a focus on obedience, order, and discipline. Often rooted in assumptions of hierarchy and power-over dynamics, it can suppress autonomy, reduce psychological safety, and hinder adaptive capacity in complex systems. While sometimes effective in crisis or high-risk settings, it contrasts with relational, inclusive, and generative approaches to leadership.

See also: Leadership Styles, Adaptive Leadership, Generative Leadership.

Authority and Power

Interrelated concepts central to leadership dynamics. Authority refers to the legitimate right to lead, often granted by role, expertise, or relational trust. Power is the capacity to influence others and shape outcomes—formally or informally—based on identity, position, relationships, or systemic structures. Effective leadership involves recognising how power operates, using authority with accountability, and navigating both responsibly to enable equity, inclusion, and collective agency.

See also: Leadership Politics, Privilege, Power Imbalance.

Autonomy

The degree of independence, self-direction, and discretion individuals or teams hold in decision-making within an organisation. Responsible autonomy is paired with accountability, ensuring that the freedom to act is aligned with shared goals, ethical standards, and responsibility for outcomes. It supports motivation, innovation, and learning, and is often associated with decentralised leadership and participative cultures.

See also: Participative Cultures, Leadership Development, Organisational Structures.

Barriers

Obstacles that hinder progress, participation, or change at individual, relational, organisational, or systemic levels. In leadership contexts, barriers may be internal (e.g., fear, bias, impostor feelings), interpersonal (e.g., conflict, exclusion), or structural (e.g., policies, hierarchies, discrimination). Recognising and addressing barriers is essential for creating equitable, psychologically safe, and adaptive environments.

See also: Bias, Marginalisation, Inclusion.

Basic Assumptions

Unconscious group behaviours identified by Wilfred Bion that influence emotional and relational dynamics often diverting attention from the primary task. Classic types include Dependency, Fight-Flight, and Pairing. Expanded concepts include Me-ness, One-ness, Bystanding, Social Defence Mechanisms, and distinctions between Work Groups and Basic Assumption Groups. Recognising these patterns helps leaders manage anxiety and maintain task focus.

See also: Primary Task, Group Dynamics, Containment, Work Group.

Bias (Unconscious/Implicit)

Hidden beliefs or attitudes that influence perception and decision-making without conscious awareness, despite good intentions. Bias can reinforce inequality, limit inclusion, and affect leadership by undermining trust, distorting judgement, and weakening team cohesion.

See also: Privilege Blindness, Intersectionality, Inclusion, Blind spots.

Big Time Bads

Deeply held, often unconscious fears and assumptions that create invisible boundaries, triggering resistance and defensive behaviours to change within individuals or organisations.

See also: Defence Mechanisms, Organisational Anxiety, Resistance to Change.

Blind Spots

Unconscious areas of perception or behaviour where individuals or groups fail to recognise their own biases, limitations, or impacts. In leadership, blind spots can hinder self-awareness, decision-making, and relational effectiveness, often perpetuating systemic inequities or conflict. Addressing blind spots requires reflective practice, feedback, and openness to diverse perspectives.

See also: Emotional Intelligence, Reflective Practice, Bias.

Burnout

A state of chronic physical, emotional, and mental exhaustion resulting from prolonged exposure to stressors such as excessive workload, lack of control, and insufficient support. It often leads to feelings of reduced competence, low self-efficacy, decreased motivation, emotional detachment, and impaired performance. Recognising and addressing burnout is essential for sustaining wellbeing, resilience, and effective leadership in complex, demanding environments.

See also: Occupational Health, Resilience, Psychological Wellbeing.

Burnout Resilience

The capacity to withstand, adapt to, and recover from prolonged stressors and workplace demands that can lead to burnout. It involves cultivating self-awareness, effective coping strategies, supportive relationships, and organisational conditions that promote psychological safety, balance, and sustainable performance. Building and supporting conditions for burnout resilience is essential for maintaining wellbeing and sustained leadership effectiveness in complex and high-pressure environments.

See also: Resilience, Psychological Safety.

Change Agents

Individuals or groups who actively facilitate, champion, and drive transformational change within organisations or systems. They possess the skills, influence, and resilience to navigate resistance, mobilise stakeholders, and embed new practices that foster innovation, inclusion, and adaptive leadership in complex environments.

See also: Change Leadership, Change Management, Transformational Leadership.

Change Fatigue

A state of exhaustion and reduced capacity to engage effectively due to prolonged or repeated organisational change initiatives. Change fatigue can result in resistance, disengagement, and decreased wellbeing, posing significant challenges to change management efforts. Recognising and addressing change fatigue is vital for sustaining momentum and resilience.

See also: Change Management, Large Scale Change, Organisational Culture.

Change Leadership

A strategic and people-centred approach that focuses on inspiring and guiding individuals and organisations through the emotional and behavioural aspects of change. Change leaders build vision, foster engagement, and address resistance by aligning culture, motivation, and communication to enable successful transitions. It bridges adaptive and technical aspects by managing the human dynamics essential for sustainable change.

See also: Adaptive Leadership, Change Management.

Change Management

A structured, technical, and process-driven discipline concerned with planning, executing, and controlling the practical steps required to implement change initiatives. It involves methodologies, tools, and frameworks to manage timelines, resources, stakeholder engagement, and risk to ensure change is delivered effectively and efficiently. Change management often supports the tactical implementation within broader adaptive or change leadership efforts.

See also: Adaptive Leadership, Change Leadership.

Clinical Leadership

The practice of applying clinical expertise and leadership skills to influence the delivery of high-quality care at various levels—from individual patient care to system-wide strategy—by integrating evidence, experience, and collaboration with stakeholders.

See also: Healthcare Leadership, Systems Leadership, Collaborative Leadership.

Co-Production – Lived Experience Involvement

A collaborative approach that actively involves individuals with lived experience—such as patients, clients, or community members—in designing, delivering, and evaluating services or interventions. It values experiential knowledge equally alongside professional expertise, fostering empowerment, shared decision-making, and more relevant, equitable outcomes within systems and organisations.

See also: Community Engagement, Participatory Leadership.

Coaching

A collaborative, goal-oriented process that supports individuals or teams in unlocking their potential, enhancing self-awareness, and developing skills to achieve personal and professional growth and enhanced performance. Rooted in active listening, powerful questioning, and reflective dialogue, coaching fosters accountability, resilience, and adaptive leadership in complex and evolving environments.

See also: Mentoring, Leadership Development, Reflective Practice.

Cognitive Analytical Therapy (CAT)

An integrative therapeutic model that maps reciprocal relationship roles ('doing' and 'feeling' positions) between individuals to understand relational patterns, dilemmas, and dynamics. Applied in leadership, CAT helps identify and repair ruptures to improve relational dynamics, communication, and organisational culture.

See also: Relational Leadership, Reflective Practice.

Collective Leadership

A relational and distributed approach to leadership where responsibility, influence, and decision-making are shared across individuals and groups. It fosters collaboration, mutual accountability, and the co-creation of vision and strategy, enabling adaptive responses and systemic change within complex, interconnected environments.

See also: Systems Leadership, Collaborative Leadership.

Commissioning and Provider Partnerships

Collaborative relationships between organisations that commission services (such as healthcare purchasers or funders) and those that deliver them (service providers). These partnerships focus on aligning goals, sharing accountability, and coordinating resources to improve service quality, equity, and outcomes within complex, integrated systems.

See also: Integrated Care Systems.

Community Mental Health Interventions

Coordinated efforts and programs designed to promote mental wellbeing, prevent mental illness, and provide support within community settings. These interventions prioritise accessibility, cultural relevance, and collaboration with local stakeholders to address social determinants of mental health and foster resilience at individual and collective levels.

See also: Public Health, Community Engagement, Socio-economic Determinants of Health.

Community of Practice

A group of individuals who share a common interest or profession and engage in ongoing collective learning, knowledge sharing, and problem-solving. Through collaboration and mutual support, communities of practice foster innovation, professional development, and the co-creation of best practices within complex organisational or systemic contexts.

See also: *Organisational Culture.*

Complex Adaptive Systems

Systems characterised by dynamic interactions, emergent behaviours, and continuous adaptation to internal and external changes.

See also: Complexity Theory, Systems Thinking, Adaptive Leadership.

Complexity Theory

A framework for understanding systems characterised by numerous interconnected components whose interactions produce unpredictable, emergent behaviours. It recognises that organisations and social systems are dynamic, nonlinear, and adaptive, requiring flexible leadership approaches that embrace uncertainty, feedback loops, and continual learning. Complexity theory informs practices that support innovation, resilience, and systemic change.

See also: Systems Thinking, Adaptive Leadership.

Conflict Navigation

The skill of addressing and transforming tension or disagreement into constructive dialogue and resolution.

Conscious-Unconscious Competence Model

A framework describing the stages of learning and skill acquisition, moving from unconscious incompetence (unaware of what one does not know), through conscious incompetence and conscious competence (aware and deliberately applying skills), to unconscious competence, where skills become automatic and integrated. This model informs leadership development by highlighting the evolving nature of self-awareness, mastery, and reflective practice.

See also: Leadership Development, Reflective Practice, Emotional Intelligence.

Containment (Psychological)

The process by which leaders or groups provide a holding environment that absorbs, regulates, and processes difficult emotions and anxieties. In leadership, containment manifests through creating safe spaces for open dialogue, managing conflict constructively, and supporting teams to navigate uncertainty and complexity without becoming overwhelmed.

See also: Holding Environment, Psychological Safety, Emotional Intelligence

Contextual Leadership

Leadership that is responsive to the political, economic, organisational, and social environment in which it occurs.

See also: Adaptive Leadership, Systems Leadership, Political Skills.

Cultural Humility

A lifelong, reflective practice that goes beyond cultural competence. It involves recognising one's own shifting privileges, acknowledging the limitations of one's perspective, and approaching others with curiosity, openness, and respect. Cultural humility centres on relationships, listens deeply, and avoids assumptions based on appearances or dominant narratives.

See also: Anti-Racism, Inclusion.

Culturally Sensitive Clinical Practice

Service that is respectful of, and responsive to, the diverse cultural backgrounds, values, beliefs, and needs of individuals and communities.

See also: Cultural Humility, Equity.

Data-Driven Decision Making

Using high-quality, ethically managed data to monitor progress, inform adjustments, support accountability, and drive continuous improvement in policy and practise.

See also: Quality Improvement.

Decolonising Psychology

Critically examining and dismantling the colonial influences embedded in psychological theories, practices, and research to promote inclusive, culturally relevant, and socially just approaches.

See also: Cultural Humility, Social Justice, Anti-Oppressive Practice, Anti-Racism.

Defensive Organisational Patterns

Recurrent behavioural and relational dynamics within organisations that serve to protect against anxiety and perceived threats but can hinder learning and adaptation. One key example is the Survival Task (a systems psychodynamic concept), where the focus shifts away from the primary task—the essential purpose or core function a system, group, or organisation must perform to survive and fulfill its reason for existence—to defensive, rigid behaviours that maintain organisational stability at the expense of effectiveness.

See also: Organisational Anxiety, Social Defences, Survival Task.

Disability

A long-term physical or mental impairment that substantially limits one or more major life activities, including work. In workplace contexts, it includes recognised conditions that require reasonable adjustments to enable full participation and access, as stipulated by equality and employment legislation.

See also: Inclusion, Equity, Reasonable Adjustments.

Distributed Leadership

A model of leadership that is not tied to hierarchy or formal authority. Instead, leadership is enacted through relationships, context, and shared responsibility, enabling all members of the ecosystem to contribute to meaningful change.

See also: Collective Leadership, Systems Leadership, Collaborative Leadership, Eco Leadership.

Diversity, Equity, and Inclusion (DEI)

A commitment to recognising and valuing differences, ensuring fair treatment, access, and participation for all, and fostering a sense of belonging in organisations.

See also: Equity, Inclusion, Anti-Oppressive Practice.

Driver Diagram

A structured visual tool used in Quality Improvement (QI) to clarify and communicate how a specific improvement goal will be achieved. It identifies the aim (desired outcome), outlines primary drivers (key factors directly influencing the aim), secondary drivers (subcomponents or enablers), and change ideas (specific actions or interventions). Driver diagrams support strategic alignment, shared understanding, and targeted action within complex healthcare and organisational systems.

See also: Quality Improvement, Systems Thinking, Change Management.

Eco-Leadership

A leadership paradigm that emphasises connectivity, ethics, and sustainability in response to complex, networked, and rapidly changing systems. Eco-leadership involves leading as part of an ecosystem, focusing on distributed influence, systemic thinking, relational intelligence, and social and ecological responsibility. It invites leaders to act as facilitators of collective intelligence and transformation within interconnected environments.

See also: Systems Thinking, Generative Leadership, Distributed Leadership.

Economic Literacy

The ability to understand and interpret economic principles, such as supply and demand, cost structures, and market dynamics within the context of service delivery. Economic literacy enables leaders to make informed decisions, advocate effectively, and design financially sustainable services.

Ecosystems of Care

A reimagining of healthcare as a living network of relationships, where services are integrated and shaped by mutual support, trust, and adaptability. This contrasts with transactional or target-driven models, highlighting care as an emergent, relational process.

See also: Integrated Care Systems, Collaborative Care, Systems Leadership, Eco Leadership

Emergent Task

New responsibilities or roles that arise in response to environmental complexity or organisational change.

See also: Primary Task, Adaptive Leadership, Complexity Theory.

Emotional Intelligence

The capacity to recognise, understand, and manage one's own emotions and those of others. It involves self-awareness, emotional regulation, empathy, and relational attunement—skills that enable effective communication, trust-building, and decision-making. In leadership, emotional intelligence is essential for navigating complexity, fostering psychological safety, and cultivating inclusive, emotionally resilient teams and systems.

See also: Psychological Safety, Adaptive Leadership, Self-Awareness.

Emotional Labour

Effort individuals invest in managing their emotions and emotional expressions to meet the expectations of their professional role or social environment. This often involves consciously adjusting outward emotions (surface acting) or internally aligning feelings with expected displays (deep acting), particularly in service-oriented or relationally demanding roles. While emotional labour can foster trust and connection, its cumulative impact, especially when unacknowledged, can lead to emotional exhaustion, disconnection, and burnout. Recognising and supporting emotional labour is essential for sustainable, compassionate, and psychologically safe leadership and workplace cultures.

See also: Burnout, Psychological Safety, Wellbeing, Empathy.

Empathy

The capacity to understand and resonate with the experiences, thoughts, and emotions of others.

- **Cognitive empathy** refers to the ability to intellectually understand another person's perspective.
- **Emotional empathy** involves feeling what others feel through emotional attunement.
- **Empathic concern** reflects a compassionate, other-oriented response—a motivation to care for or support others.

In leadership, empathy enables deep listening, inclusive engagement, and relational trust. It plays a vital role in navigating complexity, supporting wellbeing, and cultivating psychologically safe, emotionally intelligent environments.

See also: Emotional Intelligence, Relational Leadership, Psychological Safety, Emotional Labour

Ethics

The principles and values that guide decisions, behaviours, and relationships in personal, professional, and organisational life. In leadership, ethics involves navigating complex moral dilemmas with integrity, transparency, and accountability, balancing individual, collective, and systemic considerations. Ethical leadership requires critical reflection, cultural humility, and a commitment to justice, equity, and the wellbeing of others.

See also: Moral Distress, Cultural Humility, Power (in Leadership Context), Anti-Oppressive Practice, Leadership Risks, Moral Injury, Organisational Justice.

Generative Leadership

A transformative approach to leadership that focuses on creating the conditions for growth, innovation, and collective learning. Rather than directing or controlling, generative leaders foster meaning-making, dialogue, and relational trust, enabling others to think creatively, act collaboratively, and respond adaptively to complexity. It emphasises emergence, inclusion, and the co-creation of new possibilities across systems.

See also: Collective Leadership, Systems Thinking, Emotional Intelligence, Adaptive Leadership, Eco-Leadership.

Group Dynamics

The psychological and relational patterns of behaviour, communication, and emotional processes within groups that impact their ability to achieve the primary task. Drawing on Wilfred Bion's theory, group dynamics involve balancing the conscious focus on task-related work with unconscious "basic assumption" behaviours (such as dependency, fight-flight, and pairing) that can disrupt group effectiveness. Skilled leadership requires recognising and managing these dynamics to foster cohesion, containment, and productive collaboration.

See also: Primary Task, Basic Assumptions, Containment, Leadership Challenges.

Health Inequalities

Systematic, avoidable, and unjust differences in health status or access to healthcare experienced by different population groups. These disparities are driven by social determinants such as socioeconomic status, race, geography, and systemic discrimination. Addressing health inequalities requires leadership that recognises structural factors, advocates for equity, and implements inclusive policies to improve outcomes for marginalised communities.

See also: Equity, Advocacy and Policy Influence, Anti-Oppressive Practice.

Holding Environment

A psychological and relational space created by leaders or groups that provides safety, support, and containment for processing difficult emotions and complex experiences. Originating from psychoanalytic theory, a holding environment enables individuals and teams to explore uncertainty, manage anxiety, and engage in reflective practice, fostering resilience, learning, and adaptive change within organisations.

See also: Containment, Psychological Safety, Reflective Practice, Emotional Intelligence.

Horizontal Development

The expansion of knowledge, skills, and competencies within existing frameworks or roles. It involves acquiring new information and improving current capabilities, but does not fundamentally change the way a person thinks or approaches challenges. In leadership development, horizontal growth complements deeper vertical development by enhancing breadth and expertise.

See also: Vertical Development.

Human-Rights-Based Approach

A framework that integrates the norms, principles, and standards of international human rights law into policy development, organisational practices, and leadership. It prioritises the dignity, equality, and participation of all individuals, especially marginalised or vulnerable groups, ensuring accountability and non-discrimination in decision-making processes. This approach fosters empowerment and systemic change towards social justice and equity.

See also: Equity, Advocacy and Policy Influence, Anti-Oppressive Practice, Cultural Humility.

Identity and Social Identity

- **Identity** refers to the multifaceted sense of self shaped by individual experiences, social roles, cultural backgrounds, and group memberships. It influences how individuals perceive themselves and others, affecting behaviour, belonging, power dynamics, and decision-making within leadership and organisational contexts.
- **Social identity** is the aspect of identity derived from membership in social groups—such as race, gender, ethnicity, profession, or community—that shapes experiences, perceptions, and interactions within societal and organisational systems. Recognising social identity is essential for understanding diversity, equity, inclusion, and the dynamics of power and privilege in leadership.

See also: Intersectionality, Privilege, Power (in Leadership Context), Cultural Humility.

Inclusive Leadership

A leadership style that values and leverages diverse identities and perspectives to create equitable, safe, and high-performing environments. While widely promoted, the term can be vague and risks superficial use. True inclusive leadership requires ongoing reflection, cultural humility, and skilful navigation of identity and difference to address systemic inequalities and build genuine belonging.

See also: Equity, Diversity and Inclusion, Managing Difference, Identity, Cultural Humility, Psychological Safety, Leader Identity Development.

Influence and Influencing Skills

The ability to shape others' perspectives, decisions, or behaviours without relying solely on formal authority. Influencing skills include active listening, framing ideas clearly, building trust, negotiating, and aligning stakeholders. Effective influence draws on emotional intelligence, credibility, and contextual awareness to navigate power dynamics and lead change.

See also: Political Skills, Emotional Intelligence, Relational Leadership, Power (in Leadership Context).

Integrated Care Systems (ICS)

A legal framework established in England (from July 2022) to deliver coordinated health and social care through regional partnerships involving the NHS, local authorities, and voluntary/community sectors. ICS emphasises local determination, cross-organisational collaboration, and the reduction of health inequalities to improve population outcomes.

See also: Health Inequalities, Collaborative Leadership, Systems Leadership, Community Partnerships.

Intersectionality

A framework that recognises how multiple social identities (such as race, gender, class, sexuality, and ability) intersect to create unique experiences of privilege and oppression. In leadership and organisational contexts, intersectionality highlights the complexity of identity and power, urging inclusive practices that address overlapping systemic barriers and promote equity for all individuals.

See also: Identity, Social Identity, Privilege, Anti-Oppressive Practice, Cultural Humility.

Job Demands–Resources (JD-R) Model

A framework explaining how job demands (e.g., workload, emotional demands) and job resources (e.g., support, autonomy, recognition) influence employee wellbeing, motivation, and performance. The model posits that excessive demands can lead to burnout, while sufficient resources promote engagement, resilience, and sustained productivity. It guides leaders and organisations in balancing demands with resources to support workforce health and organisational effectiveness.

See also: Burnout, Work Engagement, Psychological Safety, Wellbeing at Work.

Johari Window

A model illustrating self-awareness and interpersonal communication through four domains: what is known or unknown to self and others. It helps leaders develop insight into how they are perceived, encourages mutual feedback, and expands shared understanding. By supporting openness, trust, and reflective dialogue, it enhances relational intelligence and strengthens leadership effectiveness within *teams*.

See also: Emotional Intelligence, Psychological Safety.

Large-Scale Change

A complex, organisation-wide or system-wide transformation effort that involves multiple stakeholders, processes, and cultural shifts. It requires strategic vision, collaborative leadership, adaptive capacity, and sustained engagement to navigate uncertainty and embed new ways of working across diverse teams and settings.

See also: Change Management, Adaptive Leadership, Systems Thinking, Organisational Strategy.

Leadership Concepts Overview

- **Leader**

A person, formal or informal, who exercises influence, fosters collaboration, and navigates organisational dynamics, often shaping direction amid differing or evolving goals.

- **Leader identity development**

The evolving process through which individuals come to see themselves and are recognised by others as leaders. This development involves internalising leadership roles, values, and behaviours, shaped by experiences, reflection, feedback, and social context. A strong leader identity supports confidence, authenticity, and adaptive leadership in complex environments.

- **Leaderhood**

Coined by Raelin (2003), leaderhood describes a relational, co-produced model of leadership where leadership emerges through shared meaning-making and interaction, shifting focus from individual leaders to collective processes.

- **Leadership**

A multifaceted, dynamic and relational process, with varied definitions across disciplines, involving influencing and guiding individuals or groups towards goals. While definitions differ, central themes include influencing, inspiring and enabling others, navigating complexity, fostering collaboration, and creating shared purpose. Leadership is context-specific and evolves with changing environments, requiring emotional intelligence, adaptability, and relational awareness to build trust, inclusion, and sustained impact.

- **Leadership agility**

The capacity to adapt leadership style, thinking, and behaviour in response to changing, uncertain, or ambiguous contexts. Agile leaders navigate volatility with flexibility, emotional intelligence, and situational awareness, adjusting their approach to meet emerging demands while maintaining clarity of purpose and connection with others.

- **Leadership challenges**

The complex tensions and demands leaders face while navigating uncertainty, competing priorities, and evolving contexts. These may include managing organisational change, addressing relational and identity dynamics, responding to systemic inequalities, and adapting to economic pressures such as resource constraints, cost-efficiency demands, and workforce sustainability. Effective leadership requires balancing these pressures while staying purpose-driven and people-focused.

- **Leadership development**

A deliberate and ongoing process of enhancing an individual's capacity to lead effectively across diverse and complex contexts. It involves cultivating self-awareness, emotional intelligence, strategic thinking, and relational skills through formal training, experiential learning, coaching, and reflective practice. Leadership development is dynamic, context-specific, and multifaceted, requiring attention to the unique challenges of each setting. Pitfalls include overreliance on generic programs, neglecting the importance of lived experience, and failing to adapt to evolving organisational and systemic demands.

- **Leadership Potential**

The latent capacity within individuals to grow into effective leaders, encompassing personal attributes, relational skills, self-awareness, and the ability to learn and adapt. Recognising leadership potential supports talent development and inclusive succession planning across systems.

See also: Talent Development, Leadership Development, Emotional Intelligence, Emerging Leaders.

- **Leadership Politics**

The interplay of conscious and unconscious emotional tensions, alliances, and power struggles within organisations that influence outcomes beyond formal strategy. This includes navigating complex relationships, managing competing interests, and understanding how informal dynamics shape decision-making and organisational culture.

- **Leadership Risks**

The inherent vulnerabilities and exposures faced by individuals in leadership roles include isolation, derailment from role, moral injury, and the psychological toll of making high-stakes decisions in complex, uncertain environments.

- **Leadership Style**

A leader's characteristic approach to influence, shaped by personality, context, values, and organisational culture (e.g., authoritarian, participative, transformational). Effective leaders adapt their style to meet the needs of their team and situation, balancing task focus with relational dynamics.

- **Leadership theories, models, and approaches**

- **Theories** explain why and how leadership works, providing conceptual foundations (e.g., **Transformational Leadership**, **Servant Leadership**).
- **Models** simplify and illustrate key concepts and relationships, making theories accessible (e.g., **Situational Leadership Model**, **Johari Window**).
- **Approaches** are practical methods for applying leadership in context (e.g., **Adaptive Leadership**, **Inclusive Leadership**).

Understanding these distinctions enhances reflection and flexible leadership practise.

- **Leading**

The active, relational process of enacting leadership in complex, often ambiguous settings.

- **Living Leadership**

A practice-based approach to leadership grounded in reflection, co-creation, and continuous learning from lived experience.

Management

The process of planning, organising, coordinating, and controlling resources and activities to achieve specific organisational objectives efficiently and effectively. Management typically focuses on maintaining stability, implementing systems, and ensuring operational performance. While leadership emphasises vision, influence, and change, management concentrates on execution and consistency. Effective organisational success requires the integration and balance of both management and leadership functions.

See also: Leadership, Strategic Management, Organisational Strategy, Change Management.

Marginalisation

The systemic process through which individuals or groups are pushed to the edges of social, economic, or organisational life, resulting in reduced access to resources, opportunities, voice, and power. Marginalisation often arises from intersecting identities and structural inequalities, leading to exclusion, invisibility, and disadvantage. Addressing marginalisation is critical to fostering equity, inclusion, and social justice within leadership and organisational contexts.

See also: Equity, Inclusion, Privilege Blindness, Intersectionality, Anti-Oppressive Practice.

Mentoring

A developmental relationship where experienced individuals support the growth and learning of less experienced colleagues. Mentoring emphasises insight, encouragement, and the co-construction of meaning and purpose. Central to this process are role modelling and the sharing of lived experience, which build trust, inspire learning, and foster confidence. This relationship supports skill development, reflection, and leadership progression.

See also: Coaching, Leadership Development, Reflective Practice, Supervision.

Moral Distress and Injury

The emotional and psychological harm that arises when professionals face ethical dilemmas and are unable to act in line with their values, often due to structural or leadership constraints. This experience leads to feelings of guilt, shame, or a sense of betrayal. Moral distress occurs when one knows the right action but cannot take it; moral injury reflects deeper, lasting damage to moral integrity and identity. Recognising and addressing moral distress and injury is vital for ethical practice, wellbeing, and workforce resilience.

See also: Ethics, Psychological Safety, Wellbeing, Organisational Culture.

Operational Leadership

The practice of guiding and managing day-to-day activities within an organisation to ensure effective service delivery and team performance. It involves coordinating resources, solving immediate problems, maintaining standards, job planning and supporting staff, bridging strategic goals with practical action on the ground. Unlike strategic leadership, which focuses on long-term vision and organisational direction, operational leadership deals with immediate execution. It differs from clinical leadership, which centres on clinical standards and patient care quality, and professional leadership, which emphasises the development and representation of professional roles and expertise.

See also Strategic Leadership; Clinical Leadership; Professional Leadership; Management

Organisational Anxiety

The collective, often unconscious, experience of fear, uncertainty, or threat within an organisation that influences behaviour, decision-making, and culture. It can manifest as defensive routines, resistance to change, or interpersonal tensions. Leaders who recognise and address organisational anxiety can foster psychological safety, resilience, and adaptive capacity.

See also: Social Defences in Organisations, Psychological Safety, Change Management, Leadership Challenges.

Organisational Behaviour

The study of how individuals and groups act within organisations, influenced by both conscious and unconscious processes, power structures, and social dynamics.

See also: Organisational Dynamics, Leadership, Psychological Safety, Systems Thinking.

Organisational Boundaries

The delineation between what is considered internal and external to an organisation. These boundaries define the system's focus but must remain permeable to allow interaction with key external factors such as funding, government policy, public opinion, and regulation. Maintaining clear yet adaptive boundaries is essential to prevent the organisation from becoming closed, which can lead to dysfunction and stagnation.

See also: Systems Thinking, Organisational Dynamics, Complex Adaptive Systems, Organisational Culture.

Organisational Culture

The shared values, beliefs, norms, and behaviours that shape how people within an organisation interact, make decisions, and approach their work. It influences organisational climate, identity, and performance, and can either enable or hinder change, innovation, and inclusion. Leaders shape and are shaped by culture, making cultural awareness central to inclusive, adaptive, and effective leadership

See also: Organisational Dynamics, Psychological Safety.

Organisational Development (OD)

A planned, systemic approach to improving organisational effectiveness, health, and wellbeing through interventions that foster culture change, learning, collaboration, and adaptive capacity. OD integrates behavioural science principles to support sustainable change, enhance leadership, and align organisational processes with strategic goals.

See also: Change Management, Organisational Culture, Leadership Development, Systems Thinking.

Organisational Justice

The perception of fairness within an organisation regarding decision-making processes, distribution of resources, and interpersonal treatment. It encompasses procedural, distributive, and interactional justice, influencing employee trust, engagement, wellbeing, and organisational commitment. Promoting organisational justice is vital for ethical leadership and sustaining a positive workplace culture.

See also: Psychological Safety, Equity, Organisational Culture.

Organisational Life

The complex, lived experience of individuals and groups within an organisation encompasses both formal structures and informal dynamics. Organisational life includes routines, relationships, power structures, emotions, unspoken norms, and cultural practices that shape how work is experienced and enacted. It reflects how personal, relational, and systemic forces intersect in day-to-day functioning, often influencing behaviour, morale, leadership, and change efforts beyond what is captured in formal policies or structures.

See also: Organisational Culture, Group Dynamics, Systems Psychodynamics, Psychological Safety, Organisational Anxiety, Leadership Development, Role Analysis.

Organisational Strategy

A deliberate, long-term plan developed to align resources, capabilities, and actions with the organisation's mission and environment. It guides decision-making, prioritises goals, and shapes how the organisation adapts to internal and external complexities. Effective organisational strategy integrates stakeholder perspectives, anticipates change, and fosters sustainable performance and impact.

See also: Strategic Leadership, Change Management, Systems Thinking, Adaptive Leadership.

Organisational Structures

Formal systems and frameworks that define structural tiers, organisation of functions, decision-making processes, communication channels, and accountability mechanisms within an organisation. These structures shape roles and responsibilities, influence coordination, workflow, leadership, collaboration, agility, innovation, culture, and employee engagement. Understanding organisational structures is essential for effective leadership, clear communication, strategic alignment, efficient decision-making, and successful change management.

See also: Organisational Dynamics, Leadership, Organisational Culture, Systems Thinking, Change Management.

Participative Cultures

Organisational environments in which leadership is shared rather than top-down, enabling inclusive engagement across roles, disciplines, and identities. These cultures value diverse perspectives, amplify marginalised voices, and foster collaborative decision-making, which is particularly vital in complex health and social care systems.

See also: Collective Leadership, Inclusion, Psychological Safety, Co-production, Leadership Development.

Policy Influence

The strategic actions and processes by which individuals or organisations seek to shape the development, content, or implementation of policies. This involves advocacy, coalition-building, evidence presentation, and negotiation to align policy decisions with organisational goals, values, or public interests. Effective policy influence requires understanding political contexts, power dynamics, and stakeholder interests.

See also: Advocacy, Policy Development, Organisational Strategy, Stakeholder Engagement.

Political Advisers

Individuals who work closely with elected politicians, including Prime Ministers and ministers, providing support, guidance, and strategic input. They assist in delivering political promises and managing policy implementation, often operating under high-pressure conditions with limited job security and minimal formal HR support.

See also: Political Will, Policy Influence, Leadership Politics.

Political Office

A general term for workplaces within the political system, including the offices of Members of Parliament (MPs), ministers, and the Prime Minister.

See also: Political Advisers, Political Will, Organisational Culture.

Political Skills

The ability to effectively understand, navigate, and influence organisational and social power dynamics to achieve desired outcomes. These skills differ from general interpersonal abilities by specifically focusing on strategic awareness of formal and informal power structures, adept negotiation, alliance-building, and managing competing interests. Political skills enable leaders to foster collaboration, gain support, and drive change within complex environments.

See also: Leadership Politics, Influence, Organisational Dynamics, Power (in Leadership Context).

Political Will

The collective energy, commitment, and motivation within individuals or groups necessary to initiate, support, and sustain change efforts. It is often cultivated through networking, shared accountability, and strategic advocacy.

See also: Policy Influence, Leadership Politics, Stakeholder Engagement.

Power Imbalance

The unequal distribution of influence and authority between groups or individuals—often seen between professionals and service users. In the context of psychological services, recognising and addressing these imbalances is essential to ensure that those with less power have genuine opportunities to shape the processes and decisions that affect them.

See also: Authority and Power, Advocacy, Inclusion.

Power Structures

The formal and informal distribution of authority and influence within organisations, shaped by designated roles as well as unconscious emotional dynamics such as dependency, rivalry, and fear. Understanding power structures is crucial for navigating organisational politics and fostering effective leadership.

See also: Authority and Power, Organisational Behaviour, Political Skills, Unconscious Processes.

Primary Task

The fundamental purpose or goal that defines a group's existence and is essential for its survival. It includes:

- The **formal task** as defined by the organisation or leadership,
- The **perceived task** shaped by group members' interpretations, and
- The **enacted task** reflecting what the group actually does in practice.

See also: Group Dynamics, Basic Assumptions.

Privilege Blindness

The lack of awareness or acknowledgement of one's own unearned advantages or systemic benefits linked to social identity (such as race, gender, class, or ability). This blindness can perpetuate inequities by obscuring how privilege shapes opportunities, power, and access within organisations and society. Recognising privilege blindness is a crucial step towards fostering inclusion, equity, and social justice.

See also: Bias (Unconscious/Implicit), Marginalisation, Intersectionality, Psychological Safety, Inclusion.

Professional Identity

The self-concept and sense of belonging that individuals develop in relation to their profession, shaped by values, roles, skills, and experiences. It influences how professionals perceive themselves, their responsibilities, and their relationships within organisational and societal contexts. A strong professional identity supports confidence, ethical practice, and ongoing development.

See also: Identity, Leader Identity Development, Reflective Practice.

Project Management

The discipline of planning, executing, and overseeing specific, time-bound initiatives to achieve defined objectives within scope, time, and resource constraints. It involves coordinating tasks, managing risks, engaging stakeholders, and ensuring deliverables meet quality standards. Effective project management supports organisational goals by facilitating structured change and innovation.

See also: Change Management, Organisational Strategy, Risk Management, Stakeholder Engagement.

Psychological Contract

The unwritten, implicit set of expectations and beliefs between an individual and their organisation regarding mutual obligations, roles, and rewards. This contract shapes trust, engagement, and motivation, influencing how employees interpret fairness and respond to organisational changes. Breaches in the psychological contract can lead to dissatisfaction, reduced commitment, and turnover.

See also: Organisational Justice, Trust, Employee Engagement, Organisational Culture.

Psychological Practice in Health Services

The application of psychological principles and methods to support users' mental health and wellbeing, as well as to enhance the wellbeing and effectiveness of healthcare workers and the functioning of healthcare services.

See also: Psychological Professions, Wellbeing, Occupational Health, Organisational Development.

Psychological Professions

A broad term encompassing all health and care roles that apply psychological knowledge and skills across diverse settings. This includes a wide range of practitioners involved in assessment, intervention, consultancy, and leadership, as defined by frameworks such as the NHS England Psychological Professions Taxonomy. Applied Psychologists are registered professionals who have completed accredited training in psychology and are qualified to apply psychological theories, methods, and evidence-based practices across various domains, including clinical, counselling, educational, health, forensic, occupational, academic, and organisational settings.

Psychological Safety

A shared belief within teams or organisations that it is safe to take interpersonal risks, such as speaking up, asking questions, or admitting mistakes, without fear of humiliation, punishment, or rejection. Psychological safety fosters open communication, learning, innovation, and collaboration, and is critical for effective leadership and resilient organisational cultures.

See also: Organisational Culture, Trust, Inclusion, Wellbeing at Work, Containment.

Psychologically Informed Leadership

An approach that applies psychological insights—such as human behaviour, motivation, emotional intelligence, and relational dynamics—to enhance leadership effectiveness. It supports deeper self-awareness, stronger relationships, psychologically safe cultures, and more adaptive, inclusive, and impactful organisational leadership.

See also: Emotional Intelligence, Psychological Safety, Systems Thinking, Leadership Development.

Psychologist Entrepreneurs

Practitioner psychologists who apply their clinical, behavioural, and systemic expertise to develop innovative services, private practices, or social enterprises. They combine psychological knowledge with business acumen to address unmet needs and create value-driven ventures that promote wellbeing and social impact.

Psychosocial Demands at Work

The psychological and social aspects of the work environment that require sustained cognitive, emotional, or interpersonal effort. These demands include workload pressure, role ambiguity, interpersonal conflicts, and emotional labour, which can impact employee wellbeing, job satisfaction, and performance. Effective management of psychosocial demands is essential for fostering healthy, productive workplaces.

See also: Workplace Stress, Emotional Labour, Wellbeing, Occupational Health, **J***ob Demand–Resource (JD-R) Model, Burnout, Workplace Stress.*

Quality Improvement (QI)

A systematic, continuous process aimed at enhancing services, processes, and outcomes within organisations. QI involves identifying areas for improvement, testing changes through iterative cycles, measuring impact, and embedding successful innovations to increase effectiveness, efficiency, and safety. It is widely used in healthcare to optimise patient care and organisational performance.

See also: Driver Diagram, Change Management, Systems Thinking.

Racism and Anti-Racism

- **Racism** – A system of oppression based on race or ethnicity, manifesting through individual behaviours, institutional policies, and societal structures that create and perpetuate unequal access to power, resources, and opportunities. Racism sustains marginalisation and exclusion across multiple levels of society and organisations.

- **Structural racism** – The embedded and systemic nature of racial inequities within social, economic, and political institutions. This form of racism is maintained through laws, policies, and cultural norms that systematically disadvantage certain racial or ethnic groups.
- **Antiracism** – A proactive and sustained commitment to identifying, challenging, and dismantling racism in all its forms—individual, institutional, and structural. Antiracist leadership involves not only recognising the impact of racial inequity but actively transforming policies, practices, and power dynamics to create inclusive, equitable environments. It requires critical self-reflection, cultural humility, and collective responsibility.

See also: Privilege, Bias (Unconscious/Implicit), Marginalisation, Equity, Inclusion, Racism, Cultural Humility.

Reasonable Adjustments

Changes or accommodations made to remove barriers that disadvantage individuals with disabilities, health conditions, or neurodivergence, ensuring equitable access, participation, and contribution in workplace or service environments. Mandated by legislation such as the UK Equality Act 2010, these may include physical modifications, flexible schedules, communication support, or adapted expectations.

See also: Disability, Psychological Safety, Occupational Health, Workplace Discrimination, Power Imbalance.

Reflective and Reflexive Practice

Professional approaches involving critical self-examination to enhance learning and practice. Reflective practice reviews past experiences to improve future actions, while reflexive practice deepens awareness by exploring 'self in context' *(How do who I am, my context, and my power impact this situation and others?)*, and how personal biases and assumptions shape understanding and decisions. Both foster ongoing growth, ethical leadership, and adaptability.

See also: Professional Identity, Leadership Development, Emotional Intelligence, Psychologically Informed Leadership, Self in Role.

Relational Leadership

An approach to leadership that emphasises the quality and dynamics of relationships between leaders and followers, recognising leadership as a co-created, interactive process. It prioritises trust, empathy, dialogue, and mutual influence, fostering connection and collective purpose. Relational leadership supports psychological safety, inclusion, and adaptability within complex organisational systems.

See also: Collective Leadership, Emotional Intelligence, Psychological Safety.

Renaissance Leadership

A holistic leadership approach that blends courage, compassion, personal growth, and systems thinking to navigate complexity with authenticity and purpose. Inspired by the Renaissance ideal of integrated knowledge and creativity, it emphasises relational depth, adaptability, and the cultivation of wisdom to lead meaningful, values-driven change in uncertain environments.

See also: Adaptive Leadership, Values-Based Leadership, Systems Thinking, Emotional Intelligence.

Resilience

The capacity to adapt, recover, and thrive in the face of adversity, stress, or change. It involves psychological flexibility, emotional regulation, and maintaining wellbeing despite challenges. While resilience is vital for sustained performance and organisational wellbeing, its misuse occurs when organisations overemphasise individual responsibility, ignoring systemic pressures that strain resilience. This can unfairly shift the locus of control onto individuals, overlooking organisational factors that contribute to stress and burnout.

See also: Psychological Wellbeing, Burnout Resilience, Organisational Culture, Systems Thinking.

Resistance to Change

The emotional or behavioural pushback by individuals, groups, or systems when confronted with change. It is often driven by fear, uncertainty, perceived threats to identity, power, or established norms, and can manifest as avoidance, criticism, or disengagement. Understanding resistance is essential for adaptive leadership, enabling leaders to engage with underlying concerns, build trust, and support meaningful transition.

See also: Organisational Change, Adaptive Leadership, Psychological Safety, Organisational Anxiety, Change Fatigue.

Role Analysis

A reflective process that explores the expectations, behaviours, and influences shaping an individual's professional role. It helps distinguish between personal identity, organisational demands, and external factors, clarifying responsibilities and boundaries. By enhancing self-awareness and understanding of relational dynamics, role analysis supports task focus, psychological safety, and effective leadership.

See also: Self in Role, Role Theory, Professional Identity, Group Dynamics, Task and Sentient Boundaries.

Role Theory

A conceptual framework that examines how individuals understand, enact, and negotiate the expectations and behaviours associated with their social and organisational roles. It explores how roles shape identity, influence interactions, and affect performance, wellbeing, and group dynamics. Role conflict and ambiguity can undermine effectiveness and psychological safety.

See also: Roles and Boundaries, Professional Identity, Group Dynamics, Psychological Safety.

Roles and Boundaries

Clearly defined expectations, responsibilities, and limits associated with individual positions or job descriptions within organisations. They are essential for ensuring clarity, accountability, effective collaboration, and managing both emotional and task-related demands. Well-maintained roles and boundaries support psychological safety and help prevent role conflict or burnout.

See also: Organisational Structures, Accountability, Psychological Safety, Role Theory.

Self in Role

The dynamic interplay between an individual's personal identity, values, and experiences and their professional role. Insight into the origins of thoughts, emotions, and behaviours, distinguishing what arises from personal identity, professional role, or other influences. Understanding their impact on the primary task helps maintain appropriate boundaries, stay task-focused, and respond adaptively within organisational contexts. This process aligns closely with Role Analysis, which examines these dynamics to clarify role expectations and improve effectiveness.

See also: Role Analysis, Professional Identity, Role Theory, Leadership Development, Emotional Intelligence.

Social Constructionism

A theoretical perspective asserting that knowledge, meanings, and realities are co-created through social interactions, language, and shared understandings rather than existing as objective facts. It emphasises how social contexts, power relations, and cultural narratives shape perceptions, identities, and organisational practices. In leadership and psychology, social constructionism encourages critical reflection on how meanings and behaviours are negotiated and sustained within groups and systems.

See also: Discourse Analysis, Power Dynamics, Cultural Humility.

Social Defences

Organisational rituals, structures, or norms that function to protect individuals and groups from anxiety and emotional distress. While these defences can provide temporary stability, they may also hinder adaptation, innovation, and effective change by perpetuating defensive behaviours and limiting open engagement with challenges. Understanding social defences is crucial for leaders aiming to foster psychological safety and organisational learning.

See also: Organisational Anxiety, Defensive Organisational Patterns, Containment, Systems Psychodynamics.

Social Justice

The pursuit of equity, fairness, and the protection of human rights within society. It involves addressing systemic inequalities, dismantling barriers related to race, gender, class, disability, and other social identities, and promoting inclusive participation and access to resources. In leadership and organisational contexts, social justice underpins ethical practice and transformative change towards more equitable and inclusive environments.

See also: Equity, Inclusion, Anti-Oppressive Practice, Cultural Humility.

Socioeconomic Determinants of Mental Health

Social and economic factors—such as income, education, employment, housing, and social support—significantly influence individual and community mental wellbeing. These determinants affect access to resources, levels of stress exposure, and opportunities for recovery, contributing to mental health inequalities and shaping public health and organisational strategies.

See also: Health Inequalities, Social Justice, Community Mental Health, Social Determinants of Health.

Staff Retention and Turnover

Staff retention refers to an organisation's ability to keep employees, promoting stability and engagement, while staff turnover denotes the rate of employee departure and replacement. High turnover can signal issues like burnout or poor leadership, making effective leadership and a supportive culture essential for maintaining workforce wellbeing and service quality.

See also: Burnout, Organisational Culture.

Stakeholder Engagement

The ongoing process of identifying, involving, and collaborating with individuals or groups who have an interest in or are affected by an organisation's decisions, activities, or outcomes. Effective stakeholder engagement fosters transparency, trust, shared understanding, and co-creation, supporting better decision-making and sustainable change.

See also: Co-production

Strategic Leadership

The capability to envision, influence, and guide an organisation or system toward long-term goals by aligning resources, people, and processes with a clear strategy. It involves anticipating future challenges, fostering innovation, and balancing short-term demands with sustainable impact. Strategic leaders create direction, inspire commitment, and navigate complexity to achieve organisational success.

See also: Systems Leadership, Change Management, Organisational Strategy.

Strategic Vision Translation

The process of converting a high-level strategic vision into clear, actionable goals, plans, and behaviours within an organisation. This involves communicating purpose, aligning teams, and embedding the vision into daily operations to ensure coherence between long-term aspirations and frontline practice.

See also: Strategic Leadership, Change Management, Implementation Science, Leadership Agility, Organisational Strategy.

Supervision

A structured, reflective professional relationship in which a more experienced practitioner supports the development, accountability, and well-being of another individual. Supervision fosters critical reflection on practice, ethical decision-making, and skill enhancement, often balancing both managerial and developmental functions. It differs from mentoring and coaching by its formal oversight and focus on professional standards within clinical, counselling, or organisational contexts.

See also: Mentoring, Coaching, Reflective Practice, Leadership Development.

Survival Task

A defensive organisational pattern that arises when overwhelming anxiety or perceived threat diverts attention from the primary task, resulting in rigid behaviours, misplaced priorities, and diminished effectiveness. This response serves to protect the system but can inhibit adaptive functioning and goal achievement.

See also: Primary Task, Basic Assumptions (Bion), Anti-Task, Organisational Anxiety, Resilience, Containment, Sentient Boundaries.

Systemic Approach

A perspective that emphasises the interconnectedness and interdependence of elements within a whole system. It enables leaders to move beyond siloed thinking, recognise how changes in one part impact others, and anticipate unintended consequences. Closely related to Systems Thinking, it supports analysing structures, relationships, and dynamics to navigate complexity and promote adaptive, holistic solutions in organisations and communities.

See also: Systems Thinking, Complexity Theory, Organisational Development, Systems Leadership.

Systems Leadership

A leadership approach focused on influencing and mobilising multiple interconnected stakeholders and organisations within complex systems. It involves seeing the whole system, fostering collaboration across boundaries, and enabling collective action to address systemic challenges. Systems leaders embrace complexity, promote adaptive change, and cultivate environments of psychological safety and shared purpose.

See also: Systemic Approach, Complexity Theory, Adaptive Leadership, Collective Leadership, Collective Leadership, Collective Leadership, Leadership Agility.

Systems Psychodynamics

An approach integrating open systems theory and psychoanalytic concepts to understand how conscious and unconscious emotional, motivational, and behavioural dynamics interact within organisational structures, roles, and boundaries. It helps leaders understand how unconscious group dynamics affect performance and decision-making.

See also: Organisational Dynamics, Basic Assumptions, Containment, Leadership Development.

Talent Development

Intentional efforts to nurture and cultivate leadership potential through mentoring, challenging assignments, and reflective practice. It supports both vertical development (deepening mindset and complexity) and horizontal development (broadening skills and knowledge), enabling individuals and organisations to adapt and thrive in complex environments.

See also: Leadership Development, Mentoring, Vertical Development, Reflective Practice, Workforce Planning, Mentoring.

Talent Management

Strategic organisational practices for attracting, developing, retaining, and deploying individuals with leadership potential. It aligns workforce capability with long-term goals and supports inclusive succession planning and leadership sustainability.

See also: Workforce Planning, Leadership Development, Organisational Strategy.

Task and Sentient Boundaries

Key organisational concepts that distinguish between the boundaries related to accomplishing work objectives (task boundaries) and those managing emotional and relational dynamics within groups (sentient boundaries). Task boundaries define roles, responsibilities, and processes essential for achieving goals, while sentient boundaries regulate interpersonal interactions and help contain anxiety and stress. Anti-task behaviours arise when unconscious group dynamics divert attention away from the primary task, often as a defence against discomfort or conflict, undermining group effectiveness. Effective leadership involves balancing task and sentient boundaries while recognising and managing anti-task behaviours to maintain focus, psychological safety, and group cohesion.

See also: Basic Assumptions (Bion), Containment, Psychological Safety, Role Theory.

Technology-Enabled Change

Organisational transformation driven by the adoption and integration of digital, data-driven, or automated technologies. This change often necessitates shifts in organisational culture, workflows, professional roles, and leadership approaches, requiring both technical expertise and human-centred leadership to navigate complexities and foster innovation.

See also: Organisational Change, Innovation, Leadership Agility.

Thought Leadership

The ability to shape professional discourse, influence public or policy debates, and elevate psychology's visibility through original insights and strategic advocacy. Its unique feature serves as a catalyst for change by generating and disseminating innovative ideas that challenge existing paradigms and open new possibilities. Thought leaders confidently share expertise, empower others, and create inclusive platforms for diverse voices to inspire innovation and drive meaningful collective progress.

See also: Professional Influence, Leadership Communication, Social Justice.

Transformation

A profound and systemic process of change that alters the core purpose, values, culture, and direction of an organisation or system. Unlike transactional change, which focuses on incremental improvements, transformation involves reimagining structures, identities, and mindsets to respond adaptively to complex internal or external challenges. Transformational processes require courageous leadership, psychological insight, and active engagement with uncertainty, resistance, and learning.

See also: Transformational Change, Change Leadership, Adaptive Leadership, Leadership Development, Organisational Culture, Strategic Leadership, Innovation, Psychological Safety.

Transactional and Transformational Change

Two distinct but complementary types of organisational change:

- **Transactional change** involves operational improvements and adaptations to structures, systems, processes, and work climate that support strategic goals without altering the organisation's core purpose or identity. It focuses on incremental, day-to-day management and is common in many NHS initiatives.
- **Transformational change** entails deep, systemic shifts requiring a redefinition of the organisation's mission, strategy, leadership, and culture in response to external forces. This change fundamentally reshapes organisational direction and purpose and is led by formal leadership, such as major policy shifts or funding model reforms in the NHS.

Understanding both forms is critical for effective change management and leadership in complex systems.

See also: Change Management, Strategic Leadership, Organisational Development, Systemic Change.

Transactional Business Skills

Practical competencies such as negotiation, operations management, effective communication, and data-informed planning that underpin efficient organisational functioning. These skills enable leaders and teams to manage day-to-day processes, resources, and stakeholder interactions critical for achieving operational goals.

See also: Strategic Leadership, Organisational Management, Data-Driven Decision Making.

Triad of Awareness

A leadership model based on concepts popularised by Daniel Goleman that emphasises three interconnected domains of awareness essential for effective leadership:

- **Self-awareness**: Understanding one's own emotions, strengths, and limitations.
- **Social awareness**: Recognising and empathising with the emotions and perspectives of others.
- **Wider systemic awareness**: Perceiving the broader organisational and environmental context, including systemic dynamics and cultural factors.

This triad supports leaders in making informed, adaptive decisions and fostering relational and systemic insight.

See also: Emotional Intelligence, Systems Thinking, Leadership Development.

Trust

A foundational belief in the reliability, integrity, and benevolence of individuals or organisations. Trust enables open communication, collaboration, and risk-taking, and is critical for building psychological safety, effective leadership, and a positive organisational culture. The erosion of trust undermines engagement and adaptive capacity.

See also: Psychological Safety, Organisational Culture, Leadership.

Uncertainty Management

The skill of navigating ambiguity, incomplete information, and shifting circumstances while maintaining clarity of purpose, relational engagement, and containment for teams and organisations.

See also: Adaptive Leadership, Complexity Theory, Psychological Safety, Change Management, Leadership Agility, Containment.

Unconscious Processes

Hidden psychological mechanisms, including defence mechanisms, projections, and repressed emotions, that operate below conscious awareness to influence individual and group behaviours, relationships, and decision-making. Recognising these processes is essential for leaders to understand underlying dynamics, manage anxiety, and foster healthier organisational cultures.

See also: Systems Psychodynamics, Defence Mechanisms, Group Dynamics, Organisational Behaviour.

Vertical Development

The deepening of leadership capacity characterized by expanded perspective-taking, enhanced emotional maturity, and an increased ability to navigate complexity, ambiguity, and paradox. This development transforms how leaders think and make meaning, enabling more adaptive and systemic approaches to challenges. Vertical development can be fostered through reflective practice, action enquiry, challenging stretch experiences, coaching, and sustained engagement with complex real-world situations that push cognitive and emotional boundaries.

See also: Horizontal Development, Leadership Development, Adaptive Leadership, Complexity Theory.

Wellbeing

A holistic state encompassing emotional, mental, and social health, where individuals experience positive emotions, effective coping, meaningful relationships, and a sense of purpose and fulfilment. Psychological wellbeing supports resilience, productivity, and overall quality of life. It is influenced by personal, organisational, and societal factors, including the management of workplace stress and burnout. Interrelated concepts include:

- **Stress** is the body's and mind's response to demands or pressures, which can be motivating but harmful if excessive or unmanaged.
- **Burnout** is a prolonged state of physical, emotional, and mental exhaustion resulting from chronic workplace stress, marked by overwhelm, cynicism, and reduced efficacy.
- **Occupational health** is the multidisciplinary field dedicated to promoting and maintaining employees' physical, mental, and social wellbeing by addressing risks such as stress and burnout through prevention and support.

Understanding these interrelated concepts is essential for fostering psychological wellbeing in individuals and organisations.

See also: Occupational Health Stress, Burnout Resilience, Psychological Safety, Workplace Stress.

Whole Community Partnership

An inclusive and intentional approach to engaging all parts of the community—regardless of age, background, language, visibility, or access—to ensure services reflect and serve the full spectrum of societal needs. This approach emphasises equity, connection, and shared responsibility for collective wellbeing, fostering collaboration between organisations, leaders, and community members.

See also: Community Engagement, Co-production, Social Justice, Inclusive Leadership, Co-Production, Inclusive Leadership, Community Mental Health.

Workforce Planning, Development, and Transformation

An organised and strategic process focused on building the skills, knowledge, and capacity of staff to meet current and future service needs. This approach supports both workforce and organisational sustainability to deliver high-quality services. It encompasses education, supervision, leadership development, and strategic workforce planning to adapt effectively to evolving organisational demands.

See also: Talent Development, Leadership Development, Organisational Change.

Work Groups

Task-focused groups that collaborate to achieve shared goals. In contrast to basic assumption groups, work groups remain reality-oriented, manage anxiety constructively, and support reflective, adaptive functioning within organisations.

See also: Basic Assumption Groups, Group Dynamics, Containment, Reflective Practice.

Working Relationships

Professional connections and collaborative dynamics among individuals, teams, and stakeholders. Effective working relationships underpin trust, clear communication, shared purpose, and successful change implementation within organisations.

See also: Collaboration, Trust, Stakeholder Engagement, Relational Leadership.

Workplace Discrimination and Bullying

Unfair or unequal treatment of individuals or groups in employment based on characteristics such as race, gender, disability, religion, age, or sexual orientation. This encompasses direct and indirect bias or prejudice within organisational processes. It also includes hiring, promotion, treatment, and retention—as well as behaviours of bullying that undermine equity, psychological safety, and inclusion.

See also: Inclusion, Equity, Bias (Unconscious/Implicit), Marginalisation, Psychological Safety.

Workplace Stress

The psychological and physiological response to work-related demands and pressures that exceed an individual's coping capacity. While manageable stress can motivate and enhance performance, excessive or chronic workplace stress contributes to burnout, health problems, and reduced job satisfaction. Effective organisational and leadership strategies are needed to monitor and mitigate workplace stress.

See also: Burnout, Occupational Health, Psychological Wellbeing.

Young Leaders

Early-career professionals who demonstrate leadership potential, initiative, and influence within organisations or communities. Supporting young leaders involves providing mentorship, development opportunities, and inclusive platforms to nurture diverse future leadership and innovation.

See also: Leadership Development, Talent Development, Mentoring, Emerging Leaders.

Thematic Index for Glossary of Terms

Adaptive and Systems-Informed Leadership

Explores leadership approaches and mindsets that embrace complexity, systemic thinking, and adaptive change to navigate dynamic organisational environments.

- Adaptive Leadership
- Change Leadership
- Change Management
- Complexity Theory
- Resistance to Change
- Strategic Leadership
- Systems Leadership
- Systemic Approach
- Systems Thinking
- Technology-Enabled Change
- Uncertainty Management

Anti-Oppression and Equity

Focuses on practices and concepts that promote fairness, challenge systemic inequalities, and foster inclusive environments across social and organisational contexts.

- Anti-Oppressive Practice
- Cultural Humility
- Decolonising Psychology
- Equity
- Inclusion
- Intersectionality
- Marginalisation
- Power Imbalance
- Privilege
- Privilege Blindness
- Racism and Anti-Racism
- Social Justice

Clinical, Professional, and Psychological Identity

Addresses the formation and negotiation of professional roles, identities, and social belonging in complex organisational systems.

- Identity
- Leader Identity Development
- Professional Identity
- Role Analysis
- Roles and Boundaries
- Role Theory
- Self in Role
- Social Identity

Emotional Intelligence and Relational Depth

Covers self-awareness, empathy, emotional regulation, and relational leadership skills crucial for effective and psychologically safe leadership.

- Containment (Psychological)
- Emotional Intelligence
- Empathy
- Reflective and Reflexive Practice
- Relational Leadership
- Self-Awareness

Ethics, Values, and Moral Practice

Encompasses the ethical foundations, values alignment, and moral challenges intrinsic to responsible leadership and organisational practice.

- Ethics
- Moral Distress and Injury
- Values-Based Leadership

Group and Organisational Dynamics

Explores conscious and unconscious group behaviours, organisational culture, defences, and psychological safety mechanisms that influence collective functioning.

- Anti-Task
- Basic Assumptions
- Group Dynamics
- Organisational Anxiety
- Organisational Behaviour
- Organisational Culture
- Organisational Defensiveness
- Social Defences
- Survival Task
- Systems Psychodynamics
- Task and Sentient Boundaries
- Team Functioning
- Work Group

Influence, Power, and Politics

Examines how power dynamics, political skills, and influence operate within organisations to shape decision-making and leadership outcomes.

- Authority and Power
- Influence

- Leadership Politics
- Political Advisers
- Political Skills
- Political Will
- Power Structures

Innovation and Strategic Change

Includes concepts related to fostering innovation, strategic vision, and effective change processes at organisational and system levels.

- Co-production
- Digital Transformation
- Implementation Science
- Innovation
- Strategic Vision Translation
- Thought Leadership

Leadership Concepts and Development

Core ideas and processes that define leadership practice, identity, and growth across contexts.

- Leader
- Leading
- Leaderhood
- Leadership Development
- Leadership Identity Development
- Leadership Values / Values-Based Leadership
- Leadership Politics
- Leadership Agility
- Leadership Communication (referenced under Thought Leadership / Professional Influence)
- Renaissance Leadership
- Strategic, professional, clinical, and operational leadership

Learning and Leadership Growth

Focuses on development pathways, mentoring, coaching, and processes that cultivate leadership potential and capability over time.

- Horizontal Development
- Leadership Development
- Leadership Potential
- Mentoring
- Supervision
- Talent Development and Management
- Vertical Development
- Young Leaders

Organisational Effectiveness and Delivery

Addresses operational frameworks, project execution, quality improvement, workforce planning, and inclusive organisational practices.

- Autonomy
- Driver Diagram
- Project Management
- Quality Improvement (QI)
- Reasonable Adjustments
- Stakeholder Engagement
- Strategic Leadership
- Workforce Planning, Development, and Transformation

Policy, Advocacy, and Public Engagement

Concerns mechanisms and strategies for shaping policies, advocacy efforts, and engaging diverse communities and stakeholders.

- Advocacy
- Policy Development
- Policy Influence
- Political Office
- Professional Influence
- Whole Community Partnership

Psychological Concepts in Organisational Contexts

Highlights psychological mechanisms, contracts, professions, safety, and unconscious processes relevant to organisational life and leadership.

- Containment (Psychological)
- Defence Mechanisms
- Psychological Contract
- Psychological Practice in Health Services
- Psychological Professions
- Psychological Safety
- Psychologically Informed Leadership
- Unconscious Processes

Stress, Burnout, and Workplace Wellbeing

Focuses on the causes, manifestations, and resilience strategies related to occupational stress, burnout, and employee wellbeing.

- Burnout
- Burnout Resilience
- Job Demand–Resource Model
- Occupational Health
- Psychological Wellbeing
- Resilience
- Stress
- Wellbeing
- Workplace Discrimination and Bullying
- Workplace Stress

Theoretical Perspectives and Frameworks

Provides foundational theories and conceptual frameworks that underpin the understanding of leadership, organisations, and social dynamics.

- Leadership Theories, Models, and Approaches
- Social Constructionism
- Systems Psychodynamics
- Triad of Awareness

- Jahari Windows
- Conscious and Unconscious Competence
- Resource-Demand Model

Workforce Engagement and Inclusion

Encompasses workforce participation, diversity, inclusion efforts, and strategies to support engagement and retention in organisational settings.

- Community Engagement
- Co-production
- Emerging Leaders
- Employee Engagement
- Inclusion
- Staff Retention and Turnover
- Working Relationships
- Participative Cultures

Index

Note: Page references in *italics* represents figures; Page references in **bold** represents tables.

For Product Safety Concerns and Information please contact our EU representative GPSR@taylorandfrancis.com Taylor & Francis Verlag GmbH, Kaufingerstraße 24, 80331 München, Germany